Manual Mobilization of the Joints

Joint Examination and Basic Treatment

Volume I

The Extremities

by Freddy M. Kaltenborn
in collaboration with
Olaf Evjenth,
Traudi Baldauf Kaltenborn,
Dennis Morgan, and Eileen Vollowitz

8th Edition 2014

Published and distributed by
Norli: Oslo, Norway

Also distributed by
OPTP: Minneapolis, Minnesota, USA

Published 2014 and distributed by:
Norli, Universitetsgaten 24, N-0162 Oslo, Norway

Also distributed by:
OPTP, PO Box 47009, Minneapolis, MN 55447, USA

First Edition	*Manual Therapy for the Extremity Joints*, 1974 Revised and translated from Norwegian by Barbara Robinson P.T.
Second Edition	*Manual Therapy for the Extremity Joints*, 1976
Third Edition	*Mobilization of the Extremity Joints*, 1980 Revised by Dennis Morgan, P.T., O.M.T.
Fourth Edition	*Manual Mobilization of the Extremity Joints*, 1989 Edited by Dennis Morgan, D.C., P.T., O.M.T.
Fifth Edition	*Manual Mobilization of the Joints, Volume I: The Extremities*, 1999 Edited by Dennis Morgan, D.C., P.T., O.M.T. and Eileen Vollowitz, P.T., O.M.T.
Sixth Edition	*Manual Mobilization of the Joints, Volume I: The Extremities*, 2002 Edited by Eileen Vollowitz, P.T., O.M.T. Reprinted with revisions, 2007
Seventh Edition	*Manual Mobilization of the Joints, Volume I: The Extremities*, 2011 Edited by Eileen Vollowitz, P.T., O.M.T.
Eighth Edition	*Manual Mobilization of the Joints, Volume I: The Extremities*, 2014 Edited by Eileen Vollowitz, P.T., O.M.T.

This book is a companion volume to:
Manual Mobilization of the Joints, Volume II, The Spine, 2012 (ISBN 978-82-7054-200-0)

Volume I - The Extremities

ISBN 978-82-7054-201-7

Foreword to the 8th edition

It is personal honor to be asked to write a foreword for what is a classic in manipulative therapy.

Freddy Kaltenborn can legitimately be described as the first clinical scientist in physical therapy. He like so many before him recognized that manipulation worked but that did not satisfy him – he wanted to know why. His inquiry took him to visit the "greats" of the era including physicians James Cyriax, James Mennell, Albert Cramer and Alan Stoddard to name just a few. He also collaborated with basic scientist Michael MacConnaill. Kaltenborn combined his studies with practice and teaching, the three elements needed to produce a master clinician.

Today manipulative therapy is under threat by those who with limited clinical skills and who rarely posses mastery, teach to our students only that which is recent and is evidence based, and neglect that the fundamentals of evidence based practice also include the teachings of the master clinician – and Kaltenborn is the master clinician.

In addition we are in danger of loosing a vast richness of practice if our researchers continue to tackle the easy aspects of manipulative therapy in order to gain a publishable paper while ignoring those clinical skills and outcomes that challenge research. Their efforts at reductionism result in simplistic approaches such as clinical prediction rules which further results in a dumbing down of generations of clinical knowledge and skills. When thrust techniques are taught without an adequate appreciation of the underlying fundamentals and without students having attained basic non-thrust manipulative skills, our patients will be the ones who suffer by being denied the skilled care they deserve.

Kaltenborn in this text brings focus to the fundamentals. The concepts that he developed with colleagues focus on the arthrokinematics of joints. They are well thought out, tried and tested and will endure.

Only with a true appreciation of the scientific basis of our work can today's young clinicians be inspired to the excellence that will ensure the quality of care that inspired the development of orthopaedic and manipulative as specialty fields.

Thank you Freddy Kaltenborn, my teacher, mentor and friend, for this enduring contribution to our profession. Your work will live on forever in these pages and in the hands of every master clinician.

Stanley V. Paris P.T., O.M.T., Ph.D.
President, University of St. Augustine
2014

Foreword to the 3rd edition

Professor Kaltenborn has honoured me by asking me to write a Foreword to this book. I do so gladly for two reasons: our long friendship, and the nature and scope of his work.

For some 60 years I have watched the expansion of orthopaedic surgery after the First World War, and that of physical (or orthopaedic) medicine after the Second. Manual Therapy is the child of both, and is rapidly becoming a part of nonspecialized medicine and, of course, of physiotherapy. It is of special value to the rural practitioner, who can now often treat his or her patients in a way that would formerly have needed a journey to some distant town at considerable expense in time and money. Its value for physiotherapists needs no stressing.

The book describes each test and mobilization in simple but precise language reinforced by the numerous clear photographs. What I especially like about it is its marriage of functional anatomy to clinical practice. I do not say this because of the references to part of my own work in arthrology; and ask the reader to believe me. Yet, after all, the most important part of anatomical research and teaching is that which can be used for the relief of human ills.

To comfort always, to alleviate often, to cure sometimes: these are the three aims of the healer. Professor Kaltenborn will help them to be achieved in fuller measure.

I salute his book and say to it:

Go, little book; and, in each distant part
Whereto you go, enlarge the healer's art!

M.A. MacConaill
Professor in Anatomy, Cork, Ireland
Referenced in Gray's Anatomy: Arthrology, 1980

About this book

Kaltenborn wrote this book in the belief that manual joint evaluation, mobilization, and manipulation skills are important for all practitioners of orthopedic medicine and manipulative therapy, and that hands-on training should begin early in entry-level professional educational programs.

This textbook introduces manual extremity joint evaluation, mobilization, and manipulation techniques with an emphasis on the application of biomechanical principles. This textbook and its companion *Manual Mobilization of the Joints, Volume II: The Spine*, are intended for beginning manual therapy practitioners. These books are also useful for practitioners who did not receive Kaltenborn-Evjenth OMT training during their professional education and must now learn these basic skills through continuing education courses and residencies.

New in the 8th Edition

The Convex-Concave Rule introduced by Kaltenborn over four decades ago, has been widely misunderstood. In this edition Kaltenborn revisits the concept to clarify its use and misuse.

This edition presents basic manipulative thrusts, both in theory and practice, in addition to conventional non-thrust mobilization techniques. Kaltenborn refined and developed these thrust techniques over decades of practice and believes them to be the safest way for student practitioners to develop manipulative skill.

Techniques are presented with new color photographs and a companion video DVD in which Kaltenborn demonstrates each technique. Teachers of Kaltenborn-Evjenth OMT may notice subtle differences in grip and patient positioning compared with previous editions. These should be considered additional options for delivery of the technique rather than a replacement method, keeping in mind that grip and body position change depending on the momentary needs of both patient and practitioner.

Acknowledgments

Each time I publish a new edition of this book I say it will be my last. With each publication I believe I have finally and fully explained the basis for my clinical thinking. Yet each edition stimulates more discourse among my colleagues and students. Concepts I assumed were generally agreed upon and understood, I discover instead to be sources of discord and confusion. And so I must write again and again, each time expanding and clarifying what seems so simple in patient treatment, yet has been so difficult to explain in words. I am grateful for this continued dialog, as it makes me both a better teacher and a better practitioner.

This book would not exist were it not for the interest and efforts of my collaborators and colleagues. Many spent long hours in discussions and careful editing of my drafts. I thank my many colleagues and former students from all over the world who made many valuable suggestions

I would especially like to thank my collaborators. My collaboration with Olaf Evjenth now spans nearly 50 years. I thank him for his creativity, patience, and loyalty in developing and refining our concept. I am indebted to Dennis Morgan and Eileen Vollowitz for their friendship and significant contributions to my practice and written work over the past 30 years. Their patience, insight and talent putting my thoughts into words has been invaluable. Last but not least, I thank my wife Traudi Baldauf Kaltenborn for her love and support over the last 40 years. She continues to provide professional advice and technical support and brings me calm and focus when I most need it. I could never have accomplished so much without her, nor would I have been blessed with such a satisfying and long life.

Freddy M. Kaltenborn, 2014

About the author

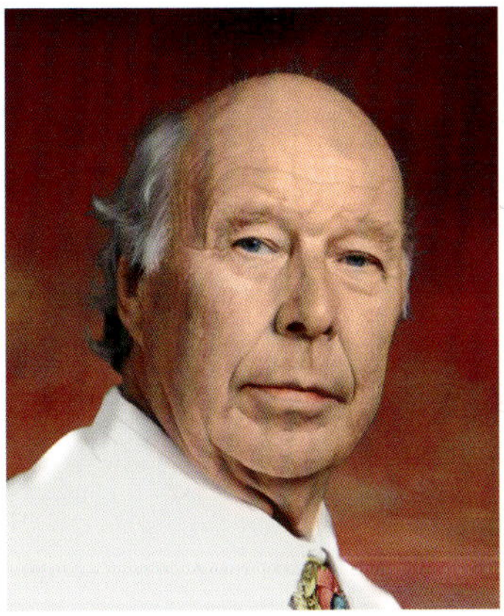

Kaltenborn's career began as a physical educator and athletic trainer in Norway in 1943 and later in Germany in 1945. His education included joint mobilization and sport massage, which soon became the focus of his professional life. In 1949 he became certified in physical therapy, and from 1952 to 1954 he apprenticed in London with Dr. James Mennell and Dr. James Cyriax to study orthopedic medicine. Kaltenborn was certified by Cyriax to teach orthopedic medicine in 1955. Upon return to his native Norway, Kaltenborn worked to incorporate his diverse professional experiences into his own manual therapy system and to teach his concepts to clinicians there.

In 1958 Kaltenborn was certified as a chiropractor by FAC, the German medical association (Forschungs- und Arbeitsgemeinschaft für Chiropraktik). Kaltenborn taught both chiropractic and his own methods to FAC medical doctors between 1958 and 1962. By 1962 the FAC had incorporated Kaltenborn's concepts to such an extent, that they changed their professional name from "Chiropraktik" to "Chirotherapy." Kaltenborn continued to provide instruction to FAC physicians until 1982.

Kaltenborn started his osteopathic studies at the British School of Osteopathy in 1958 and at the London College of Osteopathy in 1962 where he was mentored by Dr. Alan Stoddard. Kaltenborn was approved as an osteopathic instructor in 1971. Between 1977 and 1984 Kaltenborn taught as a professor at the Michigan State University College of Osteopathic Medicine in the USA.

Kaltenborn was certified in orthopedic medicine and manipulative therapy by the International Seminar of Orthopaedic Medicine/Manipulative Therapy (ISOMMT) in 1973.

Kaltenborn practiced orthopedic medicine and manipulative therapy in his native Norway for thirty-two years, from 1950 to 1982. During that time he instructed countless physical therapists, medical doctors, and many osteopaths and chiropractors in manual treatment methods. He introduced manual therapy to Norwegian physical therapists and was instrumental in developing manual therapy education and certification standards there. Together with Norwegian medical doctors, Kaltenborn also brought the benefits of manual therapy to the attention of the Norwegian national health care system, which by 1957 had recognized the effectiveness of manual therapy by reimbursing skilled manual therapy services performed by physical therapists and medical doctors at twice the rate of other physical therapy treatments.

Throughout his professional career, Professor Kaltenborn campaigned tirelessly for the creation of international educational standards and certification in manual therapy. He was a founding member of the International Federation of Orthopaedic Manipulative Therapists (IFOMT), now a subgroup of the World Confederation of Physical Therapists (WCPT). Professor Kaltenborn contributed to the creation of IFOMT's first manual therapy education and certification standards, the first such standards to be recognized by an international professional organization.

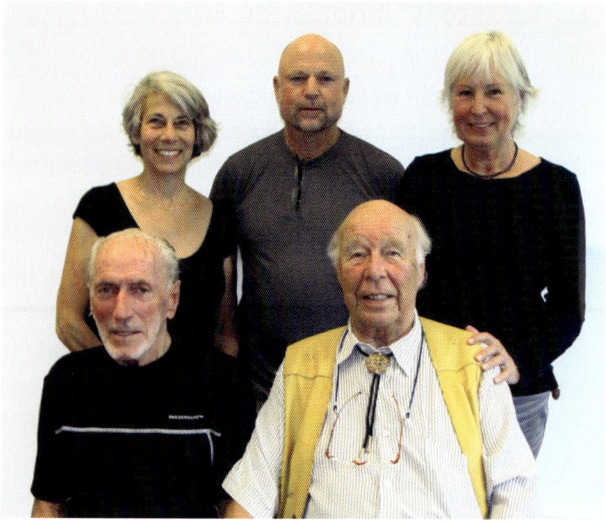

The author with his collaborators for this book:
(sitting, from right) Freddy Kaltenborn, Olaf Evjenth
(standing, from right) Traudi Baldauf Kaltenborn, Dennis Morgan, Eileen Vollowitz.
Finland 2011

Table of Contents

■ Introduction 1

Overview 2

Special features of the Kaltenborn-Evjenth Concept 4

PRINCIPLES

1. Extremity joint movement 9

Joint anatomy 9

Articular surfaces 9

Bony connections 9

The joint complex 12

Reference positions 13

Anatomical planes of reference 13

Anatomical axes of reference 14

Three-dimensional joint positioning 15

Zero position 15

Resting position 15

How to find the resting position 16

Momentary resting position 17

Nonresting positions 17

Close-packed position 18

Bone and joint movement 18

Bone rotation 19

Standard bone movements 19

Combined bone movements 21

Joint roll-gliding associated with bone rotation 22

Joint roll-gliding 22

Abnormal roll-gliding 23

Bone translation 25

Joint play associated with bone translation
(see *Chapter 2: Translatoric joint play*) 25

2. Translatoric joint play 27

Kaltenborn treatment plane 28

Translatoric joint play movements 29

Traction 29

Compression 29

Gliding 29

Determine the direction of restricted gliding 30

Direct method (Glide test) 30

Indirect method (Kaltenborn Convex-Concave Rule) 31

Grades of translatoric movement 32

The "slack" 32

Normal grades of translatoric movement (Grade I - III) 33

Pathological grades of translatoric movement 35

3. Tests of function 37

Assessing quantity of movement 37

Measuring quantity of movement 38

Manual classification of rotation movement (Class 0 - 6) 38

Abnormal range of movement 39

Assessing quality of movement 39

Quality of movement to the first stop 39

End-feel and quality of movement after the first stop: 40

Normal physiological end-feel 41

Pathological end-feel 42

Elements of function testing 43

Active and passive bone rotation movements 43

Differentiating articular from periarticular dysfunction 45

Differentiating muscle shortening from muscle spasm 47

Passive translatoric joint play movements 47

Traction and compression tests 48

Gliding tests 48

Resisted movements 49

Differential diagnosis of pain in a muscle synergy 50

Passive soft tissue movements 51

Physiological soft tissue movements 51

Accessory soft tissue movements 51

Additional Tests 52

4. OMT evaluation 53
Goals of the OMT evaluation 53
Physical diagnosis 53
Common characteristics of somatic dysfunction 54
Indications and contraindications 56
Intra-articular restrictions 57
Extra-articular and peri-articular restrictions 58
Diagnostic traction-manipulation 58
Contraindications to manual therapy 58
Measuring progress 60
Elements of the OMT evaluation 61
Screening examination 62
Detailed examination 65
Medical diagnostic studies 71
Diagnosis and trial treatment 71

5. Joint mobilization 73
Using grades of translatoric movement 74
Non-thrust mobilization 75
Pain-relief mobilization (Grade I-IISZ non-thrust) 75
Pain-relief traction mobilization 75
Vibrations and oscillations 76
Relaxation mobilization (Grade I - II non-thrust) 76
Relaxation-traction mobilization 76
Stretch mobilization (Grade III non-thrust) 77
Stretch-traction mobilization 78
Stretch-glide mobilization 79
Stretch mobilization treatment progression 80
Thrust Mobilization (Grade III thrust) 84
End-feel suitable for manipulation 85
Pre-manipulative stretch test 86
Manipulative thrust technique 87
Manipulative thrust treatment progression 92
Pre-manipulative procedures 92
Progression of manipulative treatment 92
Post-manipulative procedures 93

Avoiding negative outcomes with manual treatment 93
How much treatment is enough? 93
Risks of rotation mobilization 94
Risks of joint compression 95

6. Supplemental OMT treatment 97

Treatment for symptom control 98
Treatment to increase mobility 99
Treatment to limit movement 105
Supportive devices 106
To inform, instruct, and train 107

TECHNIQUE

7. Manual technique principles 111

Applying manual techniques 112
Objective 112
Starting position 113
Therapist's position 113
Patient's position 113
Joint position 114
Hand placement and fixation/stabilization 115
Grip 115
Therapist's stable hand 116
Therapist's moving hand 117
Procedure 117
Mobilization procedure 118
Manipulation procedure 118

8. Fingers ... **121**
Functional anatomy and movement ... 122
Finger examination scheme ... 125
Finger techniques ... 126
9. Metacarpals ... **135**
Functional anatomy and movement ... 136
Metacarpal examination scheme ... 140
Metacarpal techniques ... 141
10. Wrist ... **151**
Functional anatomy and movement ... 152
Wrist examination scheme ... 156
Wrist techniques ... 157
11. Forearm ... **173**
Functional anatomy and movement ... 174
Forearm examination scheme ... 177
Forearm techniques ... 178
12. Elbow ... **191**
Functional anatomy and movement ... 192
Elbow examination scheme ... 195
Elbow techniques ... 196
13. Shoulder ... **201**
Functional anatomy and movement ... 202
Shoulder examination scheme ... 204
Shoulder techniques ... 206
14. Shoulder girdle ... **215**
Functional anatomy and movement ... 216
Shoulder girdle examination scheme ... 222
Shoulder girdle techniques ... 224
15. Toes ... **233**
Functional anatomy and movement ... 234
Toe examination scheme ... 236
Toe techniques ... 237
16. Metatarsals ... **247**
Functional anatomy and movement ... 248
Metatarsal examination scheme ... 250
Metatarsal techniques ... 250

17. Foot and ankle 253

Functional anatomy and movement 254

Foot examination scheme 258

Ankle examination scheme 259

Foot and ankle techniques 262

18. Leg 279

Functional anatomy and movement 280

Leg examination scheme 282

Leg techniques 283

19. Knee 287

Functional anatomy and movement 288

Knee examination scheme 291

Knee techniques 292

20. Hip 309

Functional anatomy and movement 310

Hip examination scheme 312

Hip techniques 314

REFERENCE

Terminology 325

Upper extremity joint and muscle chart 330

Lower extremity joint and muscle chart 332

Convex-concave table 334

Bibliography 335

AFTERWORD

Manual therapy education 339

Traction thrust techniques for student practitioners 342

Recommendation to abandon rotatory joint techniques 343

Evidence-based treatment 344

History of the OMT Nordic System 345

Introduction

Orthopedic medicine specializes in the diagnosis and treatment of arthro-neuro-muscular conditions.[1] Orthopedic Manipulative Therapy (OMT) is a specialty within the practice of physical medicine. A large component of OMT involves the evaluation and treatment of the joint complex (i.e., the physiological joint). If the patient examination reveals joint dysfunction, particularly decreased range of motion (i.e., hypomobility), the joint mobilization techniques described in this book are often effective.[2]

The OMT Nordic System is the result of many years of collaboration between physical educators, athletic trainers, physical therapists, and physicians, first in the Nordic countries between 1954 and 1970, and later worldwide. The OMT Nordic System incorporates information and experience from ancient and folk medicine, sports medicine, traditional physical therapy, orthopedic medicine, chiropractic, osteopathy, and the further innovations of the many therapists who have practiced manual therapy techniques.

Kaltenborn introduced the OMT Nordic System in 1954 with joint testing and treatment only. Initially the system was known as "Manual Therapy ad modum Kaltenborn." In 1968, Freddy Kaltenborn and Olaf Evjenth began their decades-long collaboration to develop the system as we know it today, the OMT Nordic System, Kaltenborn-Evjenth Concept.

The methods presented in this book focus primarily on manual joint testing and basic treatment techniques for the extremity joints, which represents just one component of the OMT Nordic System.

1 In recent years, orthopedic medicine has become known as "manual medicine" or "neuromusculoskeletal medicine."

2 Information about stabilization treatments for joint hypermobility can be found in other textbooks.

■ Overview

OMT Nordic System, Kaltenborn-Evjenth Concept

The Kaltenborn approach to joint testing and mobilization presented in this book is part of the larger scope of OMT Nordic System practice.

I. Physical Diagnosis (biomechanical and functional assessment)

A. Screening exam
An abbreviated exam to quickly identify the region where a problem is located and focus the detailed examination

B. Detailed exam

*1. **History***
Narrow diagnostic possibilities; develop early hypotheses to be confirmed by further exam; determine whether or not symptoms are arthro-neuro-muscular and treatable with OMT. Includes present episode, past medical history, related personal history, family history, review of systems.

*2. **Inspection***
Further focus the exam. Includes posture, shape, skin, assistive devices.

*3. **Tests of function***

a. **Active and passive bone rotation movements**: *Identify location, type, and severity of dysfunction. Includes standard-anatomical-uniaxial movements and combined-functional-multiaxial movements.*

b. **Passive translatoric joint play movements**: *Further differentiate articular from nonarticular lesions; identify directions of joint restrictions. Includes traction, compression, and gliding.*

c. **Resisted movements**: *Test neuromuscular integrity and status of associated joints, nerves and vascular supply.*

d. **Passive soft tissue movements**: *Differentiate joint from soft tissue dysfunction and the type of soft tissue involvement. Includes physiological movements, accessory movements.*

e. **Additional tests:** *Includes coordination, speed, endurance, functional capacity assessment ...*

*4. **Palpation***
Includes tissue characteristics, structures.

*5. **Neurologic and vascular examination***

C. Medical diagnostic studies
Includes diagnostic imaging, lab tests, electro-diagnostic tests, punctures.

D. Diagnosis and trial treatment

II. Treatment

A. To relieve symptoms (most often pain)

1. Immobilization

- General (e.g.,bed rest); Specific (e.g., bracing, splinting, casting, taping)

2. Thermo-Hydro-Electro (T-H-E) therapy

- *Ice, heat, laser, TENS, etc.*

Kaltenborn's Manual Mobilization: Volumes I and II →

3. Joint mobilization

a. Non-thrust Grade I - II Pain-relief mobilization

Grade I-II mobilizations in the momentary resting position;
Intermittent manual traction, vibrations, oscillations

4. Special procedures

- *Acupuncture, acupressure, soft tissue mobilization, etc.*

B. To increase mobility

1. Soft tissue mobilization

a. Passive soft tissue mobilization

- *Classical, functional, and friction massage, muscle stretching*

b. Active soft tissue mobilization

- *Contract-relax, reciprocal inhibition, active assisted functional massage.*

Kaltenborn's Manual Mobilization: Volumes I and II →

2. Joint mobilization

a. Non-thrust Grade I - II: Relaxation mobilization

- *Three-dimensional, pre-positioned mobilizations*

b. Non-thrust Grade III: Stretch mobilization

- *Manual mobilization in the joint resting position*
- *Manual mobilization at the point of restriction*

c. Thrust Grade III: Manipulation

- *High velocity, short amplitude, linear thrust mobilization*

3. Neural tissue mobilization

To increase mobility of dura mater, nerve roots, and peripheral nerves

4. Specific exercise

To increase or maintain joint mobility and soft tissue length and mobility

C. To limit movement

1. Specific exercise: To stabilize or limit joint movement

2. Treatments to increase movement in adjacent joints

D. Supportive devices

E. To inform, instruct, and train

Exercise and education to maintain and improve function, compensate for disability, and prevent reinjury, including MTT (medical training therapy), self-treatment (e.g., automobilization, autostabilization, autostretching, self massage), ergonomics, and self-care.

■ Special features of the Kaltenborn-Evjenth Concept

Certain special features can be identified as basic and unique in their application to the OMT Nordic System Kaltenborn-Evjenth Concept. In many cases Kaltenborn and Evjenth were the first to introduce these concepts to the physical therapy profession. Today these concepts are widely accepted and practiced by practitioners of physical medicine worldwide.

Biomechanical approach to diagnosis and treatment

Manipulative technique has changed over the past 50 years. Traditional manipulations applied long-lever rotation movements. The compressive forces produced by these long-lever rotation movements sometimes injured joints.

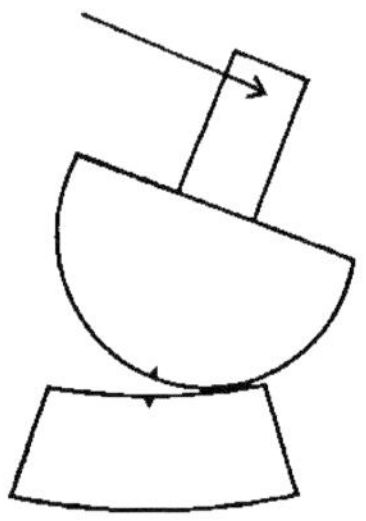

Figure I.1
Prior to 1952, practitioners used long-lever rotation techniques (i.e., passive continuation of active movements)

In the 1940s, James Mennell, M.D. introduced shorter lever rotation manipulations which reduced the possibility of injury. In 1952 Norwegian manual therapists adopted these short-lever manipulative techniques.

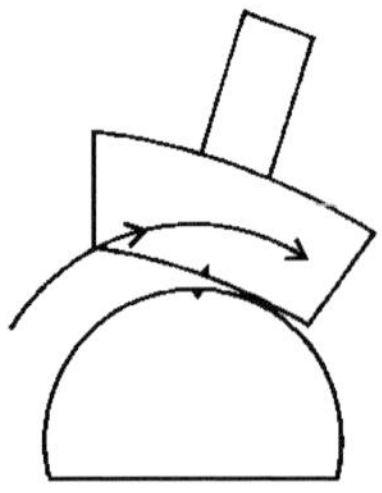

Figure I.2
In 1952, practitioners began to use short-lever rotation techniques

In 1954, Kaltenborn introduced the concept of translatoric linear bone movements. Linear translatoric traction and gliding in relation to a treatment plane reduces joint compression forces. Over the next 30 years Kaltenborn worked to incorporate translatoric joint movements into a comprehensive joint evaluation and treatment approach. These techniques reduced the need for high-risk short-lever rotation mobilizations. By 1979, Evjenth and Kaltenborn had refined these techniques to eliminate rotatory forces in extremity joint treatment, and by 1991, had accomplished the same for spinal manipulations.

Biomechanical principles form the core of the analysis and treatment of arthro-neuro-muscular conditions:

» Translatoric treatment in relation to the Kaltenborn Treatment Plane allows for safe and effective joint mobilization.

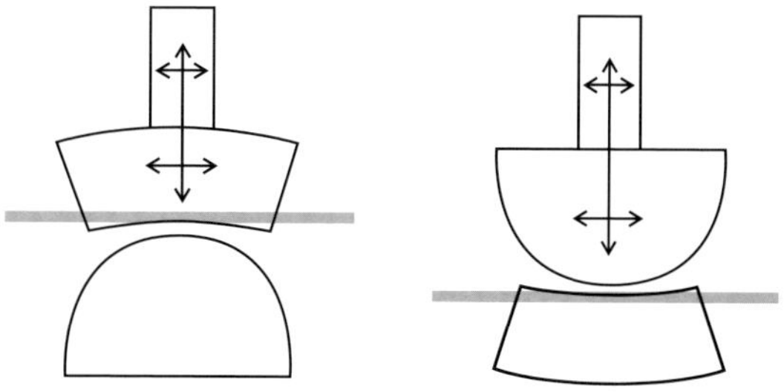

Figure I.3
In 1954, I incorporated the concept of translatoric bone movement in relation to the treatment plane

» The therapist evaluates the translatoric joint play movements of traction and gliding by feeling the amount of slack in the movement and sensing the end-feel. The therapist uses grades of movement to designate the amount of joint play movement they palpate.

» Three-dimensional joint positioning, carefully applied before a test or mobilization, refines and directs the movement.

» The Kaltenborn Convex-Concave Rule allows indirect determination of the direction of decreased joint gliding to insure normal joint mechanics during treatment.

» The therapist evaluates and treats all combinations of movements, coupled and non-coupled.

» The therapist uses specific evaluation and specific treatment, including special tests to localize symptomatic structures, and to treat hypermobility in addition to hypomobility.

Combination of techniques

The use of multiple treatment techniques, often in one treatment session, has always been part of our system. For example, techniques to improve joint mobility are often preceded by pain-relief and soft-tissue-mobilization techniques such as functional massage and muscle stretching. Self-treatment is an important part of the Nordic OMT System and may include instruction in automobilization, autostretching, autotraction, strengthening, stabilization, and coordination exercises. Advice on body mechanics and ergonomics is important to maintain improvements gained in therapy and to prevent recurrences.

Trial treatment

An experienced practitioner views any treatment procedure also as an evaluation procedure. Kaltenborn formalized this concept within his system in 1952 with the term "trial treatment," where the manual therapist confirms the initial physical diagnosis with a low-risk trial treatment as a part of the evaluation procedure.

Ergonomic principles for the therapist

Kaltenborn-Evjenth OMT emphasizes good *therapist* body mechanics. An example of this was Kaltenborn's development in the 1950's of the first pneumatic high-low adjustable treatment table designed for manual physical therapy practice. Nordic OMT practitioners have since developed a number of treatment techniques and tools for efficiency and safety, including mobilization and fixation belts, wedges, and articulating tables.

PRINCIPLES

1 Extremity joint movement

Joint anatomy

Articular surfaces

Classical descriptions of joint surfaces as "plane" or "spheroid" are terms of convenience and not completely accurate. No joint surface is perfectly flat or part of a cylinder, cone, or sphere. In reality, all joint surfaces have a certain amount of curvature, which is not constant but changes from point to point. MacConaill's classification of joint surfaces more accurately reflects this reality. He describes joint surfaces as either ovoid or sellar.

Ovoid joint surfaces (*Figure 1.1a*) can be either convex or concave in all directions and are similar to a piece of egg shell, in that their surfaces are of a constantly changing angular value.

Sellar or saddle surfaces (*Figure 1.1b*) are inversely curved with convex and concave surfaces situated at right angles to each other.

Figure 1.1 Classification of joint surfaces (after MacConaill)

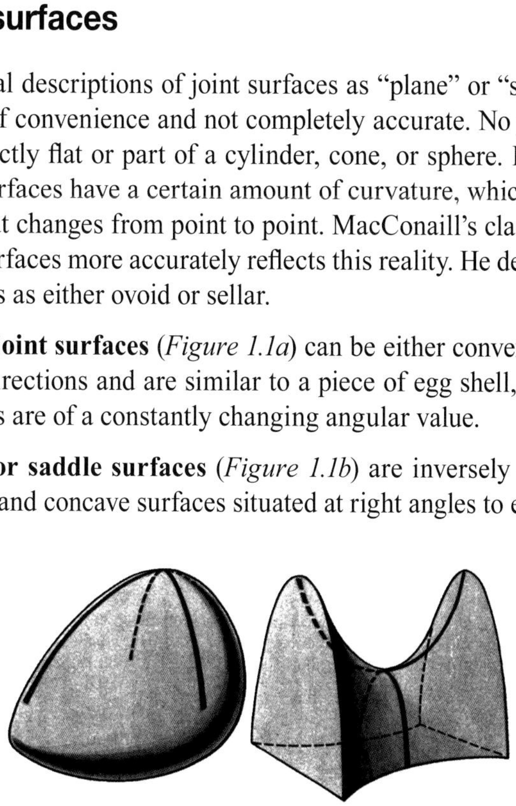

a. Ovoid surface *b. Sellar surface*

Bony connections

In most joint positions the articular surfaces are not fully congruent. The incongruence of joint partners is due to the differences in curvature of the articular surfaces, e.g., the convex partner is more curved (smaller radius of curvature) than its concave joint partner.

Joints have traditionally been classified only by their morphology and mechanical characteristics. In more recent years, MacConaill developed a more useful classification of joints based on the type of bone movement allowed at each joint. In the following pages we review both.

A conventional classification of joints

Bony connections are conventionally classified according to their morphology. Synovial joints are further classified according to their mechanical characteristics.

Conventional Classification of Joints

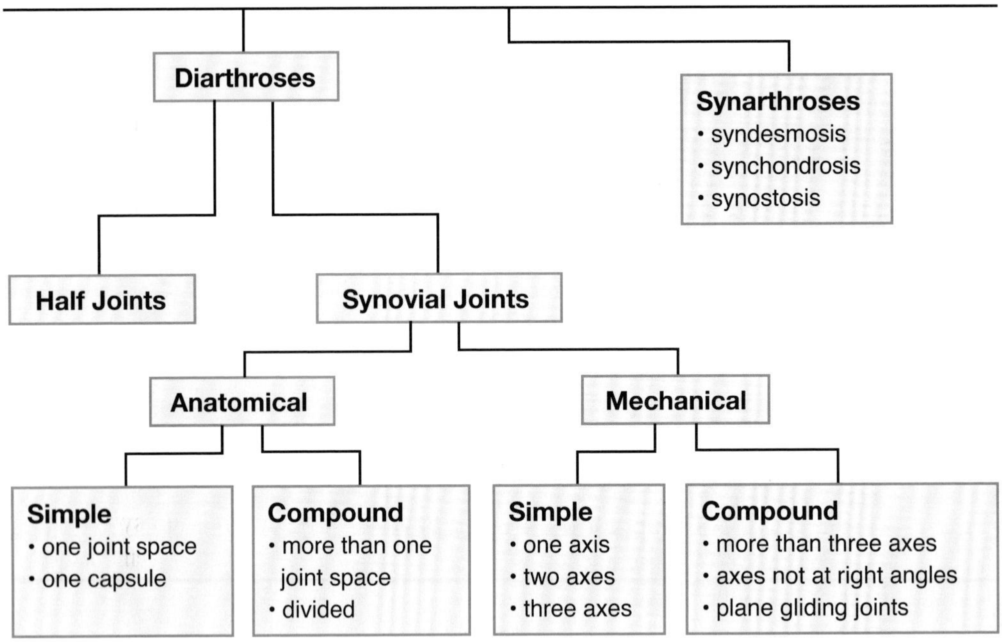

Bony connections are first classified as either synarthroses or diarthroses.[1]

Synarthroses are named according to the type of tissue that connects them:

» Syndesmosis: fibrous tissue

» Synchondrosis: cartilage

» Synostosis: bone

Diarthroses are classified as synovial and half joints (e.g., symphysis, uncovertebral joints).

» Synovial joints with less than 10° of movement are called amphiarthroses.

1 Since most diarthroses are synovial joints and there are very few half joints in the human body, many people use the term "synovial joints" synonymously with "diarthroses."

Synovial joints are classified as anatomical or mechanical, simple or compound joints.

» **Anatomically simple** joints have only one joint space.

» **Anatomically compound** joints have:
  - More than one joint space, divided by a meniscus or articular disc.

» **Mechanically simple** joints have one, two or three axes which are situated at right angles to each other:
  - One Axis: ginglymus (hinge) and trochoid (pivot)
  - Two axes: ellipsoid, sellar (saddle)
  - Three axes: spheroid (enarthroses, ball and socket)

» **Mechanically compound** joints have:
  - More than three axes
  - Axes not situated at right angles to each other
  - Very flat joint surfaces without the usual axes

MacConaill's classification of joints

MacConaill describes four structural classifications of synovial joints which are correlated with the types of bone movements and the degrees of freedom allowed at each articular pair:

» **Unmodified ovoid**: (art. spheroidea), ball and socket, triaxial, e.g., hip and shoulder joints

» **Modified ovoid**: (art. ellipsoidea), ellipsoid, biaxial, e.g., metacarpophalangeal (MCP) joints

» **Unmodified sellar**: (art. sellaris), saddle, biaxial, e.g., first carpometacarpal joint

» **Modified sellar**: (art. ginglymus), hinge, uniaxial, e.g., interphalangeal joints

The joint complex

Anatomical joint

The anatomical joint consists of two articular surfaces (joint partners) with its extra-articular joint capsule and ligaments and intra-articular tissues. For differential diagnosis, Cyriax classifies these structures as "inert (non-contractile) structures."

Figure 1.2a
Anatomical joint

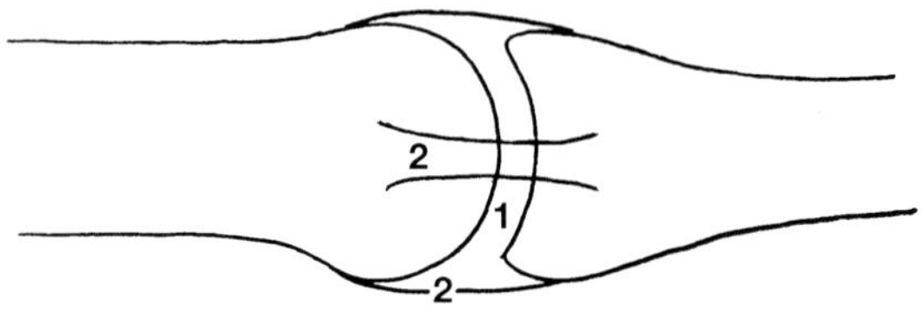

1. Intra-articular joint structures
2. Extra-articular joint structures

Physiological joint

The physiological joint, also called the "joint complex," describes the anatomical joint plus all the periarticular soft tissues, including muscles, connective tissues, nerves, blood vessels, lymph and skin. For differential diagnosis, Cyriax classifies the neuromuscular tissues within the physiological joint, including muscles, tendons, tendon insertions and innervation, as "contractile structures."

Figure 1.2b
Physiological joint

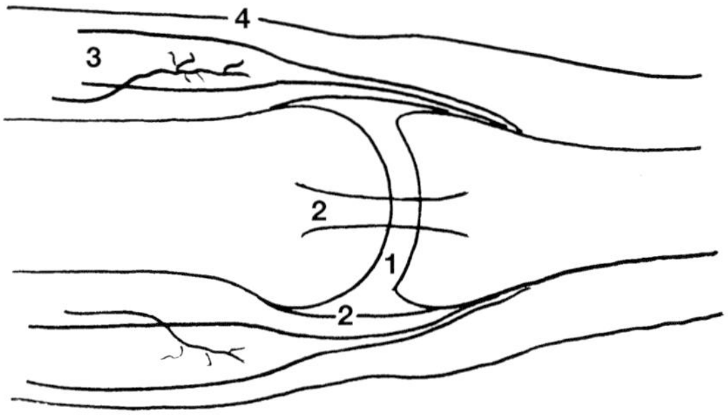

Articular:	*1. Intra-articular joint structures*	*Anatomical Joint*	*Physiological Joint*
	2. Extra-articular joint structures		
Periarticular:	*3. Neuromuscular tissues*		
	4. Skin and soft tissues		

From a clinical perspective, all joint movement involves the entire joint complex, and all joint mobilization techniques affect the entire joint complex (i.e., the physiological joint).

Reference positions

Anatomical planes of reference

The body is traditionally divided into three anatomical (cardinal) planes that are situated at right angles to each other and intersect at the body's center of gravity. These planes of reference are used for describing and measuring anatomical bone movements.

The median plane divides the body symmetrically into right and left halves and all planes parallel to this are called *sagittal* planes. Planes dividing the extremities into right and left halves are called *dorsal-ventral, dorsal-palmar,* or *dorsal-plantar* planes.

The frontal plane divides the body into anterior (ventral) and posterior (dorsal) halves. Planes dividing the extremities into anterior and posterior halves are called medial-lateral, radial-ulnar, or tibial-fibular planes.

The transverse plane or horizontal plane divides the body into *cranial* and *caudal* halves and the extremities into *distal* and *proximal* halves.

Figure 1.3 Anatomical planes of reference

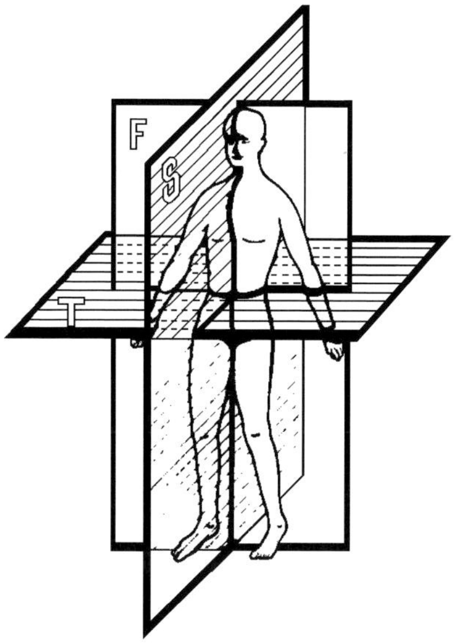

■ Anatomical axes of reference

The anatomical axes lie at the intersection of two anatomical planes and anatomical bone movements take place around these axes.

The **frontal axis** lies at the intersection of the frontal and transverse planes and runs from right to left. In the extremities, this axis is called *transverse, medial-lateral, radial-ulnar, or tibial-fibular (Figure 1.4a)*.

The **sagittal axis** lies at the intersection of the sagittal and transverse planes and runs in a dorsal-ventral direction. In the extremities, this axis is called *dorsal-ventral, dorsal-palmar, dorsal-plantar*, or *posterior-anterior* (*Figure 1.4b*).

The **longitudinal (vertical) axis** lies at the intersection of the sagittal and frontal planes and runs in a cranial-caudal direction. In the extremities, this axis passes through a part of a bone such as the neck of the femur or the entire length of a bone, for example, the shafts of the humerus and clavicle (*Figure 1.4c*).

Figure 1.4
Anatomical axes (after MacConaill)

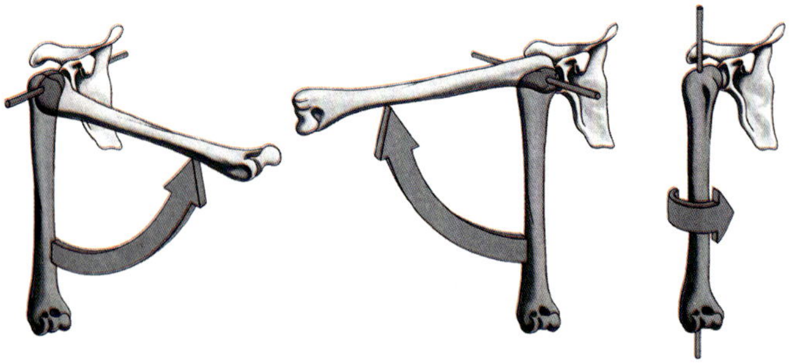

a. Frontal Axis *b. Sagittal Axis* *c. Longitudinal Axis*

During active and passive movements the mechanical axis does not remain stationary due to the joint's changing radius of curvature. The constantly changing curvature and the lack of congruency allows roll-gliding to occur in all joints. Since the axis for movement does not remain stationary, we use the term Instantaneous Axis of Rotation (IAR) to emphasize this fact. Normally the IAR is located on the convex side of the joint.

■ Three-dimensional joint positioning

The effectiveness of joint evaluation and mobilization treatment can be enhanced by placing the joint specifically in one, two, or three planes. For practical purposes, we classify joint positions into five categories:

» Zero position[1]

» Resting position (Least-packed position)[2]

» Momentary resting position

» Nonresting positions

» Close-packed position

■ Zero position

All joint range of motion measurements are taken from the zero starting position, if possible. The range of motion is measured with a goniometer on both sides of zero. For example, a movement of thirty degrees flexion and ten degrees extension is written: flexion/extension 30-0-10. However, if there is limitation of movement, with movement only possible on the flexion side of zero, both figures are written on the left side of zero as in flexion/extension 30-10-0.

■ Resting position

The resting position (least-packed position) is the joint position (usually three-dimensional) where articular structures are most lax and allow the greatest range of joint play. With many joint conditions, this position is also the patient's position of comfort (symptom-relieving posture) affording the most relaxation and least muscle tension.

Uses of the resting position

» To evaluate joint play through its range of motion, including end-feel, and diagnostic manipulations.

» To treat symptoms with Grade I-II traction-mobilization within the slack.

» To treat hypomobility with Grade II relaxation-mobilization or Grade III stretch-mobilization and manipulations.

» To minimize secondary joint damage due to long periods of immobilization associated with casting and splinting.

---

1 This book uses the internationally accepted zero position originally described by Cave and Roberts in 1936, and later by Chapchal (1957) and Debrunner (1966).

2 MacConaill referred to the "resting position" as the "least-packed position."

How to find the resting position

Example: MCP Joint

1) Begin your exploration of the resting position by positioning the joint in a typical resting position according to established norms. For example, the normal resting position for the MCP is slight palmar flexion and slight ulnar flexion. If you observe that the patient presents with an atypical resting position (e.g., holding their fingers in marked ulnar flexion), then begin your exploration there.
2) In this approximate resting position, apply several gentle Grade II traction joint play tests to the first stop, feeling for the ease and degree of movement.
3) Reposition into slightly more or less flexion/extension and apply the traction tests again until you locate the position with the greatest ease and degree of movement. Maintain this position as you proceed to the next step.
4) Repeat the traction tests with subtle repositioning into more or less abduction/adduction and apply the traction tests again until you locate the position with greatest ease and degree of movement. Maintain this flexion/extension and abduction/adduction position as you proceed to the next step.
5) Repeat the traction tests with subtle repositioning into more or less rotation (internal and external) until you find the position with the greatest ease and range of movement in <u>all three dimensions</u>.

   This is the resting position for this patient.

Comments

- Experienced practitioners may speed their exploration of the resting position with simultaneous joint positioning in multiple planes.
- The direction of the final traction test (see #5 above) establishes the orientation of the treatment direction for traction-mobilization and the line of drive for traction-manipulation. The Treatment Plane lies at a right angle to it.
- The resting position may vary considerably among individuals.

Momentary resting position[1]

The momentary resting position may vary considerably from the true resting position due to pathological changes and as a response to therapeutic intervention. The momentary resting position is used in special circumstances when it is impossible, difficult, or impractical to use the true resting position. For example, in the presence of joint pathology or pain the therapist positions the joint where there is least soft tissue tension or where the patient reports least discomfort (i.e., antalgic position). In such cases the momentary resting position is used for initial evaluation and treatment.

Joint play is easiest to palpate in a joint's momentary resting position where the joint capsule, ligaments, and muscles are most lax.

The therapist determines the momentary resting position using the same technique for finding the normal resting position. The momentary resting position will display somewhat less ease and range compared with the true resting position. Careful observation of the patient's habitual posture can give the therapist an approximate regional posture from which to begin exploration of the momentary resting position.

■ Nonresting positions

Many subtle joint dysfunctions only become apparent when the joint is examined in a position other than the resting position. It may then be necessary to treat the joint in this *nonresting* position.

Nonresting positions are also used to increase or decrease soft tissue tension to focus examination and facilitate treatment. Positioning a joint to decrease soft tissue tension can be helpful when mobilizing structures belonging to the "anatomical" joint. Positioning the joint to increase soft tissue tension may be useful when stretching peri-articular soft tissues.

Since nonresting positions allow less joint play, more skill is required to perform techniques safely in these positions. Novice practitioners applying stretch mobilizations in nonresting positions are more likely to overstretch and cause injury. Stretch-mobilization treatment in positions other than the resting position are considered "advanced" in our system and should be introduced to students only after they demonstrate competence with resting position mobilizations.

---

1 In earlier editions the momentary resting position was called the "actual resting position." The term "actual resting position" continues in use in some countries.

Close-packed position

The close-packed position is characterized by the following criteria:

- The joint capsule and ligaments are tight or maximally tensed.
- There is maximal contact between the concave and convex articular surfaces. For example, the shoulder is close-packed when it is positioned in maximal abduction and external rotation (*Figure 1.5a*).
- Articular surface gliding is maximally reduced and traction results in only minimal joint separation.

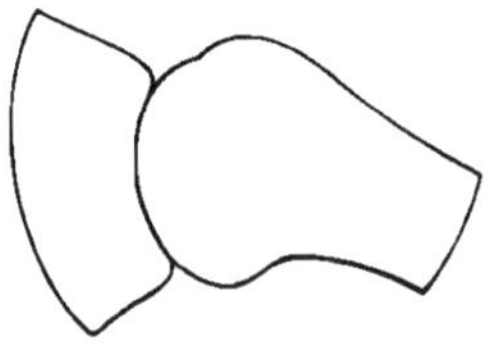

Figure 1.5a
Close-packed position

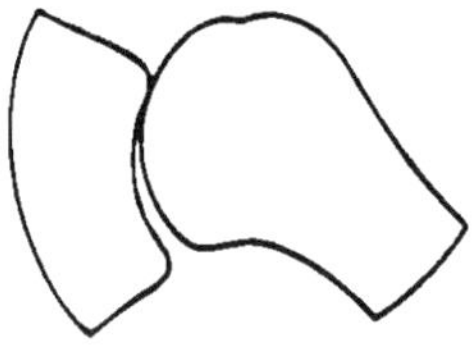

Figure 1.5b
Resting position

Joint play testing and mobilization are difficult to perform at or near the close-packed position.

Bone and joint movement

Bone movements produce associated joint movements. The relationship between a bone movement (osteokinematics) and its associated joint movements (arthrokinematics) forms the basis for many orthopedic manual therapy (OMT) evaluation and treatment techniques.

Two types of bone movements are important within the OMT Nordic System:

- **Rotation:** Curved (angular) movement around an axis
- **Translation:** Linear (straight-lined) movement parallel to an axis in one plane

Bone rotation produces the joint movement of roll-gliding.

Bone translation produces the linear joint play movements of traction, compression, or gliding in relation to the Kaltenborn Treatment Plane. From a mechanical perspective translations can be curved or linear, however *only* linear translations are used in Nordic System OMT.

Conventional movement therapies utilize bone rotations that produce roll-gliding movements within a joint. Roll-gliding movements are a combination of "curved gliding" and "rolling" movements.

The term "translation" in this text refers *only* to linear translations in relation to the Kaltenborn Treatment Plane.

Bone movements	***Resulting joint action***
Rotation (angular movement)	**Roll-gliding**
- Standard (anatomical, uniaxial)	
- Combined (functional, multiaxial)	
Translation (linear movement)	**Translatoric joint play**
- Longitudinal bone separation away from the treatment plane	- Traction
- Longitudinal bone approximation towards the treatment plane	- Compression
- Transverse bone movement parallel to the treatment plane	- Gliding

■ Bone rotation

From a mechanical viewpoint, both active and passive movements occurring around an axis are rotations of bone.

There are two types of bone rotations:

» Standard, uniaxial (MacConaill's "pure, cardinal swing")

» Combined, multiaxial (MacConaill's "impure arcuate swing")

Standard bone movements

Standard bone movements are bone rotations occurring around one axis (uniaxial) and in one plane. Standard movement is called "anatomical" movement when the movement axis and the movement plane are in anatomical (or cardinal) planes.

Anatomical bone movements beginning at the zero position are useful for describing and measuring test movements. They provide a standardized method for communicating examination findings that can be reproduced by other health care professionals. Anatomical movements of the bones in the three cardinal planes are described below.

Sagittal plane movements around a frontal axis

- **Flexion from zero**: movement occurs with the help of the flexor muscles and begins from the zero position.
- **Extension to zero**: movement occurs with the help of the extensor muscles from a flexed position back to the zero position.
- **Extension from zero**: extension movement continues past the zero position.
- **Flexion to zero**: movement occurs with the help of the flexor muscles from the above described extended position.
- **Palmar** and **dorsiflexion** in the hand, and **plantar** and **dorsi-flexion** in the foot, describe movements around a transverse axis.

Figure 1.6 Sagittal plane movements

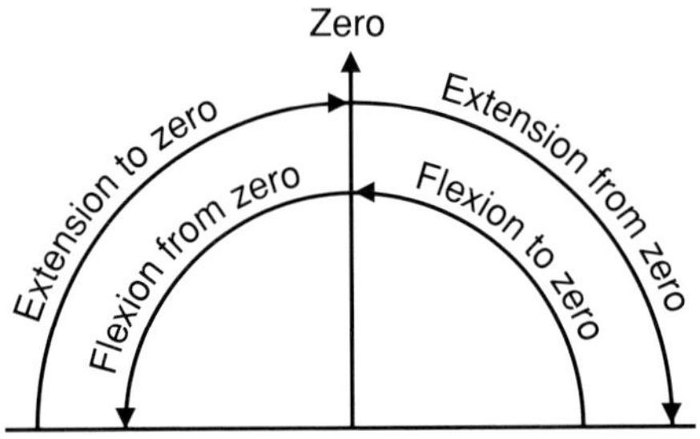

Frontal plane movements around a sagittal axis

- **Right and left side bending**: trunk or spinal movements occur in the frontal plane.
- **Abduction**: movements are away from the median or sagittal planes.
- **Adduction**: movements are towards the median or sagittal planes.

In the extremities, abduction and adduction movements are usually described relative to the regional anatomy, for example radial and ulnar flexion of the wrist.

Transverse plane movements around a longitudinal axis

The term "rotation" is used to describe movement of a bone around its longitudinal (vertical) axis or to an axis parallel to a longitudinal axis. A similar movement, "torsion" describes movement of bones in relationship to each other around an axis approximately parallel to their longitudinal axes, for example pronation and supination of the forearm.

» **Right and left rotation**: trunk or spinal movements in the transverse plane

» **Medial and lateral rotation**: movement of the extremities around longitudinal axes of bones

Combined bone movements

Bone movement that occurs simultaneously around more than one axis (multiaxial) and in more than one plane is called combined, or functional movement. For example, simultaneous knee extension with rotation is a combined movement. These movements do not occur purely in cardinal planes and around stationary axes, but rather in oblique or diagonal directions. Combined movements represent most of the movements we carry out during daily activities. Manual therapists often examine combined movements in order to reproduce a patient's chief complaint and to analyze mechanisms of injury.

Combined movements are further classified as coupled and noncoupled movements according to the degree and nature of movement ease possible when flexion/extension, abduction/adduction and internal/external rotation are combined in various ways.

» **Coupled movements** have the greatest ease (greatest range of movement and softest end-feel), for example, knee extension with external rotation.

» **Noncoupled movements** have less ease (less range of movement and a harder end-feel), for example, knee extension with internal rotation.[1] These movement distinctions are primarily applicable to spinal motion and are covered in more detail in the book Manual Mobilization of the Joints, Volume II: The Spine.

1 Prior to 1992, coupled movement was called "physiological" movement and noncoupled movement was called "nonphysiological" movement. The terms were changed because "nonphysiological" movement was sometimes misinterpreted as abnormal movement, when in fact it simply identified another pattern of normal combined movements with different range and end-feel characteristics.

■ Joint roll-gliding associated with bone rotation

Joint roll-gliding

In a healthy joint, functional movement (i.e., bone rotation) produces joint roll-gliding. Roll-gliding is a combination of rolling and gliding movement which takes place between two joint surfaces. Relatively more gliding is present when joint surfaces are more congruent (i.e., flat or curved), and more rolling occurs when joint surfaces are less congruent.[1]

Rolling occurs when new equidistant points on one joint surface come into contact with new equidistant points on the surface of its bony joint partner. Rolling is possible between two incongruent curved surfaces (i.e., surfaces of unequal radii of curvature). As illustrated below, a convex surface can roll on a concave surface (*Figure 1.7a*) or vice versa *(Figure 1.7b*).

The direction of the rolling component of joint roll-gliding is always in the direction of the bone movement.

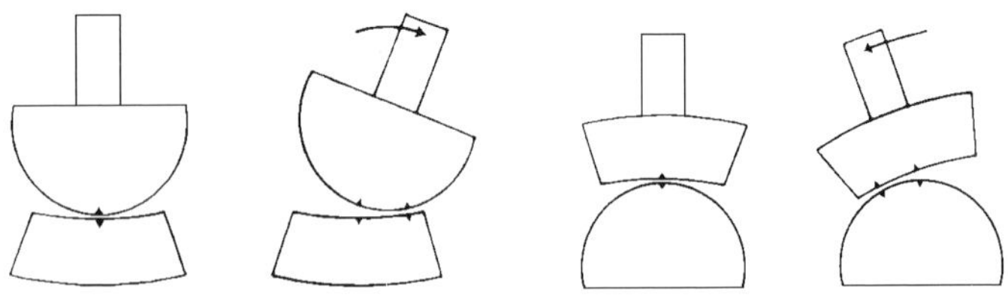

Figure 1.7a
Rolling convex surface

Figure 1.7b
Rolling concave surface

Gliding occurs when the same point on one joint surface comes into contact with new points on the surface of its bony joint partner. Pure gliding is the only movement possible between flat or congruent curved surfaces. Since there are no completely curved congruent or purely flat joint surfaces in the human body, pure gliding does not occur.

1 Joint "gliding" is called joint "sliding" by some authors.

The arthrokinematic direction of the gliding component of joint roll-gliding depends upon whether a concave or convex articular surface is moving.

Gliding direction of a concave joint surface

If a concave surface moves, joint gliding and bone movement are in the same direction. In this case, the distal aspect of the moving bone and its concave articular surface are on the same side of the axis of movement.

Figure 1.8
Gliding direction of a concave surface

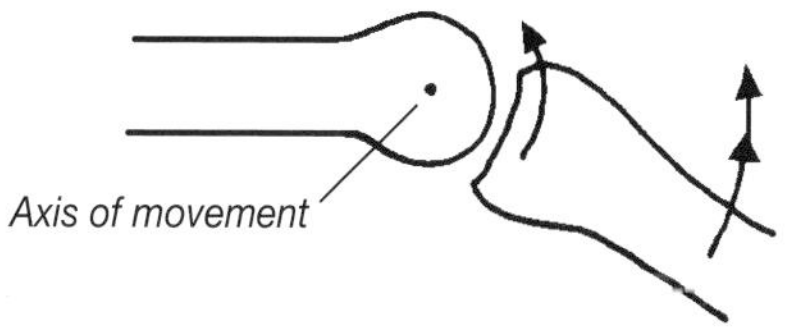

A concave surface glides (single arrow) in the same direction as the bone movement (double arrow)

Gliding direction of a convex joint surface

If a convex joint surface moves, joint gliding and distal bone movement are in opposite directions. In this case, the distal aspect of the moving bone and its convex articular surface are on opposite sides of the axis of movement.

Figure 1.9
Gliding direction of a convex surface

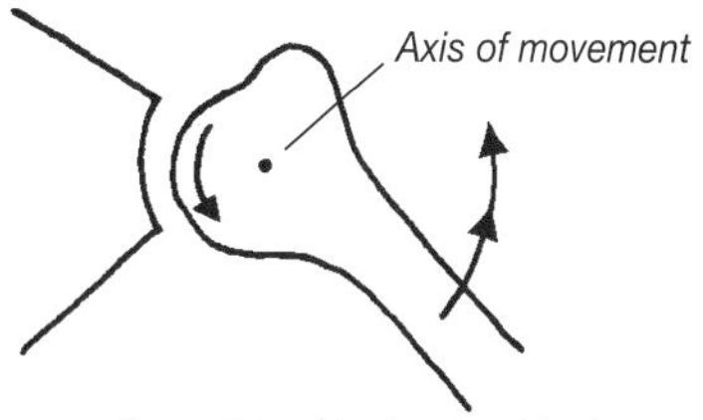

A convex surface glides (single arrow) in the opposite direction of the bone movement (double arrow)

Abnormal roll-gliding

With symptomatic movement restrictions (i.e., hypomobility) normal joint roll-gliding is often disturbed and joint gliding is impaired. If joint rolling occurs without its associated gliding, the instantaneous axis of movement shifts to an abnormal location. This in turn can cause a joint rolling movement to produce a damaging concentration of forces in the joint or strain periarticular soft tissues.

Normally, the axis of movement lies within the convex joint partner. With pathologic hypomobility the axis of movement shifts to the location of the tissue that is limiting the movement. A bone rotation with an abnormal axis of movement can compress and pinch intra-articular structures on the same side toward which the bone is moving, which can cause injury. At the same time, on the side opposite the bone movement tissues can be overstretched.

Joint rolling movements in the absence of gliding can produce damaging forces in a joint.

We avoid the use of bone rotation techniques in the presence of joint hypomobility due to the damaging forces that can occur. These high-risk treatments include long-lever rotation techniques (*Figure 1.10a)* and short-lever techniques applied parallel to an articular surface (*Figure 1.10b*).

Figure 1.10

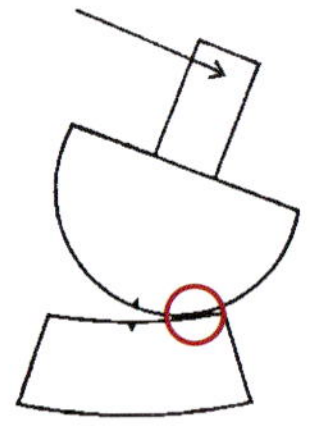

Figure 1.10a

Joint compression from forced passive bone rotation moving a convex surface through a long lever.

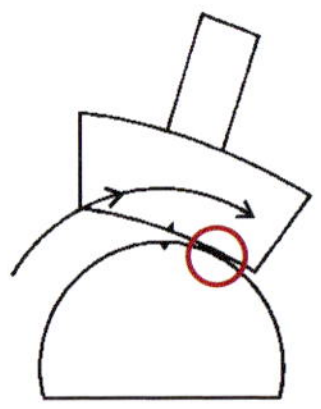

Figure 1.10b

Joint compression from forced passive bone rotation moving a concave surface through a short lever parallel to a convex surface.

Highly congruent joints, whether flat or curved, are relatively more affected by impaired gliding. An important goal in the Nordic System approach to OMT is to restore the gliding component of roll-gliding to normalize movement mechanics.

If bone rotation techniques are used in supplemental treatments (for example, soft tissue stretching), the practitioner must first examine the underlying joints to insure that the simultaneous joint gliding component occurs in an appropriate degree and direction for the technique and that the axis of movement is in a normal location. If joint gliding is restricted or the movement axis is abnormal, the movement should be stopped immediately and the appropriate treatment applied to restore joint gliding.

■ Bone translation

Bone translation in OMT is a linear movement of a bone *along* a defined axis in its respective plane. During pure translation of a bone, all parts of the bone move in a straight line, equal distances, in the same direction, and at the same speed. Bone translation can be performed only in very small increments.

Depending on the direction of the movement, bone translation can be described as parallel movement along a particular axis.

Longitudinal Axis Bone Translation

» **Separation** of adjacent joint surfaces, pulling them away from each other

» **Approximation** of adjacent joint surfaces, pushing them toward each other

Sagittal Axis Bone Translation

» **Ventral-Dorsal Gliding:** parallel movement of adjacent bones in relation to each other in a ventral or dorsal direction

Frontal Axis Bone Translation

» **Lateral Gliding**: parallel movement of adjacent bones in relation to each other to the right or left

In contrast to bone rotation, translation of the bone is not normally under voluntary control, but occurs as a consequence of external (e.g., passive movement) forces on the body.

■ Joint play associated with bone translation

Bone translations produce isolated traction, compression, or gliding joint play movements *in relation to the treatment plane*. These translatoric joint play movements are essential to the easy, painless performance of active movement (see *Chapter 2: Translatoric joint play*).

Figure 1.11
Translatoric joint play

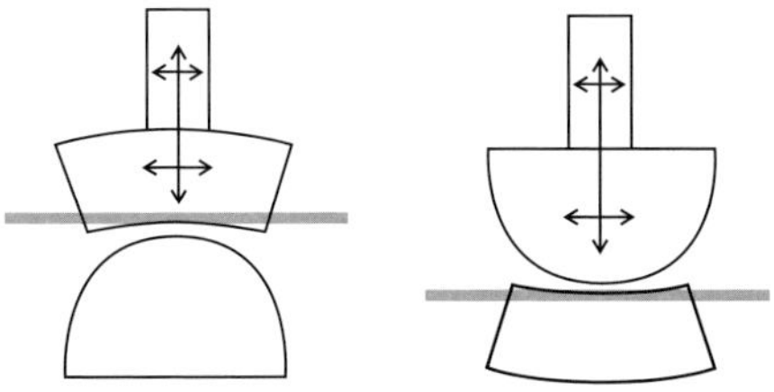

Notes

2 Translatoric joint play

In every joint there are positions in which looseness or slack in the capsule and ligaments allows small, precise accessory joint movements to occur as a consequence of internal or external forces on the body. While these accessory joint movements are not under direct voluntary control, they are essential to the easy and painless performance of all active movements.

Linear translatoric accessory joint movements are defined as "joint play."[1] Translatoric joint play movements are used in both evaluation and treatment. Translatoric traction, compression and gliding joint play movements are used to evaluate joint function. Translatoric gliding and traction mobilizations are used to restore joint play.

Figure 2.1
Directions of translatoric joint play

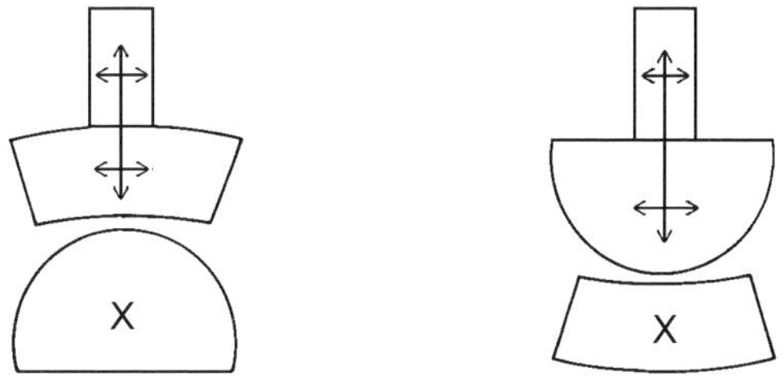

Figure 2.1a
The concave joint surface moves in relation to the stationary convex surface

Figure 2.1b
The convex joint surface moves in relation to the stationary concave surface.

The purpose of joint mobilization is to restore normal, painless joint function. In restricted joints, this involves the restoration of joint play to normalize the roll-gliding that is essential to active movement.

1 In the Nordic OMT System, the term "joint play" refers only to translatoric (linear) accessory joint movement. We do not use the term "joint play" to describe a curved accessory joint movement. We caution against the use of curved accessory joint movements in both examination and treatment. Curved joint movements carry greater risk of injury to the patient. Linear movements are safer and in many cases more effective.

■ Kaltenborn treatment plane

Joint play testing and joint mobilization techniques move a bone parallel to, or at a right angle to, the Kaltenborn treatment plane.[1]

The treatment plane passes through the joint and lies at a right angle to a line running from the axis of rotation in the convex bony partner, to the deepest aspect of the articulating concave surface. For practical purposes, you can quickly estimate where the treatment plane lies by imagining that it lies on the concave articular surface.

Figure 2.2 Treatment plane orientation

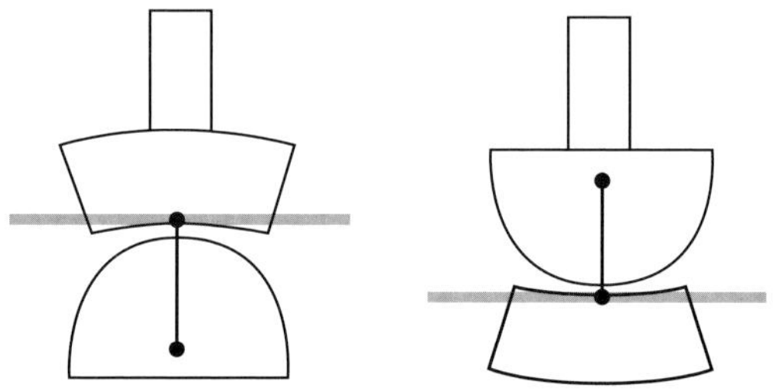

The Kaltenborn Treatment Plane lies on the concave articular surface.

The treatment plane remains with the concave joint surface whether the moving joint partner is concave or convex.

Figure 2.3 Treatment plane orientation and movement

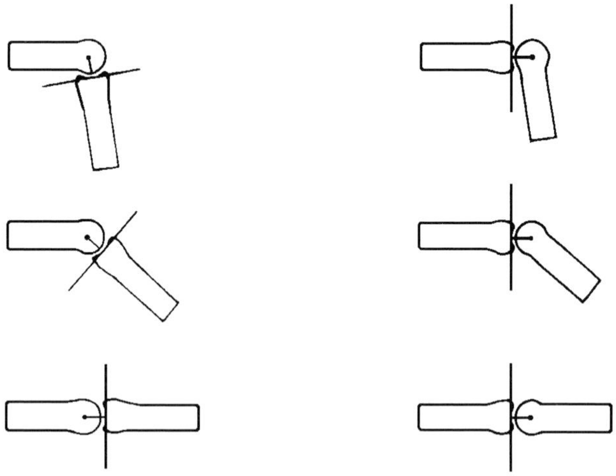

A
The treatment plane moves with the concave joint partner.

B
The treatment plane remains essentially stationary when the convex joint partner moves.

1 Kaltenborn first described the treatment plane concept in 1954 as the "joint plane" and later as the "tangential plane." The term "treatment plane" was coined by Dennis Morgan D.C., P.T. in the 1970's while collaborating with Kaltenborn on his writing.

■ Translatoric joint play movements

The translatoric joint play movements used in the Kaltenborn-Evjenth OMT system are traction, compression, and gliding. Traction, compression, and gliding joint play movements are defined in relation to the treatment plane.

Traction

Traction is a linear translatoric joint play movement that separates (pulls apart) joint surfaces at a right angle to the treatment plane.

Figure 2.4
Traction

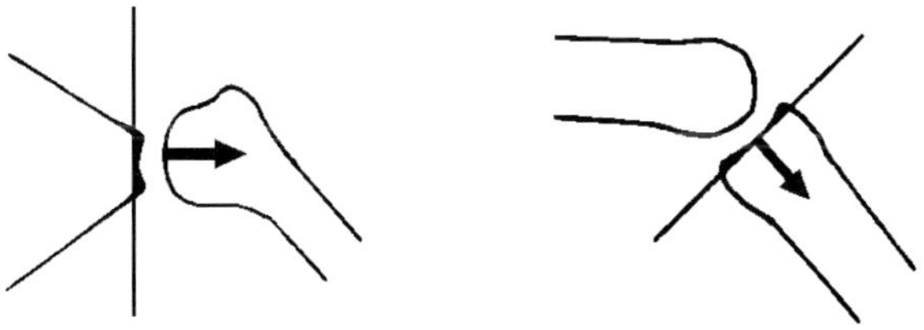

Bone movement at a right angle to and away from the treatment plane results in traction (separation) of joint surfaces.

Compression

Compression is a linear translatoric joint play movement that approximates (presses together) the joint surfaces at a right angle to the treatment plane. Joint compression can be useful as an evaluation technique to differentiate between articular and extra-articular lesions.

Figure 2.5
Compression

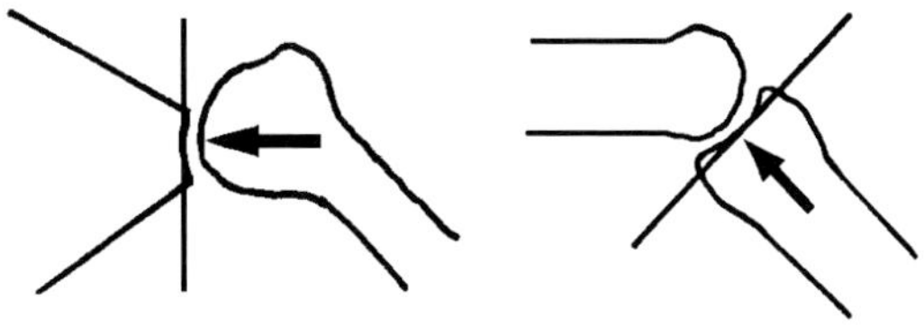

Bone movement at a right angle to and towards the treatment plane results in compression of joint surfaces.

Gliding

Translatoric gliding is a joint play movement *parallel to the treatment plane*. Translatoric gliding is possible over a short distance in all joints because curved joint surfaces are not perfectly congruent.

Translatoric gliding movements are always accompanied by the simultaneous application of a Grade I traction.

Figure 2.6

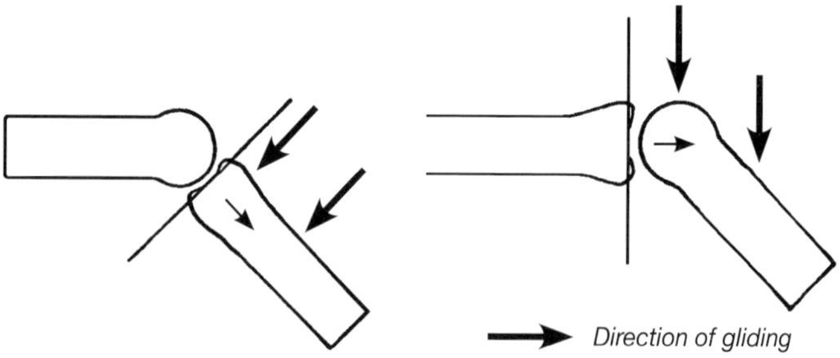

Translatoric gliding parallel to the treatment plane resulting in translatoric gliding in the joint

Instead of using the expression "translatoric gliding," we sometimes omit the word "translatoric" or replace it with a word indicating the direction of the gliding movement. For example, we say "dorsal glide" instead of "translatoric dorsal gliding." This describes translatoric gliding of a joint in a dorsal direction as a result of passive, linear displacement of a bone with a simultaneous traction component.

■ Determine the direction of restricted gliding

There are two ways to determine the direction of restricted joint gliding. The direct method, a glide test, is the most important and is frequently used for assessment both before and after a treatment intervention. A glide test utilizes direct palpation (feeling) of gliding movements in the joint. The indirect method, the Kaltenborn Convex-Concave Rule, is deduced based upon arthrokinematic principles of movement and used when accurate palpation is not possible.

■ Direct method (Glide test)

Glide tests give the most accurate information about the direction, degree and nature of a gliding restriction. A glide test is performed with a passive translatoric gliding movement. Joint gliding, including assessment of end-feel, is tested in all directions.

Skilled clinicians who possess the ability to elicit and feel precise joint gliding movements, rely primarily on glide tests to assess movement restrictions in a joint.

■ Indirect method (Kaltenborn Convex-Concave Rule)

There are conditions for which glide tests cannot be used, for example, in the presence of severe pain or spasm, or in a joint with a very small range of movement (e.g., amphiarthroses or marked hypomobility). In such cases, the Convex-Concave Rule can be used to deduce the direction of decreased joint gliding. The Convex-Concave Rule is also helpful for clinicians not yet experienced enough to feel gliding movement and end-feel with direct testing.

CONVEX → OPPOSITE   CONCAVE → SAME

The Convex-Concave Rule is based upon the arthrokinematic relationship between normal bone movement (bone rotations) and the corresponding joint movement (joint roll-gliding). The therapist first determines which bone movements are decreased and whether the moving joint partner is convex or concave, and then applies the Convex-Concave Rule to deduce the direction of decreased joint gliding.

Convex Rule: In bones with a *convex* joint surface, a bone movement restriction (e.g., shoulder abduction) is likely to be associated with a gliding restriction in the *opposite* direction (e.g., caudal glide of the humeral head on the glenoid fossa).

Figure 2.7a
Convex Rule

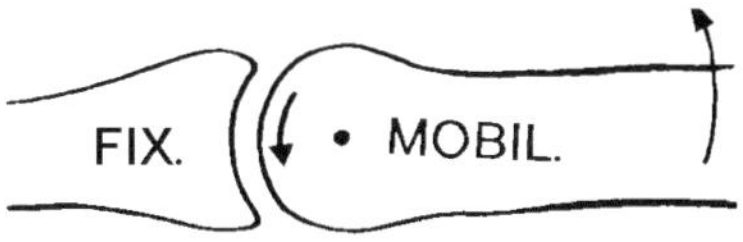

CONVEX RULE → OPPOSITE

Concave Rule: In bones with a *concave* joint surface, a bone movement restriction (e.g., finger extension) is likely to be associated with a gliding restriction in the *same* direction (i.e., dorsal glide of the distal phalanx bone).

Figure 2.7b
Concave Rule

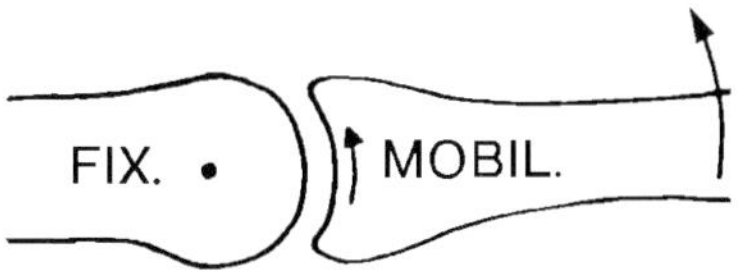

CONCAVE RULE → SAME

Grades of translatoric movement

The translatoric movements of traction and gliding are divided into three grades. These grades are determined by the amount of joint slack (looseness and resistance) in the joint that you feel when performing passive joint play movements.

The "slack"

The term "slack," when used as a nautical expression, describes the looseness of a rope as it hangs between a boat and a dock or post. As the boat moves away from the post, the expression "taking up the slack" is used to describe tightening of the rope.

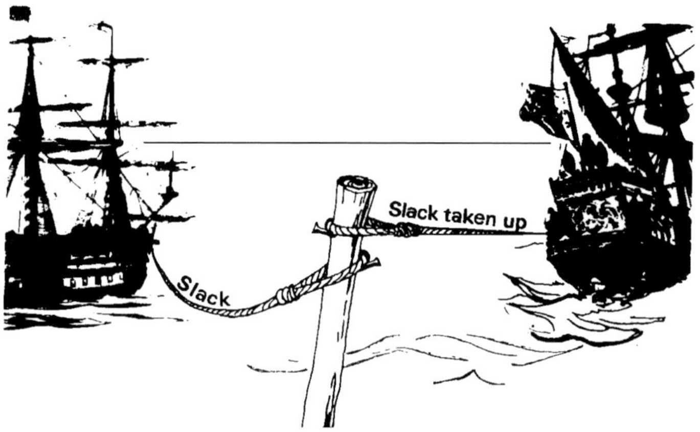

Figure 2.8
The "Slack"

All joints have a characteristic amount of joint play movement before the tissues crossing the joint tighten. The amount of movement present may be of very short amplitude, but it is normally present and possible to produce. This looseness or slack in the capsule and ligaments is necessary for normal joint function. The slack is taken up when testing and treating joints with gliding or traction. When gliding is performed, the slack is taken up in the direction of joint gliding; when traction is performed, the slack is taken up in the direction of traction.

The ability to correctly perform grades of movement depends on the manual therapist's ability to feel slackness in the joint and when tissues crossing the joint become tightened. Many factors influence the feel of joint slack being taken up, including the particular anatomy of the joint being moved, the size of the joint, the amount of soft tissues crossing the joint, the speed and smoothness of the movement, and the skill with which you perform the movement.

■ Normal grades of translatoric movement

The practitioner's ability to correctly perform translatoric movements depends on skill in feeling when there is slack in the joint and when the tissues that cross the joint become tightened. Joint play movements are greatest, and therefore easiest to produce and palpate, in a joint's *resting position*, where the joint capsule and ligaments are most lax.

Grade I "loosening" movement is an extremely small traction force which produces no appreciable increase in joint separation. Grade I traction nullifies the normal compressive forces acting on the joint.

Grade II "tightening" movement first takes up the slack in the tissues surrounding the joint and then tightens the tissues. In the *Slack Zone* (SZ) at the beginning of the Grade II range there is very little resistance to passive movement. Further Grade II movement into the *Transition Zone* (TZ) tightens the tissues and the practitioner senses more resistance to passive movement. Approaching the end of the Grade II range the practitioner feels a *marked resistance*, called the *First Stop*.

Grade III "stretching" movement is applied after the slack has been taken up and all the tissues become taut beyond the TZ. At this point a Grade III stretching force applied over a sufficient period of time can safely stretch tissues crossing the joint. Resistance to movement increases rapidly within the Grade III range.

Passive translatoric grades of movement

Figure 2.9
Grades of movement
I, II, and III

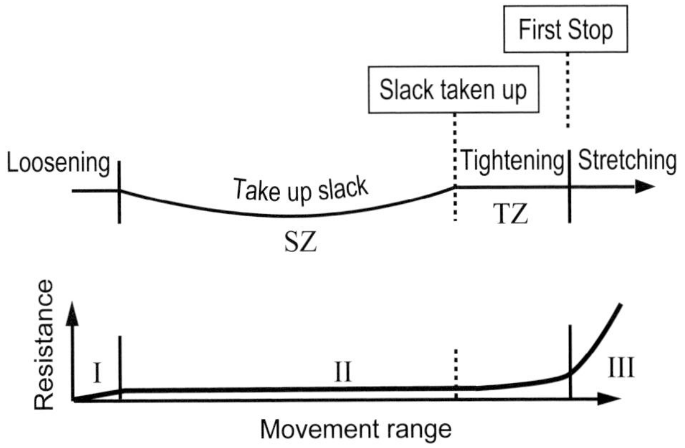

SZ = Slack Zone
TZ = Transition Zone

In the Grade I and IISZ range the therapist senses little or no resistance. In the Grade IITZ range the therapist senses gradually increasing resistance. At the first stop, the practitioner senses marked resistance as the slack is taken up and tissues become taut. Stretching occurs beyond this point. While in the diagrams below the slack in the Grade II translatoric movement range appears quite large, in reality it may be only millimeters long.

The location of the first stop can be difficult to feel. There is not an absence of resistance suddenly followed by an abrupt stop; rather, there is a Transition Zone (TZ) of increasing resistance that may build slowly or quickly. The therapist will notice some increasing resistance immediately before the marked resistance of the first stop.

Mobilization for pain relief takes place in the SZ range and stops at the beginning of the TZ, well before the marked resistance of the first stop.

The degree of Grade IITZ and Grade III resistance varies among individuals and in various joints.

Figure 2.10
Normal variations in resistance to movement (dotted lines)

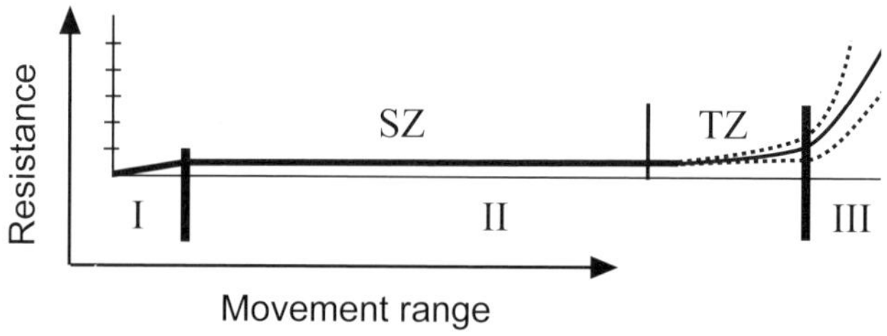

SZ = Slack Zone
TZ = Transition Zone

■ Pathological grades of translatoric movement

In the presence of joint pathology, the quality of end-feel is altered and grades of movement may be altered as well. For example, in the presence of a *marked hypomobility* the slack is taken up sooner than normal and greater force may be necessary to nullify intra-articular compression forces. In *hypermobility* the slack is taken up later than normal and less force may be necessary to achieve Grade I traction.

Figure 2.11`
Normal and pathological palpation resistance

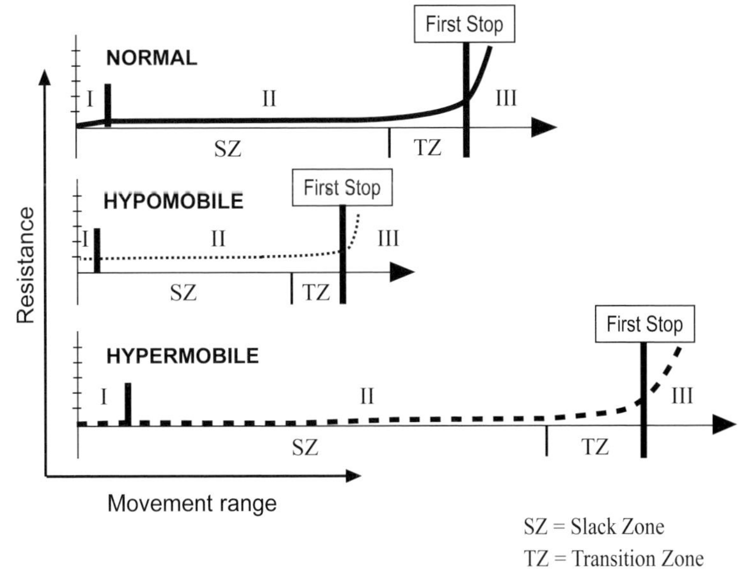

When mobilizing for pain relief, the practitioner must recognize the beginning of the Transition Zone and stop there, well before the marked resistance of the first stop is reached.

■ Notes

3 Tests of function

Tests of function are a key element within the OMT evaluation process (see *Chapter 4: OMT evaluation*).

A test of function enables the therapist to *see*, *hear*, and *feel* the patient's complaints. The constellation of symptoms and signs that emerges from tests of function can differentiate the location and nature of the pathology. For example, if the therapist can determine that a problem lies with a specific muscle or a joint, treatment can be applied specifically to that structure.

The therapist must be specific when asking the patient about changes in their symptoms during the examination. With each test procedure, the patient is asked to describe the character and distribution of their symptoms or if already existing symptoms change. It is especially important to note if a particular movement or position provokes or relieves the primary complaint for which the patient is seeking treatment.

Tests of function include systematic symptom localization procedures that correlate the provocation or alleviation of the patient's symptoms with specific movement tests that stress or relieve forces on specific anatomical structures. With manual testing skill and an in-depth knowledge of anatomy and movement, an experienced therapist can localize the source of an arthro-neuro-muscular complaint and may also be able to infer the nature and stage of the pathology. This provides a basis for the biomechanical diagnosis and a baseline for measuring treatment efficacy.

Assessing quantity of movement

Active movement with passive overpressure is the primary tool for assessment of movement quantity. The practitioner examines the range of motion for each standard and combined movement first by observing the active movement and then continuing the same movement passively with overpressure. The passive part of the movement is not started again at the zero position, but begins where the active movement stops. Passive overpressure normally reveals greater range of motion than the active movement. When passive overpressure does not move the joint further than the active movement, this may be the first indication of joint dysfunction in the differential diagnosis.

■ Measuring quantity of movement

The amount of active or passive joint movement can be measured with an instrument such as a goniometer, ruler, or other device (e.g., distance of fingertips to floor as a measurement of standard rotation spine and hip movement). Standard bone movements are measured from the zero position around their defined axes.

Manual classification of rotation movement (Class 0-to-6)[1]

In joints with little range of motion such as the carpal joints or single spinal segments, it may be impossible or impractical to measure range of motion with a goniometer. Range of motion may then be tested manually and classified using the following scale:

Hypomobility	0 = No movement (ankylosis)
	1 = Marked decrease in movement range
	2 = Slight decrease in movement range
Normal	3 = Normal
Hypermobility	4 = Slight increase in movement range
	5 = Marked increase in movement range
	6 = Complete instability

A joint can be both hypomobile in one direction and hypermobile in another.

1. The *Class 0 - 6 Scale* for manual measurement of small rotatoric movements was originally based on Stoddard's *1 - 4 Scale* and was later revised and expanded by Paris in 1977.

Abnormal range of movement

The results of movement testing may reveal **hypomobility**, defined as movement less than established norms, or **hypermobility**, defined as movement greater than established norms. A joint can be hypomobile in one direction and hypermobile in another direction.

Hypomobility or hypermobility are pathological findings only if they are associated with symptoms (for example, positive symptom provocation or alleviation tests) *and* if the associated end-feel is pathological. Hypomobility or hypermobility with a normal end-feel is usually due to a congenital structural anomaly or a normal anatomic variation and is unlikely to benefit from mobilization treatment. Range of movement tests alone cannot differentiate the nature of the dysfunction, but can implicate a capsular pattern or significant muscle shortening.

Hypomobility or hypermobility are pathological findings only if they are associated with symptoms and a pathological end-feel.

Assessing quality of movement

The ability to *see* and *feel* movement quality is of special significance, as slight alterations from normal may often be the only clue to a correct diagnosis.

Quality of movement to the first stop

Passive movement quality is first assessed from the beginning of the movement to the first stop (i.e., the first marked resistance). The movement should be free, smooth, and independent of the speed with which it is carried out. The therapist must use minimal force so as not to obscure slight deviations from normal.

It is important to evaluate the quality of a passive movement from the very beginning of the movement range. Important findings are easily overlooked if passive movement is tested only at the limit of active movement (i.e., with overpressure), since significant findings in a passive movement are often found early in the range. The therapist must be alert to slight abnormalities from the very instant he touches the patient. Deviations from normal can often be detected at the first contact or very early in the range of movement.

Passive movements can be tested at different speeds to reveal various types of restrictions. For example, slower passive movements are more likely to reveal joint restrictions, while more rapid movements can trigger abnormal muscle activity.

■ End-feel and quality of movement after the first stop

Manual assessment of the quality of movement after the first stop is called "end-feel." Manual end-feel testing is the most effective method for revealing subtle pathological joint findings, and helps the manual therapist to differentiate joint from soft tissue dysfunctions.

End-feel is the sensation imparted to the therapist's hands at the limit of the available range of movement. End-feel is tested with an additional stretch after the first stop of a *passive* movement (i.e., a test of movement *quality*). End-feel testing is not the same as overpressure applied after an *active* movement (i.e., a test of movement *quantity*).

Figure 3.1
End-feel

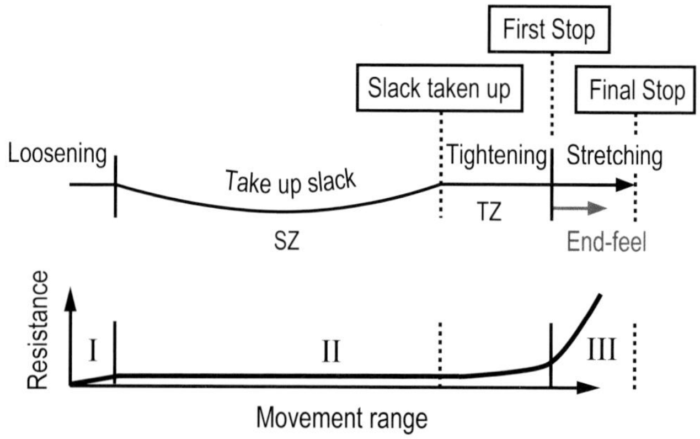

Subtle end-feel findings are easily overlooked if end-feel is tested too quickly or if an insufficient range of movement is explored. However, it is not always necessary or advisable to pursue end-feel testing through to the final stop.

End-feel can be evaluated with standard and combined passive movements and during translatoric joint play movements (i.e., joint play end-feel). It may be necessary to perform an end-feel test more than once and in multiple directions in order to thoroughly assess mobility in a joint. Skilled manual therapists repeat end-feel testing often during examination and treatment.

Normal physiological end-feel

A normal end-feel can be soft, firm, or hard depending upon the anatomical characteristics of the joint and the direction of movement tested. All three types of normal joint end-feels have an *elastic* quality to varying degrees. When the end-feel stretch is released, the joint rebounds back to the first stop or further into the slack (Grade II range).

» **Soft:** A soft end-feel is characteristic of soft tissue approximation (e.g., knee flexion) or soft tissue stretching (e.g., ankle dorsiflexion).

» **Firm:** A firm end-feel is characteristic of ligamentous or capsular stretching (e.g., medial or lateral rotation of the humerus and femur). A normal capsular end-feel is less firm (firm "-") and a normal ligamentous end-feel is more firm (firm "+"). A firm end-feel is variable among individuals depending on many factors, including the size and age of the individual and the extent of degenerative changes.

» **Hard:** A normal hard end-feel occurs when bone or cartilage meet (e.g., elbow extension and flexion).

A normal end-feel can vary among individuals depending on age, body type and build. There may also be considerable asymmetry from one side of the body to the other within an individual. The skilled OMT practitioner makes treatment decisions on the basis of abnormal quality of movement, not on published norms for movement range.

If end-feel is normal and pain-free in all directions, the joint is normal, regardless of asymmetries or deviations from established norms in range or direction of movement.

For example, joint play testing of the acromioclavicular joint may reveal that the concave joint surface of the acromion faces more medially on one side of the body and faces more laterally on the other side of the body. Or the therapist may discover that, while the patient's total range of internal rotation and external rotation is equal for both shoulders, there is 20° more external rotation on the right and 20° more internal rotation on the left with all *normal* end-feels. Such findings are likely the result of asymmetrical orientations of the glenoid fossae rather than joint pathology. Years of participation in an activity which is asymmetrical can also lead to asymmetrical adaptations in anatomical structure, for example in sports such as tennis, golf and javelin.

Pathological end-feel

A joint end-feel is abnormal when the quality of the stop is uncharacteristic for the joint being tested.

» Intra-articular swelling produces a soft resistance ("boggy" end-feel) just before or instead of the usual end-feel.

» Shortened connective tissue such as fascia, capsules and ligaments produce a firmer, less elastic end-feel.

» A hypermobile joint presents with an extended, very soft and less elastic end-feel in the hypermobile movement direction

» Scar tissue imparts a firmer, less elastic end-feel.

» Muscle guarding produces a more elastic and softer end-feel.

» Muscle spasm produces a more sudden end-feel associated with a protective rebound.

» Some end-feels are characteristic of specific pathologies. For example, a displaced meniscus can impart a "springy" end-feel and is painful.

» The patient may resist end-range movement testing or ask that the movement be stopped before reaching the "true" end-feel. This is called an "empty" end-feel. The empty end-feel is usually a protective response to severe pain or muscle spasm secondary to conditions such as fractures or acute inflammatory processes, or can be psychogenic in origin.

It is possible for the same joint to present with a normal end-feel in one movement direction and a pathological end-feel in another direction.

Some end-feels are only apparent when tested with rotation or with a specific three-dimensional movement. Indications and contra-indications for treatment based on end-feel findings only apply to the impaired movement direction. For example, a hard, inelastic end-feel only contraindicates Grade III stretch mobilization in the restricted direction.

Pathological end-feel findings can be subtle and may be apparent only to the most skilled practitioner. A symptomatic joint may appear to have normal range of movement to a student practitioner, while an experienced practitioner will discover an abnormal end-feel. A student practitioner usually needs an immediate and careful comparison with a normal joint to recognize the pathological character of an end-feel. Conversely, a student practitioner may inappropriately judge that a joint with less than expected range of movement requires treatment, while the experienced practitioner would assess a normal end-feel with no associated muscle reactivity, and would judge the joint as normal.

■ Elements of function testing

A. Active and passive bone rotation movements

Identify location, type, and severity of dysfunction.

- Standard anatomical (uniaxial) movements
- Combined functional (multiaxial) movements

B. Passive translatoric joint play movements

Differentiate articular from nonarticular lesions; identify directions of joint restrictions.

- Traction
- Compression
- Gliding

C. Resisted movements

Identify contractile lesions

D. Passive soft tissue movements:

Differentiate joint from soft tissue dysfunction and the type of soft tissue involvement.

- Physiological movements
- Accessory movements

E. Additional tests

■ Active and passive bone rotation movements

There are two general categories of bone rotation movements used for different purposes in an OMT evaluation:

1. **Standard (anatomical) movements** (e.g., flexion, extension, abduction, adduction and rotation) occur in the cardinal planes and around defined axes. They are used for measurement and to reveal asymmetries and disturbances in movement quality (for example, a painful arc). Since these movements are standard and generally recognized, they facilitate communication between therapists and physicians.

2. **Combined (functional) movements** (e.g., coupled and non-coupled movements) occur around multiple axes and in multiple planes and allow the therapist to specifically stress various tissues and structures. These movements are useful in understanding and analyzing the exact mechanism of injury and reproducing the patient's chief complaint. It is not unusual to use combined movements in order to reveal subtle lesions that could be overlooked with standard movement testing alone.

Active movement tests quickly provide a general indication of the location and type of dysfunction as well as its severity. Active movements require patient cooperation, upper and lower motor neuron integrity, and normal muscle and joint function. Since active movements stress both joints and soft tissue, positive findings can only be interpreted in light of additional tests of function, particularly passive movement testing.

During each active movement test, the practitioner observes both the quantity and quality of the movement. The practitioner notes whether the active movement is smooth or if there is angularity, asymmetry, crepitus, or other abnormality. At the same time the therapist monitors changes in the patient's symptoms or abnormal sensations, such as a painful arc. The active movement test may need to be repeated to observe from the back, the front, and the sides.

When possible, the movement achieved actively can be continued passively with gentle overpressure, moving the joint to the last stop while the patient relaxes. This is not an evaluation of end-feel movement quality, but rather a way to determine whether a joint structure is limiting the active movement. If passive overpressure produces little or no increase in the active movement range, the movement is probably limited by a joint structure.

Passive movement tests provide additional information by allowing the therapist to *feel the quality of movement and end-feel.* Sensing the type of resistance through the entire range of movement, including how the movement stops, provides valuable diagnostic information. Slight alterations from normal may be the only clue to a diagnosis.

Changes in the quantity and quality of a passive movement can be due to lesions within the joint or in the surrounding tissues. Careful examination of passive movements allows the therapist to detect hypomobility, hypermobility, an abnormal movement axis, a painful arc, a capsular pattern, and muscle shortening. Specific passive movements are also used to test neural tension and mobility. It is possible to differentiate between lesions involving contractile and non-contractile elements by comparing the results of active and resisted tests to various types of passive movements.

As with all examination procedures, the therapist must correlate the provocation, alleviation, or alteration of symptoms with precise movement and position changes, and compare the results with accepted norms or with the same movement in the opposite joint.

Painful arc

Pain occurring anywhere in the range of active and/or passive movement which is preceded and followed by no pain is called a painful arc, according to Cyriax. A painful arc implies that a pain-sensitive tissue is being squeezed between or moved over hard structures. Deviations from the normal path of movement may be an attempt by the patient to avoid such pain. It is important to note such deviations in order to not overlook a painful arc.

Capsular pattern

If the entire capsule is shortened, we find what Cyriax calls a "capsular pattern." A capsular pattern manifests as a characteristic pattern of decreased movements in a joint. When describing the capsular pattern, a series of three or four movements are listed in sequence: the first movement listed is proportionally most decreased, the second movement listed is next decreased, and so on. For example, the capsular pattern for the shoulder is "external rotation-abduction-internal rotation." This denotes that external rotation is proportionally the most decreased movement, abduction the next decreased, and internal rotation the least decreased movement.

A capsular pattern is usually present when the entire capsule is affected (e.g., inflammatory arthritic conditions). However, limitation of movement due to capsular shortening does not necessarily follow a typical pattern. For example, only one part of a capsule may be shortened due to trauma, surgery, inactivity, or some other localized lesion of the capsule. In these cases, limitation of movement will be evident only with movements that stretch the affected part of the capsule. During each active and passive movement test, the patient is asked to specifically describe abnormal sensations or changes in their symptoms. The patient should describe the character and distribution of pain or if already existing symptoms change with each test procedure. It is especially important to note if a particular movement provokes the same symptom the patient complains of during daily activities.

Differentiating articular from peri-articular dysfunction

Cyriax provides one model for distinguishing contractile (e.g., muscle) lesions from noncontractile (e.g., joint) lesions by comparing responses to various tests of active and passive movement. Cyriax divides musculoskeletal structures into contractile and noncontractile elements for diagnostic purposes. The contractile elements consist of the muscle with innervation and its tendons and attachments. Noncontractile elements include all other structures such as bones, articular surfaces, joint capsules, ligaments, bursae, fasciae, dura mater, nerve roots, blood vessels, lymph and skin.

Noncontractile Dysfunction (adapted from Cyriax)

» Active and passive movements produce or increase symptoms and are restricted in the same direction and at the same point in the range.

Example: Active and passive external rotation of the shoulder is painful and/or restricted at the same degree of range.

» Passive joint play movements produce or increase symptoms and are restricted.

» Resisted movements are symptom free.[1]

Contractile Dysfunction (adapted from Cyriax)

» Active and passive movements produce or increase symptoms and are restricted in opposite directions.

Example: Active external rotation of the shoulder is painful and restricted as the affected muscle contracts; passive external rotation is pain free and shows a greater range of movement; passive internal rotation is painful as the affected muscle is stretched.

» Passive joint play movements are normal and symptom-free.[2]

» Resisted movements produce or increase symptoms.[1]

While Cyriax's differentiation process produces clear findings in many musculoskeletal lesions of the extremities, interpretation of findings can be less clear in some pathologies, such as with the presence of subtle contractile tissue lesions, in cases where a significant inflammatory process produces pain during a resisted test, or when the muscle contraction produces symptomatic joint compression in underlying dysfunctional joints. Therefore, joint dysfunction must be confirmed with joint testing. For example, traction-alleviation and compression-provocation tests can confirm a suspected joint dysfunction.

---

1 According to Cyriax, resisted movements produce symptoms only in the presence of a contractile lesion. In practice these examination findings are not always clear since a resisted muscle contraction also produces loads on underlying joint structures and associated soft tissues..

2 According to Cyriax, passive joint play movements produce symptoms only in the presence of a joint lesion. In practice these examination findings are not always clear since the soft tissues surrounding the joint may affect its pliability, mobility, and elasticity with palpation.

If it is determined that a joint structure is involved, the OMT evaluation is focussed on more specifically identifying the nature and location of the joint dysfunction so that the practitioner can select a more specific, and thus more effective, treatment approach.

Differentiating muscle shortening from muscle spasm

A skilled practitioner can usually differentiate between muscle connective tissue shortening and muscle guarding based on the nature of the stop. A shortened, tight muscle imparts a firmer, less elastic end-feel, while muscle guarding produces a more elastic and softer end-feel that is sometimes accompanied by spasm and increased muscle reactivity.

Student practitioners may make the same differentiation based on the patient's response to a specific muscle relaxation maneuver. For example, in the case where a patient's hamstrings limit a straight-leg-raise movement, the practitioner positions the limb at the limit of available motion and then performs a "hold-relax" muscle relaxation maneuver on the hamstrings. In the relaxation period immediately following the muscle contraction, muscle guarding or spasm will relax sufficiently to allow some elongation of the muscle and the straight-leg-raise range will increase. A tight muscle with connective tissue shortening will not allow movement into the range without additional sustained stretching.

■ Passive translatoric joint play movements

Testing the quantity and quality of joint play, including end-feel, is always a part of the examination of extremity joints.

Joint play is evaluated using traction, compression, and gliding in all directions in which a joint is capable of moving. During each joint play test, the practitioner asks the patient if symptoms change during the movement and notes whether the quantity or quality of the movement is abnormal.

Joint play range of movement is greatest in the resting position of the joint and therefore easiest to feel in this position. An experienced manual therapist can also evaluate joint play outside the resting position, where typically a smaller range of movement makes the movement more challenging to palpate.

There are two ways to test joint play:

1. Fixate one joint partner and move the other through the fullest possible range of joint play movement. Feel for changes in the resistance to the movement through Grade II, past the first stop, and into Grade III for end-feel. Determine whether there is normal movement quality through the range and if there is hypomobility or hypermobility.
2. Apply vibrations, oscillations, or small amplitude joint play movements while palpating the joint space. Apply no fixation or stabilization. This method of joint play testing is primarily used for spinal and sacroiliac joint testing.

Traction and compression tests

Since traction often relieves and compression often aggravates joint pain, these joint play movements help determine if an articular lesion exists. Resisted movements produce some joint compression, so it is important to test joint compression separately and before resisted tests.

It is important to test joint compression separately and before resisted tests, since resisted movements also produce joint compression.

If the patient has symptoms with traction tests in the normal resting position, use three-dimensional positioning to find a position of greater comfort (i.e., the momentary resting position) and evaluate the patient's response to traction.

If a joint compression test produces the patient's complaints, you may need to limit other evaluative techniques that produce joint compression loads. For example, resistive tests usually increase joint compression forces.

If compression tests in the resting position are negative, and if no other function tests provoke or increase the patient's complaint, the practitioner may also need to explore compression tests in various three-dimensional positions. In some subtle joint dysfunctions, this may be the only way to locate a patient's lesion.

Gliding tests

Examination of translatoric joint play gliding movements helps further differentiate articular from extra-articular lesions, since gliding primarily tests structures belonging to the anatomical joint. Gliding movements are also important for determining the specific direction of a joint movement restriction. Gliding movements are first tested in the resting position. If the practitioner suspects a joint lesion and gliding tests in the resting position are negative, the practitioner may also need to explore gliding movements in various positions outside the resting position.

Resisted movements

Resisted tests simultaneously evaluate neuromuscular integrity, the contractile elements, and, indirectly, the status of associated joints, nerves, and vascular supplies.

According to Cyriax, a resisted test must elicit a maximal muscle contraction while the joint is held still near its mid-position (resting position). Not allowing movement during a resisted test will help eliminate the joint as the source of pain; however, a certain amount of joint compression and gliding is inevitable. To exclude pain arising as a result of joint dysfunction, compression tests should be performed before the resisted test. Therefore, if compression tests provoke pain, resisted tests are of limited value.

Cyriax interprets resisted tests in the following ways:

Painful and strong	=	minor lesion of a muscle or tendon
Painful and weak	=	major lesion of a muscle or tendon
Painless and weak	=	neurological lesion or complete rupture of a muscle or tendon
Painless and strong	=	normal

There are three general methods of performing resisted tests: manual muscle testing (standard positions and methods); machines (e.g., tensiometers and various isokinetic testing devices); and specific functional maneuvers (e.g., proprioceptive neuromuscular facilitation techniques).

When testing large muscles with manual resistance, the potentially strong muscle contractions are best controlled if the practitioner induces the force. The patient should resist your attempt to move them ("Hold") in response to your instruction, "Don't let me move you." The patient should not try to push or pull against you, nor should you instruct them to "Push" or "Pull."

Differential diagnosis of pain in a muscle synergy

Several muscles usually act together in a synergy to perform a particular movement. All muscles which normally function in a synergy contract regardless of joint position. Electromyographic studies have shown that muscle activity is not significantly affected by changes in joint position. Therefore, conventional manual strength testing performed from various positions cannot reliably differentiate the source of musculotendinous pain.

To identify a specific muscle or tendon responsible for a patient's pain, the examiner selectively elicits or prevents contraction of a specific muscle or group of muscles.

There are three ways to identify a specific contractile tissue giving rise to pain in a muscle synergy:

1) Test a muscle's secondary function in the same joint

If one muscle in a joint movement synergy has a secondary function not shared by the other muscles in the synergy, it can be selectively tested. For example, if resisted knee flexion is painful, further examination of resisted lateral and medial leg rotation may identify the specific muscle causing the pain. If lateral rotation is painful and medial rotation is not, then it is likely that the biceps femoris is injured and not the other knee flexors which medially rotate the leg.

In the chapters on joint techniques, the secondary functions of relevant muscles are included in the examination schemes as "Other functions."

2) Test a muscle's secondary function at an adjacent joint

A muscle or tendon can be selectively stressed if it is the only muscle in a synergy which functions at another joint. For example, pain with resisted shoulder flexion can be due to a lesion in one of several muscles in a synergy producing this movement. If resisted elbow flexion produces the same pain, then the biceps is implicated as it is the only muscle which can produce both shoulder and elbow flexion.

3) Test using reciprocal inhibition

Selectively relaxing a muscle may be useful as a differential diagnostic procedure. This technique uses the concept of "reciprocal inhibition" to prevent a muscle from contracting in synergy with other muscles during a movement. This is accomplished by resisting the antagonist of the muscle to be eliminated at the same time as the test movement is resisted.

An example illustrating this procedure is the differentiation between muscles extending the wrist and those extending the fingers. To eliminate the wrist extensors and test the finger extensors, the examiner resists palmar flexion at the wrist and finger extension simultaneously; the resisted wrist palmar flexion will inhibit contraction of the wrist extensors. To eliminate the finger extensors and test the wrist extensors, finger flexion and wrist extension are resisted simultaneously; a reflex relaxation of the finger extensors is accomplished by resisting finger flexion.

■ Passive soft tissue movements

Soft tissues are examined similarly to joints, using passive movements to assess the quantity and quality of movement and pain.

There are two major types of passive soft tissue movements: physiological and accessory movements.

Physiological soft tissue movements

Test soft tissue length and end-feel by moving a limb or bone so that muscle attachments are moved maximally apart (lengthened). It is often necessary to use combined movements to achieve full tissue lengthening. Soft tissue end-feel testing during lengthening is particularly important to help differentiate joint from soft tissue dysfunction and to determine the type of soft tissue dysfunction. For example, muscle guarding will have a less firm end-feel than a muscle contracture.

It is not unusual for joint structures to limit movement before a position of muscle stretch can be attained, for example, when a muscle crosses more than one joint, or in the presence of chronic joint disorders with associated degenerative changes. Muscle length testing requires that you be knowledgeable about muscle functions, muscle attachments, and muscle relationships to each joint they cross.

Accessory soft tissue movements

Examination of accessory soft tissue movement tests the elasticity, mobility, and texture of soft tissues. Accessory soft tissue movement cannot be performed actively, but is tested by passively manipulating soft tissues in all directions. Skillful technique can help pinpoint localized changes in soft tissue texture due to, for example, scar tissue, edema, adhesions, and muscle spasm.

Muscle play is an accessory soft tissue movement. Muscle play testing involves manually moving muscles in transverse, oblique, and parallel directions in relation to the muscle fibers. A passive lateral movement of muscle is one example of muscle play.

■ Additional tests

Additional examination procedures may be necessary, including assessment of coordination, speed, endurance, functional work capacity, and work site ergonomic evaluations. These exams do not always have to be complicated, expensive, or require special equipment in order to give valid, useful and important information.

4 OMT evaluation

Goals of the OMT evaluation

The OMT evaluation is directed toward three goals:

1. **Physical diagnosis**. To establish a physical, or biomechanical, diagnosis.
2. **Indications and contraindications.** To identify indications and contraindications to treatment.
3. **Measuring progress.** To establish a baseline for measuring progress.

For example, translatoric joint play including end-feel is assessed in all directions prior to manual joint mobilization. The results of these skilled manual tests may be used to confirm the diagnosis, screen for contraindications, determine whether a joint is suitable for mobilization, or serve as a baseline for measuring progress.

The emphasis of an OMT evaluation varies depending on the purpose of the patient visit and the setting in which the manual therapist practices.

Physical diagnosis

Indications for treatment by manual therapy are based more on the physical diagnosis than on the medical diagnosis.

The skilled manual therapist can *hear* (via the patient history) and *see* and *feel* (via the physical exam) a patient's physical diagnosis.

The physical diagnosis is based on a model of somatic dysfunction that assumes a highly interdependent relationship between arthro-neuro-muscular symptoms and signs.[1] In the presence of somatic dysfunction there is a correlation between the patient's arthro-neuro-muscular signs and the production, increase, or alleviation of symptoms during a relevant examination procedure.

1 The concept of somatic dysfunction was originally used by osteopaths to reflect the many interrelated somatic aspects of a arthro-neuro-muscular dysfunction.

Arthro-neuro-muscular conditions that respond well to treatment by manual therapy typically present with a clear relationship between signs and symptoms. An OMT evaluation that reveals no correlation between signs and symptoms may indicate that the patient's problem originates from outside of the arthro-neuro-muscular system and that mechanical forms of treatment such as manual therapy are less likely to help.

Common characteristics of somatic dysfunction

Symptoms

- pain, weakness, stiffness, numbness, headache, dizziness, nausea, etc.

Signs

A. Soft tissue changes
   - altered tissue tension, elasticity, shape, texture, color, temperature, etc.

B. Functional changes
   - impaired strength, endurance, coordination
   - impaired mobility:
     - joints (e.g., hypomobility or hypermobility)
     - soft tissues (e.g., contractures)
     - neural and vascular elements (e.g., entrapment syndromes, neural tension signs)

OMT examination techniques are designed to reveal the subjective and objective manifestations of somatic dysfunction. The practitioner must be able to distinguish between them in order to administer appropriate treatment. For example, a patient's inability to straighten the knee may be due to pain or soft tissue contractures, peripheral neuropathy, intra-articular swelling, primary muscle disease, lumbar radiculopathy, or an internal derangement.

The OMT practitioner makes three major differential diagnostic decisions in the evaluation of a somatic dysfunction:

1. Determine whether a problem is primarily in the anatomical joint or associated soft tissues, including neural structures (e.g., the physiological joint).
2. Decide if joint hypomobility or hypermobility is present.
3. Determine whether treatment should be directed toward pain control or biomechanical dysfunction.

A manual therapist skilled in mobility testing can often palpate a somatic dysfunction before it can be medically diagnosed. For example, symptoms of nontraumatic origin (usually pain) associated with arthroses, discopathies, or segmental pain syndromes with radiating pain are often associated with a palpable alteration in movement quality, for example, an abnormal end-feel. In the early stages of pathology, this subtle alteration in movement quality may be palpable long before there is restriction in range of movement and before the pathology is apparent on diagnostic imaging studies.

The role of the manual therapist in making a physical diagnosis varies in different practice settings. Most often a referring physician establishes a medical diagnosis that implicates the musculoskeletal system and rules out serious pathology that might mimic a musculoskeletal disorder. In this case, the manual therapist typically omits the organ system review and family history from the OMT evaluation. Emphasis is on the more detailed biomechanical and functional assessment necessary to identify the structures involved (refinement of the medical diagnosis) and the functional status of their involvement (the physical diagnosis).

The manual therapist confirms the initial physical diagnosis of somatic dysfunction with a low-risk trial treatment as an additional evaluation procedure. For example, a traction mobilization or manipulation is the most common trial treatment for a joint hypomobility. If the trial treatment does not alleviate symptoms or if symptoms are worsened, further evaluation is necessary.

The physical diagnosis is further refined through ongoing assessments of each subsequent treatment. The results of these reassessments are an ongoing part of the evaluation process.

■ Indications and contraindications

Mobilization, including manipulative thrust treatments, are based on a specific biomechanical assessment of joint hypomobility and hypermobility.

» Class 0 ankylosed joints are not treated with joint mobilization or manipulation.

» Class 1 hypomobile joints with marked movement restriction should not be manipulated, however, when associated with a suitable end-feel, non-thrust manual mobilization techniques are often effective.

» Class 2 hypomobile joints with a mild movement restriction and a suitable end-feel, may be good candidates for both non-thrust mobilization and manipulative thrust techniques.

» Class 3 joints with normal range and end-feel should not be stretched or manipulated.

» Class 4 and 5 hypermobile joints should not be stretched or manipulated. Mobilization treatments, if used, should be limited to the Grade I and II ranges. These joints often benefit from stabilizing treatments and movement reeducation directed toward normalizing joint function and movement.

» Class 6 unstable joints (e.g., dislocation; ligamentous laxity with instability) may require surgical intervention.

In cases where a joint is restricted in one direction (e.g., flexion) and hypermobile in another direction (e.g., extension), mobilization may be indicated for the restricted flexion and contraindicated for the hypermobile extension.

In most cases, an end-feel suitable for mobilization is also associated with limited range of motion. It is possible for the range-of-motion to appear normal, but present with symptoms and an abnormal end-feel. Conversely, there are joints with reduced range of motion which are asymptomatic and present with a normal end-feel. These are normal anatomical variations frequently mistaken as joint restrictions by student practitioners.

Joints with reduced range of motion that are asymptomatic and present with a normal end-feel, are normal anatomical variations and should not be stretched in an attempt to increase range of motion.

Normalization of the end-feel is an important objective for stretch-mobilization and manipulation. In a restricted joint, normalization of the end-feel often moves the abnormal first stop from a shortened range to a normal range.

It is impossible for students of manual therapy to determine when to stretch or manipulate, and when not to stretch or manipulate, until they develop the palpation sensitivity required to accurately assess joint end-feel. Pathological end-feel findings can be subtle and may be apparent only to the most skilled practitioner. A symptomatic joint may appear to have normal range of movement to the student practitioner, while the experienced practitioner will discover an abnormal end-feel with a slight movement restriction.

Intra-articular restrictions

Intra-articular joint restrictions present with a pathological end-feel that is less elastic, more firm, and appears earlier in the range than in a normal joint. The pathological end-feel is judged to be less elastic if the movement does not rebound back to its first stop when the testing pressure is released. The end-feel will be quite firm, or "almost" hard (e.g., "Firm ++").

Joint manipulation is generally the most effective treatment for a Class 2 intra-articular joint hypomobility. A manipulative thrust can have a mechanical effect on releasing the hypomobile joint.

A Grade III stretch mobilization can also be effective for intra-articular restrictions, and is recommended especially in cases where the joint presents with a Class 1 restriction that has too little movement freedom to tolerate a manipulative thrust. However, no matter how skillfully a mobilization is applied and no matter how long or how often the treatment, mobilization by its very nature has limitations in efficacy. Many joint conditions that do not respond to mobilization treatment, can be successfully treated with specific manipulation.

In patients who cannot yet tolerate examination or specific treatment with a biomechanically significant force, treatment utilizing within-the-slack (Grades I-IISZ) mobilizations and other palliative modalities can provide short-term symptomatic relief. These symptom-control treatments are primarily used as a temporary measure to prepare a patient to tolerate further specific examination or more intensive treatment (for example, a Grade III stretch-mobilization or traction-manipulation) that can produce a more lasting effect.

Extra-articular and peri-articular restrictions

When joint movement is limited by shortened extra- or peri-articular connective tissues, stretch mobilization targeting the joint and other stretching techniques that specifically target the restricted tissues are recommended.

When the hypomobility involves muscle spasm in the absence of tissue shortening, relaxation mobilizations in the Grade I - II range can help reduce muscle reactivity. A manipulative thrust may also relax the muscle spasm with a neurological effect.

Diagnostic traction-manipulation

A *hyper*mobile joint locked in a positional fault can present as a *hypo*mobile joint. It is often not possible to differentiate a locked hypermobile joint from a hypomobile joint with passive motion testing. A trial treatment with traction-manipulation can "unlock" the positional fault and reveal the underlying hypermobility.

Contraindications to manual therapy

No treatment performed on a living subject is guaranteed to be free of risk or complications. Conscientious patient evaluation and appropriate selection of techniques minimize the potential risks of manual treatment.

Contraindications to manual therapy are relative and depend on many factors, including the vigor of the technique, the medical and physical diagnoses, the stage of pathology, the relationship between specific musculoskeletal findings such as joint play range of movement and joint play end-feel, and the patient's symptoms. In other circumstances good professional judgment limits the use of any manual contact technique, for example, in the case of patient resistance to treatment or unwillingness to cooperate.

Grade I and II "within-the-slack" mobilizations are seldom contraindicated, however many contraindications exist for Grade III stretch mobilization and manipulation.

General contraindications to Grade III stretch mobilization and manipulation relate primarily to health problems that reduce the body's tolerance to mechanical forces and therefore increase the risk of injury from stretch mobilization treatment. For example:

- pathological changes due to neoplasm, inflammation, infections, or osteopenia (e.g., osteoporosis, osteomalacia)
- active collagen vascular disorders
- massive degenerative changes
- loss of skeletal or ligamentous stability (e.g., secondary to inflammation or infection or after trauma)
- certain congenital anomalies
- anomalies or pathological changes in vessels
- coagulation factors (e.g., hemophilia)
- dermatological problems aggravated by skin contact and open or healing skin lesions

In the presence of excessive joint play (hypermobility), stabilizing (limiting) measures are indicated and Grade III stretch mobilization and manipulation is contraindicated.

Grade III stretch mobilization and manipulation are contraindicated in joints with active inflammation. However, the presence of a progressive inflammatory disease, such as rheumatic disease, is not an absolute contraindication. During a quiescent stage of illness when the joint involved is not inflamed, a joint can often be safely stretched beyond its slack.

Specific contraindications to Grade III stretch mobilization techniques include:

- decreased joint play with a hard, nonelastic end-feel in a hypomobile movement direction
- increased joint play with an extended, very soft, and less elastic end-feel in a hypermobile movement direction
- pain and protective muscle spasm during mobilization

Screening tests may identify conditions that contraindicate specific mobilization techniques and should be completed prior to treatment.

General contraindications for manipulation are the same as for Grade III stretch mobilization, and relate primarily to health problems that reduce the body's tolerance to mechanical forces. In addition, traction-manipulation is contraindicated in the following cases:

» Decreased joint play with a hard, nonelastic end-feel (e.g., "bone-to-bone" stop).

» Increased joint play with an extended, very soft, and less elastic end-feel (e.g., hypermobile joint).

» Pain or protective muscle spasm during traction testing or mobilization (e.g., empty end-feel).

The most critical contraindication for manipulation may be the practitioner's level of skill and the extent of their clinical acumen. The high-velocity thrust of a manipulation is applied so quickly, the patient cannot interrupt it with a protective reaction or reflex. Advanced thrust procedures require a high level of skill and knowledge to apply safely and should only be applied by well-trained and certified practitioners.

■ Measuring progress

The practitioner determines the efficacy of manual therapy treatment through the reassessment of key signs and symptoms using valid and reliable measures for pain and functional impairment. A relevant sign is one that is reproducible and related to the patient's chief complaints. That is, the sign improves as the patient's symptoms improve, and the sign worsens as the patient's symptoms worsen.

Improvement in the range of restricted joint gliding is one of the most useful findings for reassessment after treatment by stretch-mobilization and manipulation. Since the roll-gliding in all joint movements begins with a short initial gliding motion before the rolling component commences, it is important to determine the specific direction of decreased gliding for reassessment purposes, even if the stretch-mobilization or manipulation treatment is in a traction direction. If there is a distinct, easy-to-feel joint play restriction in a particular direction, this movement direction can be used as a key sign to monitor treatment efficacy.

■ Elements of the OMT evaluation

Through the physical examination the manual therapist correlates the patient's signs with their symptoms. A relationship between musculoskeletal signs and symptoms suggests a mechanical component to a problem that should respond well to treatment by manual therapy.

OMT evaluation

A. **Screening exam:** An abbreviated exam to quickly identify the region where a problem is located and focus the detailed examination.

B. **Detailed exam:**

1. **History:** Narrow diagnostic possibilities; develop early hypotheses to be confirmed by further exam; determine whether or not symptoms are musculoskeletal and treatable with OMT.
   - Present episode
   - Past medical history
   - Related personal history
   - Family history
   - Review of systems
2. **Inspection:** Further focus the exam.
   - Posture
   - Shape
   - Skin
   - Assistive devices
   - ADL
3. **Tests of function:** Differentiate articular from extra-articular problems; identify structures involved (see *Chapter 3*).
4. **Palpation**
   - Tissue characteristics
   - Structures
5. **Neurologic and vascular examination**

C. **Medical diagnostic studies:** Diagnostic imaging, lab tests, electro-diagnostic tests, punctures

D. **Diagnosis and trial treatment**

The constellation of signs and symptoms revealed during the physical examination implicates the nature and stage of pathology and forms the basis of a treatment plan. For instance, before treating a patient who is unable to straighten a knee, the practitioner must first determine if the limitation is due to pain (e.g., lumbar radiculopathy), hypomobility (e.g., soft tissue contracture, intra-articular swelling, a meniscal block, nerve root adhesion), weakness (e.g., peripheral neuropathy, primary muscle disease), or a combination of these disorders.

■ Screening examination

The screening examination is an abbreviated exam intended to quickly identify the region of the body where a problem is located. It serves to define or focus additional examination and in some cases leads to a diagnosis and immediate treatment. The screening exam leads to one of the following three things:

» **A diagnosis** may be made if the physical signs are obvious, correlate well with the history and confirm your initial impressions;

» **Further detailed examination** may follow if insufficient data is collected and a diagnosis cannot be made;

» **Contraindications** to further examination or treatment may be uncovered and lead you to refer the patient to an appropriate specialist.

For experienced manual therapists, there is no set sequence in which to perform screening examination procedures. The circumstances surrounding each particular problem determine how much and in which order the examination should proceed.

Be careful not to over-examine, aggravate the patient's condition, or cause unnecessary pain during the screening examination. On the other hand, make sure the examination is thorough enough to gather all important information.

You must plan the examination from the very moment you meet the patient. And you must be prepared to modify your screening plan spontaneously based on emerging information during the process.

In practice, the screening exam is usually brief and results in either a provisional diagnosis or a further, more detailed examination. It should give you a good idea of the type of problem and where it exists. If the diagnosis is still unclear or you wish to confirm your impressions, examine the patient further in the detailed examination.

Screening examination skills require mastery of the detailed examination in addition to much thought and clinical experience. We therefore recommend that student practitioners first follow and master the detailed examination before relying heavily on screening examination findings.

Student practitioners should first master the detailed examination before relying heavily on screening examination findings.

Components of the screening examination

Begin the screening exam by interviewing the patient for a brief history of the problem. You need enough information to determine where in the body to begin examination and which examination procedures will be most useful. A skillful examiner quickly gets the patient to describe their problem and the immediate circumstances preceding the onset. This brief history, if skillfully gathered and interpreted, can give you a description of the patient's symptoms and functional limitations, define the anatomical location of the problem, and identify any precautions.

Inspection begins from the very moment you meet the patient and start taking the history. Note static postures, respiration, and antalgic positions. The region to be examined should be visible so you can see swelling, discoloration, deformities, and skin changes. Observe the patient moving for valuable clues to the type and severity of their dysfunction. For example, watch how the patient gets up to move from the waiting room to the exam room and undress. These observations may lead you to ask further questions of the patient and guide you in planning further examinations.

The physical testing component of the screening examination varies, depending on the information obtained from the history. Use **active** and, if necessary, **passive movement** to further define the anatomical location and mechanical nature of the dysfunction. The emphasis in the screening exam is on the interpretation of active movements. Try to anticipate which movements will be painful so that they are not the first movements you test. If you provoke symptoms early or often in the examination you may make the rest of the exam difficult or impossible to interpret.

Use selected **resisted movements** to quickly screen muscle strength and the status of contractile elements and nerve supply. Since active, passive, and resisted movements can provoke symptoms, they give clues as to the structures at fault and the origin of symptoms. Perform additional **symptom localization** screening tests if you need to more clearly identify mechanical aspects of the problem.

The goal of **superficial palpation** in the screening exam is to quickly identify obvious changes in the characteristics of soft tissues or underlying joints. Palpation may confirm information obtained in the history or observed during inspection or active movements. Unsuspected information may also be uncovered which may require additional examination. For example, you might suspect neurological dysfunction if the patient does not feel your touch or is hypersensitive to palpation.

Superficial palpation sometimes leads to more specific examination using **passive joint and soft tissue movement** tests. Accessory joint mobility, stability, and pain are assessed with joint play movements. Passive soft tissue movements help assess the quality and texture of muscles, tendons, ligaments, and other soft tissues.

A **neurological or vascular exam** may be performed at any time during the screening exam, especially if some potentially serious condition is suspected which contraindicates further examination or treatment. For example, the patient may describe symptoms that suggest central nervous system pathology. In that case you might begin the screening examination with a neurological examination before any other test.

■ Detailed examination

A good patient history will often narrow diagnostic possibilities, however, an appropriate physical examination is still necessary to confirm the diagnosis.

Components of the detailed examination

1. History
2. Inspection
3. Tests of function (see Chapter 3)
4. Palpation
5. Neurological and vascular examination

History

During the history, you begin forming early hypotheses which subsequently must be confirmed or eliminated by further examination. In this way the history guides you in planning an appropriate physical examination.

a. Present episode
b. Past medical history
c. Related personal history
d. Family history
e. Review of systems

After obtaining the history, you should have in mind a list of possible diagnoses. If the history is clear and you are confident in the diagnosis, the physical exam may be brief and directed to confirm your impressions. On the other hand, if the history is vague or confusing, multiple possible diagnoses must be explored. In this case the detailed exam must be broader in order to explore more possibilities.

If the physical examination does not confirm your initial impressions, proceed to further and more detailed questioning of the patient.

Present Episode

Obtain a complete description of all the patient's complaints and the events leading up to the current episode. Define any mechanical characteristics of the patient's complaint and identify cause-related or symptom-aggravating factors.

It is important to determine if the complaint is mechanical in nature. Non-mechanical symptom behavior raises the suspicion of more ominous diagnoses and may lead to a broader exam or referral to an appropriate medical specialist.

If the patient reports symptoms only during certain times, for example, in the evenings, it may be necessary to schedule the physical examination during that symptomatic period.

Symptoms (chief complaint):

- » Location: anatomical site or area of symptoms
- » Time: behavior of symptoms over a twenty-four-hour period
- » Character: quality and nature of symptoms
- » Influences: aggravating and alleviating factors
- » Association: related or coincidental signs and symptoms
- » Irritability: how easily symptoms are provoked and alleviated
- » Severity: degree of impairment and pain

History and course of complaint (chronology): Trace the chronology of relevant events leading up to the present episode.

- » Date of onset
- » Manner of onset: sudden, traumatic, or gradual
- » Pattern of recurrence: previous or usual manner of onset; related events; duration, frequency, and nature of episodes
- » Previous treatments and their effect

Past medical history

A complete medical history is especially important if you suspect the patient's problem is not musculoskeletal or mechanical in nature. Identify all major past health problems and recognize their possible relation to the patient's current complaints. Obtain the results of previous medical tests and treatments for further useful information. Remember that systemic and visceral diseases can mimic musculoskeletal disorders and their symptoms may even be temporarily alleviated with physical therapy procedures.

General health

- » General health status
- » Weight (recent weight loss or gain)
- » Last physical examination (date and results)
- » Medical tests (dates and results)
- » Treatments, including medications (date, type, and effect)
- » Major illnesses
- » Hospitalizations, operations, injuries, accidents

Habits

- » Sleep, diet, drugs (including coffee, alcohol, tobacco), activity level

Related personal history

Details about the patient's personal background and everyday environment may give insight into possible aggravating or complicating factors. Listening to a patient's typical day's or week's activities, especially occupational and recreational, often provides clear evidence as to the cause of the person's problem. Social, psychological, and financial hardships should also be considered, as they can greatly influence the success of treatment.

- » Occupation (past and present work; future job requirements)
- » Recreational activities
- » Psychosocial status, including financial hardship
- » Home environment (marital status, children ...)
- » Typical day's activities
- » Environmental factors (exposure to environmental pollutants ...)

Family history

Identify any patterns of recurring health problems in the patient's family or any possible genetic or familial conditions. Some joint and connective tissue disorders have a genetic cause or familial link.

- » Age and/or cause of parents' and grandparents' deaths
- » Hereditary, genetic and chronic diseases (parents, grandparents, siblings, children)

Review of organ systems and anatomical regions

Answers to questions about each organ system and anatomical region can uncover symptoms not previously identified. A complete review of organ systems is especially important to rule out pathologies that might mimic musculoskeletal disorders in patients who come to the physical therapist without a medical referral. It can be difficult to determine whether symptoms are of visceral or musculoskeletal origin. For example, nerve root irritation in the thoracic spine can mimic symptoms of angina pectoris and make diagnosis difficult.

- Integumentary system (skin)
- Bones, joints, muscles
- Hematopoietic system
- Immune system
- Endocrine system
- Cardiovascular system
- Respiratory system
- Gastrointestinal system
- Genitourinary system
- Nervous system
- Lymphatic system

- Head
- Eyes
- Ears
- Nose
- Throat
- Mouth
- Neck
- Breasts

Inspection

Initial observations of the patient provide information which helps you further focus the exam. For example, watch the patient get up or down from sitting or take their shoes off for clues as to the body region where a problem exists. Make a mental note as to various areas of potential dysfunction and subsequently clarify these impressions with detailed examination.

Observe the patient both in static postures (static inspection) and while moving (dynamic inspection). The dynamic inspection includes selected daily activity movements and continue during other tests of function.

- Posture: habitual, antalgic, or compensatory body positions
- Shape: general body type, changes in normal contours, deformities, swelling, atrophy
- Skin: color changes, scars, callouses, trophic and circulatory changes
- Activities of daily living: gait, dressing, undressing, getting in and out of a chair
- Assistive devices: use of cane, crutches, corsets, prostheses

Tests of function

See *Chapter 3: Tests of function.*

Palpation

Palpation progresses from superficial tissues to deep structures and reveals asymmetries and deviations. Specific palpation of nerves follows the neural pathway, particularly at the most common sites of impingement.

Compare palpation findings in weight-bearing postures (standing, sitting) with findings in non-weight-bearing postures (lying). Some subtle palpation findings may only be detectable during activity. Palpation during many tests of function, especially passive movement testing, is therefore an essential part of an OMT evaluation.

Tissue characteristics

- Temperature
- Pulses
- Thickness
- Symmetry
- Crepitus
- Moisture
- Contour and shape
- Texture
- Tenderness
- Mobility and elasticity

Structures

- Nerves
- Fat
- Muscle
- Tendon
- Ligament
- Skin and subcutaneous tissue
- Tendon sheaths and bursae
- Fascia
- Blood vessels
- Bone

Neurologic and vascular tests

Any suspicion of neurologic or vascular involvement should initially be considered a positive finding.

Neurologic tests

No single neurologic test is sufficient to determine a diagnosis. Neurologic tests overlap other tests of function and must be interpreted in light of an entire constellation of signs and symptoms. For example, reduced strength can be a by-product of muscle, joint, or neurologic dysfunction. In addition, positive findings from any nerve test that involves limb movement (particularly root tension and mobility tests) can originate from a variety of tissues, including nerves, joints, and muscles. Separately assess the joints and muscles involved in each test and consider these when interpreting findings.

- » Deep tendon reflex testing
- » Strength and fatigability testing (including repeated resisted tests)
- » Sensory testing (light touch, pinprick, vibration, and position sense)
- » Tension signs and neural mobility tests
- » Girth measurements
- » (See *Volume II: The Spine* for additional neurologic tests relevant to spinal and central nervous system examination and treatment.)

Vascular tests

- » Blood pressure
- » Pulses
- » Bruits
- » (See *Volume II: The Spine* for additional vascular tests relevant to spinal examination and treatment.)

Medical diagnostic studies

Additional medical diagnostic studies may be indicated to confirm the diagnostic hypothesis or to rule out serious pathology. The practitioner should be knowledgeable about the indications for referring the patient to a physician for these tests.

- » Diagnostic imaging (e.g., x-ray, CT scan, MRI)
- » Laboratory tests (e.g., analysis of blood and other body fluids)
- » Electrodiagnostic tests (e.g., EMG, EEG)
- » Endoscopy, arthroscopy
- » Punctures (e.g., biopsy, aspiration)

In some cases, the result of these tests may reveal an immediate need for a surgical procedure, medication, rest, or other medical intervention.

Diagnosis and trial treatment

A trial treatment is an essential evaluation tool. If examination findings implicate a joint condition which is treatable by manual mobilization, the therapist should attempt to confirm the diagnosis with a trial treatment. If the patient's response to the trial treatment is as predicted, the probability that the diagnostic hypothesis is correct is increased. In some cases several trial treatments may be required before a diagnostic hypothesis can be confirmed, for example, when the diagnosis involves shortened tissues.

Before initiating a treatment plan for manual mobilization, the therapist should be confident that the following questions have been answered:

- » Is there good correlation between the history and the physical exam?
- » What is the patient’s diagnosis? What are their problems and priorities for treatment?
- » Is there enough information to begin treatment or should the therapist reexamine the patient?
- » Should this patient be referred for further evaluation?
- » Can this patient be helped with manual mobilization? What treatments does the therapist have to offer?
- » Are there contraindications to treatment?

■ Notes

5 Joint mobilization

Joint mobilization is perhaps the most important component of OMT practice. Hands-on skill in joint mobilization enhances both diagnostic acumen and treatment effectiveness.

The mobilization techniques presented in this book evolved largely as a result of the following observations:

» One can *see* and *measure* decreased active movement of a limb and *feel* restricted joint play in the associated joint.

» Following treatment with passive translatoric movements, there is usually an increase in active movement, an increase in passive joint play, and decreased pain.

The subject of this book and the emphasis in this chapter is limited to joint mobilization and manipulation. However, it is important to remember that there are many more tools and techniques, including other manual techniques, that are integral components of OMT practice.

Manual joint mobilization

1. Non-thrust mobilization

A. Pain-relief mobilization

Non-thrust mobilization in the momentary resting position in the Grade I - IISZ range

B. Relaxation mobilization

Non-thrust mobilization in the momentary resting position in the Grade I - IITZ range

C. Stretch mobilization

Non-thrust mobilization in the momentary resting position in the Grade III range

Non-thrust mobilization from the point of restriction into the Grade III range

2. Thrust Mobilization

A. Manipulation

Thrust traction-mobilization initiated from the momentary resting position at the beginning of the restricted Grade III range

■ Using grades of translatoric movement

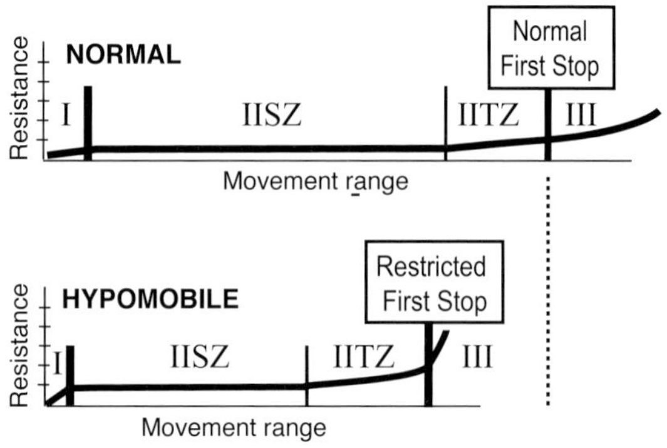

Figure 5.1a
Grades of movement for testing

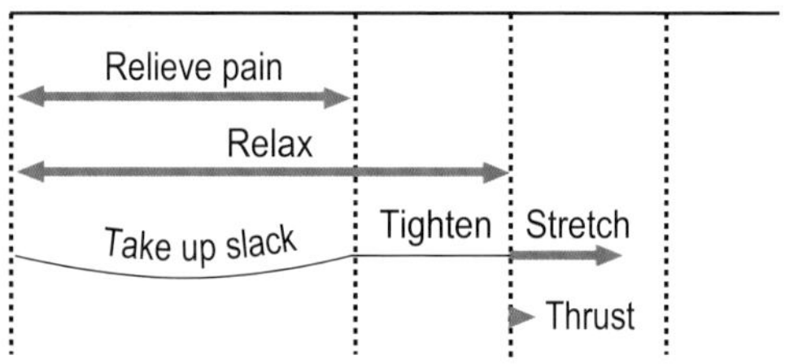

Figure 5.1b
Treatment in a restricted range of movement

Grade I

Grade I traction is not a real movement but serves to neutralize compression forces in the joint during glide tests and mobilization.

- **To relieve pain** with intermittent, vibratory, or oscillatory movements.
- **To facilitate gliding movements.** It may be necessary to increase the Grade I traction force in order to nullify a pathological increase in joint compression.

Grade II

- **To test joint play traction and glide movements.**
- **To relieve pain.** Treatment takes place within the SZ range. The therapist must recognize the beginning of the TZ and stop there.
- **To increase or maintain movement,** for example when pain or muscle spasm limits movement in the absence of shortened tissue. Relaxation mobilization can be applied within the entire Grade II range, including the TZ, as long as the mobilization stops well before the marked resistance of the first stop.

Grade III

- **To test joint play end-feel.**
- **To increase mobility and joint play** by stretching shortened tissues.
- **For manipulative thrust.** Primarily used for intra-articular restrictions.

In addition to treating the primary joint lesion, the manual therapist also evaluates and treats related areas of impaired function. For example, knee lesions can be associated with dysfunction in the tibio-fibular joint or hip; shoulder joint lesions can be associated with dysfunction in the acromio-clavicular joint and mid or lower cervical spine; hip joint lesions can be associated with dysfunction in the pelvis or lumbar spine. Remember also that peripheral joint pain can be of spinal origin (refer to the dermatome, myotome and sclerotome charts in *Volume II: The Spine*).

Non-thrust mobilization

Pain-relief mobilization

Grade I - IISZ non-thrust

If the patient has severe pain or other symptoms (e.g., spasm, paraesthesia) such that the biomechanical status of the joint cannot be confirmed or Grade III stretching techniques cannot be tolerated, treatment is directed toward symptom control. Pain-relief mobilizations are applied as *intermittent Grade I and IISZ movements in the momentary resting position.*

Mobilization for pain relief takes place in the Slack Zone (SZ) of the Grade I - II range and stops well before the marked resistance of the restricted first stop.[1] This is especially important when the biomechanical status of the joint cannot be confirmed. For example, if an undiagnosed hypermobile joint is temporarily hypomobile (i.e., locked) in a positional fault, attempts to stretch through the restriction could stress the joint.

Grade I and IISZ mobilizations, particularly intermittent traction movements, help to normalize joint fluid viscosities and thus improve joint movement when movement is restricted by joint fluids rather than by shortened peri-articular tissues.

Pain-relief traction mobilization

Intermittent Grade I and II traction-mobilizations in the Slack Zone, applied in the resting position or momentary resting position (i.e., three-dimensional positioned traction) is the initial trial treatment of choice for symptom control.

1 In some countries, practitioners refer to Grade I and II Slack Zone mobilizations for pain relief as "passive movements" and reserve the term "mobilization" for the treatment of hypomobility in Grade III.

Remember to apply mobilizations for pain relief within the Slack Zone (SZ), staying well short of the Transition Zone (TZ).

As soon as decreased symptoms allow the patient to tolerate full biomechanical testing with end-feel assessment, the focus of treatment can shift to the appropriate mobilization for hypomobility or stabilization for hypermobility.

Vibrations and oscillations

Short amplitude, oscillatory joint movements other than traction are also used for the treatment of pain. These movements are usually applied manually, but the use of mechanical devices such as vibrators may also be effective in the application of high frequency and very short amplitude movement. These movements can decrease pain and muscle spasm, therefore improving mobility without stretching tissues.

■ Relaxation mobilization

Grade I - II non-thrust

Relaxation mobilization is applied as an intermittent Grade I or II movement in the momentary resting position to decrease pain and relax muscles. It is used in cases where joint movement is limited by muscle spasm and soft tissue tone rather than by shortened tissues. Relaxation mobilization is also used as preparation for more intensive treatments (e.g., Grade III stretch mobilization) which are more effective when the patient's muscles are fully relaxed.

Relaxation mobilization differs from pain-relief mobilization in that it can be applied anywhere in the Grade I-II range, including both the Slack Zone and through the increasing resistance of the Transition Zone. It is important to differentiate relaxation mobilization from the more gentle and benign Grade I-II pain-relief traction mobilizations that are applied only within the Slack Zone.

Relaxation mobilization should not produce or increase pain.

Relaxation-traction mobilization

Relaxation-traction mobilization is applied intermittently in the momentary resting position of the joint within the Grade I and II ranges, including the Transition Zone. The joint surfaces are slowly distracted then slowly released, until the joint returns to the starting position. The joint is then allowed to rest a few seconds in the starting position before the procedure is repeated. Between each traction movement, three-dimensional positioning is readjusted to follow changes in the momentary resting position as joint tissue response allows. It may be necessary to interrupt the traction procedure and reposition the joint in different dimensions until a new momentary resting position is found. There should be a natural progression in joint position toward the true resting position of the joint.

Avoid tissue stretching by staying well within the Grade I and II ranges. Do not mobilize into the Grade III range where tissue stretching occurs. Subtly and continuously modify joint positioning, mobilization forces, and the rhythm and amplitude of the traction procedure based on the patient's response to treatment.

Evaluate the effect of these carefully graded traction forces. It is rare for Grade I or II intermittent traction to increase a patient's symptoms. There should be an immediate improvement in signs and symptoms if the treatment approach is correct.

Stretch mobilization

Grade III non-thrust

Grade III stretch mobilization is one of the most effective means to restore normal joint play. Stretching the shortened connective tissues in muscles, joint capsules and ligaments can increase and maintain mobility and delay progressive stiffness and loss of range of movement in chronic arthro-neuro-muscular disorders.

Restricted range of movement presenting with a normal end-feel is considered a normal anatomical variation, is rarely symptomatic, and is not stretched as a primary treatment. However, such "normal" joints may be stretched in order to relieve stress on a vulnerable neighboring hypermobile joint. Hypomobility presenting with a hard end-feel is characteristic of a bony limitation and should not be stretched.

Grade III stretch mobilization is indicated primarily when joint hypomobility presents with an abnormal end-feel and is related to the patient's symptoms.

In viscoelastic structures, the longer a stretch is sustained the greater and more lasting the mobility gain. *Sustain each stretch mobilization for a minimum of seven seconds, up to a minute or longer,* as long as the patient can comfortably tolerate the stretch. In larger joints, we instruct students to apply 30 to 40 seconds of stretch with the assistance of a mobilization belt. For greatest effect, continue the treatment for 10-15 minutes in a cyclic manner. It is not necessary to release tissue tension completely between stretch mobilizations. A return to the end of the Grade II range, just easing off the stretch into the Transition Zone, is adequate before repeating the process.

Poor gains in range are more commonly due to insufficient duration of stretch, rather than insufficient force. However, it is necessary to apply enough force to stretch the shortened tissue. To determine the most effective amount of force to use, the therapist should begin with forces approaching, but not exceeding, what the patient safely tolerates during daily activities. In some larger joints, for example, in the shoulder, elbow, hip and knee joints, the force of Grade III stretch traction-mobilizations can be significant.

Stretch mobilizations must be applied with care and within the patient's tolerance. Grade III mobilizations can produce a localized sensation of tissue stretching which can be uncomfortable and occasionally painful for the patient. However, Grade III stretch mobilizations should not produce or increase the patient's dominant symptoms or chief complaint.

Stretch-traction mobilization

A series of sustained Grade III stretch-traction mobilizations in the joint resting position is the recommended initial treatment for joint hypomobility. Stretch-traction mobilization is applied at a right angle to the treatment plane.

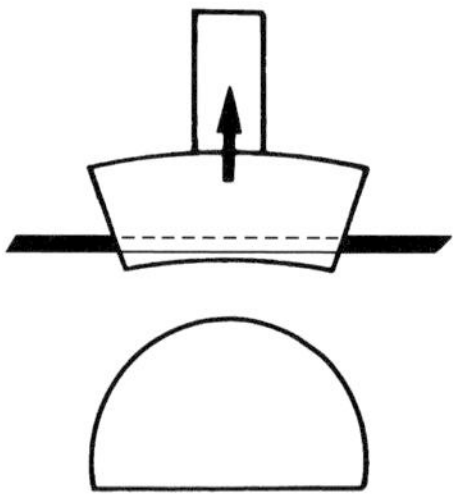

Figure 5.2
Traction at a right angle to the treatment plane

Grade III traction mobilization in the momentary resting position can stretch any soft tissue that crosses the joint and limits joint movement, including muscle connective tissues, joint capsules and ligaments. As a trial treatment, it is sufficient to apply about ten stretch-traction mobilizations. In treatment, the therapist should continue with stretch-traction mobilization and progress with the joint positioned progressively closer to the true resting position, and ultimately also in non-resting positions, as improvement allows.

Grade III traction mobilization at the point of restriction is applied with the joint positioned near the limit of range in the restricted movement direction. This maneuver will increase joint mobility primarily in the positioned direction. For example, to increase a flexion restriction, the joint is positioned at the limit of the flexion range and the stretch-traction mobilization is applied in that position. Skilled practitioners position and stretch in more than one dimension, for example, in flexion with abduction (bi-axial joint) or flexion with abduction and external rotation (tri-axial joint). Stretch-traction mobilization is progressed further into the restriction as improvement allows.

Stretch-glide mobilization

Stretch-glide mobilizations are applied parallel to the treatment plane. Glide-mobilizations produce some intra-articular compression, more so with stiffer joints. To facilitate the glide mobilization and rcducc comprcssivc forccs acting on thc joint, glide mobilization is combined with a Grade I traction movement. In joints with advanced degenerative changes or which are painful when compressed, it may be necessary to increase the traction force component in order to apply the glide-mobilization without eliciting pain.

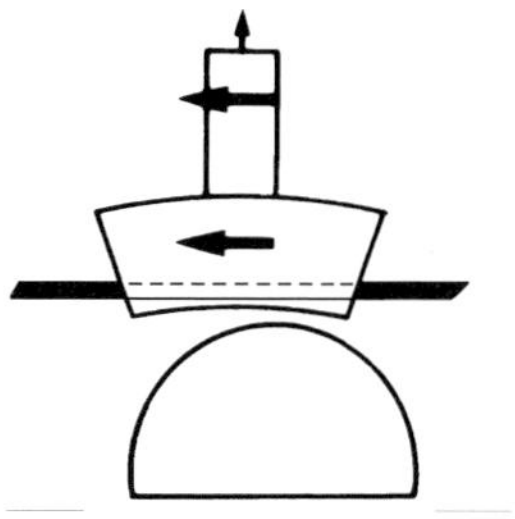

Figure 5.3
Gliding parallel to the treatment plane.

In both examples which follow, mobilization is applied to complement the direction of joint gliding according to the Convex-Concave Rule. The left joint partner is fixated (FIX) and the right partner mobilized (MOBIL).

Convex Rule: In a joint where the moving bone has a convex joint surface, bone movement in an upward direction (long curved arrow) is arthrokinematically associated with joint gliding in the opposite direction (short curved arrow). The complimentary glide-mobilization is downward in the opposite direction (two bold arrows).

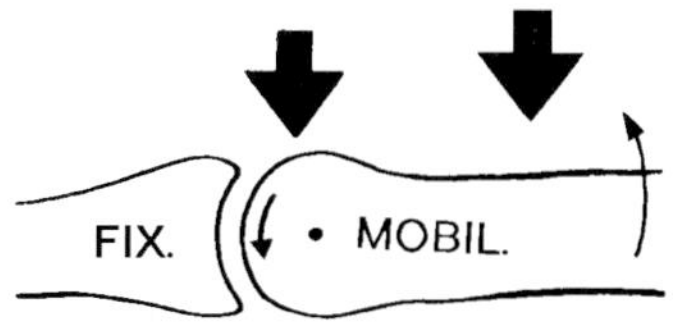

CONVEX RULE → OPPOSITE

Figure 5.4a
Treatment direction using the Convex Rule

Concave Rule: In a joint where the moving bone has a concave joint surface, bone movement in an upward direction (long curved arrow) is arthrokinematically associated with joint gliding in the same direction (short curved arrow). The complimentary glide-mobilization direction is upward in the same direction (two bold arrows).

Figure 5.4b
Treatment direction using the Concave Rule

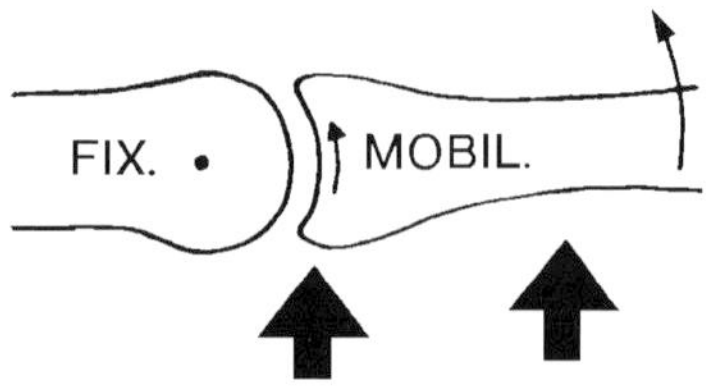

CONCAVE RULE → SAME

Joint positioning is progressed in the same way as for stretch-traction mobilization. Treatment starts in the momentary resting position and progresses toward the true resting position, with the joint gradually positioned nearer and nearer to the point of restriction as improvement allows. For best effect when the joint is positioned at the movement limit, the therapist should ease off the limit a little before applying the stretch-glide mobilization.

Stretch mobilization treatment progression

Grade III stretch mobilization treatment can continue as long as reassessment confirms increased range of movement, normalization of end-feel, and decreased symptoms. Stretch-mobilization should be discontinued when gains in the patient's symptoms and range of movement plateau and the patient can perform active movement throughout this range. Chronic cases and Class 1 marked hypomobility may require several treatment sessions before a change is apparent.

Grade III stretch-mobilizations can produce immediate improvement within the first treatment session. The therapist should see, hear, and feel a difference in the patient's dominant signs and symptoms. Lasting effects may require several treatments.

A Grade III stretch mobilization should be discontinued if it produces protective muscle guarding, severe pain, or symptoms at locations other than the site being stretched. Such a response to treatment suggests the need to reposition the patient, alter the intensity or direction of treatment, or to postpone stretch-mobilization until some healing occurs independent of treatment.

Stretch mobilization treatment direction

It is important to stretch a joint in all restricted directions in which the joint would normally move. However, stretching a joint into some movement patterns is safer, while other stretch-mobilizations have greater risk of patient injury and must be applied with skill and caution.

It is a common misunderstanding that the only effective treatment for restricted joint movement is a gliding stretch-mobilization in the direction of restriction according to the Convex-Concave Rule. In practice, the mobilization direction varies depending upon the stage and nature of the restriction.

Stretch mobilization is often successful with skillful positioning at the point of restriction combined with stretch-traction mobilization alone. In some cases, especially to treat the last degrees of restriction, it can be useful to apply stretch-glide mobilization as well.

It is rare for traction to increase a patient's symptoms. If it does, the manual therapist should:

» **Adjust joint positioning**. Continuously monitor changes in the momentary resting position and adjust the three-dimensional positioning of the joint as needed.

» **Reduce traction force.** Early in the healing process a patient may tolerate only minimal forces.

» **Correct an underlying positional fault.** A positional fault can occur in both hypomobile and hypermobile joints. It is a condition in which joint partners are in an abnormal position, most often involving a hypermobile joint stuck in an unusual joint position. While minor positional faults often correct with a Grade II or III traction mobilization, strongly fixated positional faults may require correction with a Grade III traction- or glide-manipulation.

» **Discontinue traction treatment.** In some cases, for instance with certain acute soft tissue lesions (e.g., ligamentous strain), traction treatment may be contraindicated along with any form of stretch to the injured fibers. In this case, treatment is postponed until some healing occurs. Stretch-traction treatment may also be contraindicated in cases where symptoms are produced in an adjacent hypermobile joint which cannot be adequately protected to prevent further injury during treatment.

Skilled manual therapists who possess the clinical acumen to accurately assess joint movement and end-feel with manual palpation, are able to safely progress stretch mobilization treatment based upon a joint's emerging responses to stretch mobilization techniques as they are applied. Students require a more structured approach to insure patient safety. We instruct our OMT students to carefully progress the application of stretch mobilization treatment based upon the degree of hypomobility in the presenting joint.

Class 1 hypomobility. In a joint with marked movement restriction, stretch-mobilization treatment is applied in the least-restricted joint positions and in the least restricted movement directions.

» When joint hypomobility is so marked that the joint cannot assume the true resting position, stretch mobilization begins in the momentary resting position. As joint structures gradually loosen, stretch mobilization is repeated with the joint progressively positioned closer to the true resting position. When joint hypomobility allows positioning in the true resting position, stretch mobilization begins there.

» Traction in the momentary resting position is the first treatment of choice. Once gains from traction mobilization plateau, or if stretch-traction does not produce the desired result, stretch-glide mobilization is applied in the most mobile joint play directions. If a joint is quite restricted in one direction, it may be prudent to mobilize in other directions, even in a direction opposite the restricted gliding, until the joint loosens and can tolerate stretching according to the Convex-Concave Rule.

» Stretch-glide mobilization in a severely restricted gliding direction may produce joint compression and be too painful for a patient to tolerate. In this case, treatment should revert back to Grade III stretch-traction mobilizations carefully applied in less restricted and less symptomatic positions.

» Stretch mobilization is progressed in this manner until the Class 1 hypomobility loosens sufficiently to be treated as a Class 2 hypomobility.

Class 2 hypomobility. In a joint with a slight movement restriction, the joint should be asymptomatic in the true resting position and should comfortably tolerate stretch-traction mobilization at the limit of motion.

» Stretch mobilization begins with the joint in the true resting position. As the joint loosens, stretch mobilization with traction is repeated with the joint progressively positioned further into non-resting positions, gradually progressing joint position to the various points of restriction.

» Stretch-glide mobilization can begin once the joint can safely tolerate stretch-traction mobilization at the limit of motion. The direction of the gliding movement can be in any direction a restriction exists.

» The most effective glide direction generally complements normal joint arthrokinematics according to the Convex-Concave rule. Remember that when the Concave Rule applies, for example, with the fingers, elbow, toes, and knee, the treatment plane changes with each new position of the joint partners. When the Convex Rule applies, the treatment plane does not change with each new position of the distal (convex) joint partner, but remains with the stationary proximal concave joint partner.

■ Thrust mobilization

Grade III manipulative thrust

In our experience, joint manipulation is the most effective treatment for intra-articular restrictions. Traction-manipulation can also be used as a trial treatment or as a means to release a temporarily locked joint which could mask the presence of a hypermobile joint.

A manipulative thrust is thought to have two physiological actions: A mechanical effect on intra-articular dysfunctions that the practitioner can feel, and a neurophysiological effect created by the avalanche of neurological input precipitated by the thrust.

The audible "pop" ("click" or "crack") often associated with joint manipulation is thought to be the end result of a mechanism known as cavitation. Radiographs reveal gas bubbles in the synovial fluid as the manipulation produces a vacuum (decreased pressure) within the joint. Within 0.01 seconds, these small gas bubbles combine into a larger bubble and synovial fluid rushes into the area of low pressure, causing the bubble to collapse. The collapse of the bubble is thought to produce the audible sound. The audible "pop" primarily occurs with manipulation of synovial joints. Manipulation of synchondroses (e.g., a lumbar disc joint) rarely produces a sound.

The after-effects of cavitation are thought to be therapeutic. There is an increase in the joint space for approximately 15 minutes, increased range of movement and neurological reflex muscle inhibition. These immediate effects of manipulation enhance joint function. After a successful joint manipulation, the "pop" cannot be reproduced again for 15 - 20 minutes or more.

Neither patients nor practitioners should place too much emphasis on the audible "pop". An effective joint manipulation may not produce a sound. Many joint fixations loosen without an audible sound. In many cases, the sound simply serves to make the therapist happy.

Practitioners who focus solely on creating an audible joint "pop", often resort to excessive force and nonspecific techniques using long levers, large amplitudes, and rotational movements. Repeated manipulations of this kind generally "pop" the normal joints and have little or no effect on restricted joints. Frequent manipulation of any joint can eventually lead to chronic irritation, pain, inflammation, hypermobility or symptomatic instability. Repeated rotational manipulations with long lever arms, accelerate these damaging effects.

Not all joint sounds reflect the same underlying physiology. Joint sounds can emanate from both normal and pathological joints with a variety of movements. The "crack" associated with a manipulative release of a fixated joint, is unlikely the same as the "pop" we hear when we crack our own joints. Self-manipulation rarely affects joint range of motion or pain.

There are two types of manipulation used to treat intra-articular restrictions:

1. Straight-lined (translatoric traction, translatoric gliding)
2. Curved (rotatory)

We practice manipulation as a high velocity, low amplitude, low force, straight-line impulse (thrust[1]) applied to a joint showing a suitable end-feel. The manipulation is initiated from the momentary resting position, gently tightening the slack with a translatoric movement and applying a thrust the instant the restricted first stop is met. The mechanical goal is to produce joint separation and restore the curvilinear gliding component of normal joint roll-gliding. The treatment goal is to restore normal, painless joint function. The desired effect is to move the restricted first stop to the normal first stop and to normalize the end-feel.

This book presents selected translatoric traction-manipulations only. Rotation manipulations carry significant risk of injury and are not used in Kaltenborn-Evjenth OMT. Gliding manipulations can also carry some risk of injury if applied in an unskilled manner, for example, without quickness, with large amplitude or without a traction component. Gliding manipulations are best taught only to those who have acquired the prerequisite quickness and coordination learned through the practice of safe traction-manipulations.

End-feel suitable for manipulation

Manipulation is indicated when there is a pathological end-feel that is less elastic and more firm than normal. A pathological end-feel is judged to be less elastic if the movement does not rebound back to its first stop when the testing pressure is released. The end-feel will feel quite firm or "almost" hard (e.g., "Firm ++"). One goal of manipulation is to normalize end-feel. In a restricted joint, normalization of the end-feel often moves the abnormal first stop from a shortened range toward a normal range.

1 In some countries where the terms "manipulation" or "manipulative thrust" have legal implications, the term "quick mobilization" is used.

In most cases, an end-feel suitable for manipulation is also associated with limited range of motion. It is possible for the range of motion to appear normal, but present with symptoms and a firmer end-feel suitable for manipulation. Conversely, there are joints with reduced range of motion which are asymptomatic and present with a normal end-feel. These are normal anatomical variations and should not be treated.

■ Pre-manipulative stretch test

The therapist must confirm that the patient can safely tolerate a manipulation with thorough end-feel testing during the detailed physical examination. However, in classroom settings where techniques practice is not routinely preceded by a detailed examination, a brief pre-manipulative stretch test (PMST) should be applied to insure that the joint on which the student is practicing can safely tolerate the application of a thrust.

The PMST is applied in the treatment direction at the precise location of the restricted first stop where the thrust will be applied. The stretch test must explore tissue tolerance *beyond* the expected excursion of the manipulative thrust.

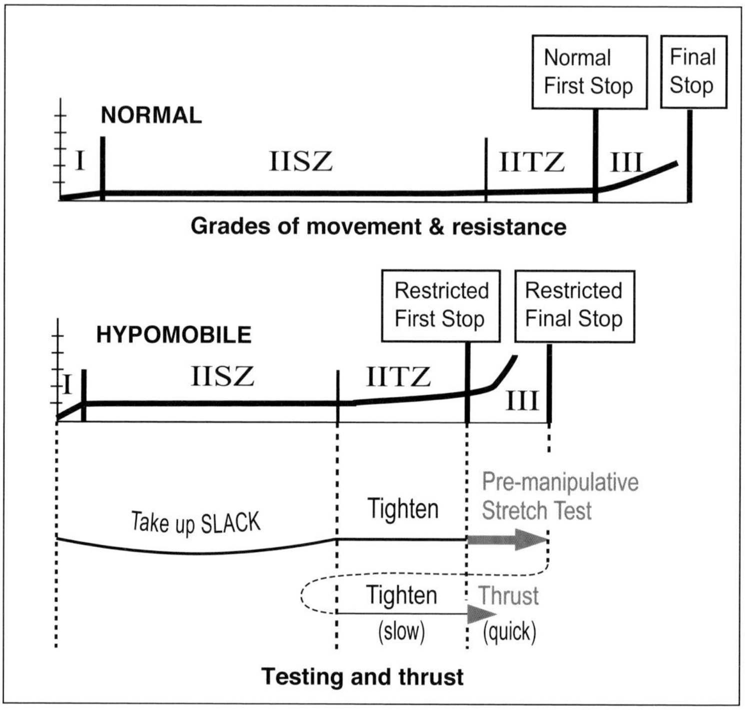

Figure 5.5
For classroom teaching of manipulation, a pre-manipulative stretch test in the direction of the line-of-drive should precede the practice of a manipulative thrust technique.

If the pre-manipulative stretch test is applied immediately prior to the manipulative thrust, the stretch must be released at least back into the Grade II Slack Zone (IISZ) before slowly taking up the slack again, this time tightening the tissues through the Grade II Transition Zone (IITZ) approaching the restricted first stop again for the application of the manipulative thrust. It is often useful to start all over again after applying the PMST in order to create a mental separation between slow stretching and a quick manipulative thrust.

When the PMST is performed immediately prior to a manipulation, it is important that it be performed *only once* and *only for a very brief duration*, so as not to elicit muscle guarding nor aggravate the patient's symptoms.

Manipulative thrust technique

At the time of the manipulation the patient should be as relaxed as possible. The same supplemental treatments used to prepare the joint in the days preceding the manipulation, can also be used immediately prior to the manipulation treatment to warm and loosen the area and facilitate relaxation.

Manipulation is contraindicated when the tissues surrounding the joint are not completely relaxed.

Place the joint in the momentary resting position

Since the momentary resting position can change from moment to moment as a result of handling, positional changes, the treatment itself, and a variety of other factors, it should be assessed immediately prior to *every* manipulative procedure. (See *Chapter 1: How to find the resting position.*)[1]

With rotational and locking techniques, there is a tendency for student practitioners to "overwind" when positioning a joint for manipulation (i.e., position the joint beyond the first stop), so that no manipulation or movement can occur. "Overwinding" not only hinders movement, but can also produce harmful compression forces in the joint and result in unintended trauma to intra-articular and extra-articular structures.

---

1 Joint positioning for manipulation begins in the momentary resting position and the joint slack is taken up from that starting point. This is in contrast to joint positioning for slow stretch-mobilization, where the starting point is often outside the momentary resting position (a "pre-stretch" position) close to the point of restriction.

Students of manipulation may not yet feel when they move a joint beyond the first stop, and thus their attempts to mobilize or manipulate will fail. Without skilled supervision these students resort to more force when instead they should be more gentle in their positioning and/or quicker with their thrust. At this stage of learning, students should limit their practice of manipulation to translatoric *traction* techniques. If students attempt more advanced manipulation techniques with special positions that "lock" joints above and below a targeted spinal segment, they often also lock the segment to be manipulated. The result is ineffective at best and can also be harmful to the patient.

Establish the line of drive

The line of drive (i.e., treatment direction) for a traction-manipulation lies at a right angle to the Treatment Plane through the concave joint partner.

Figure 5.6

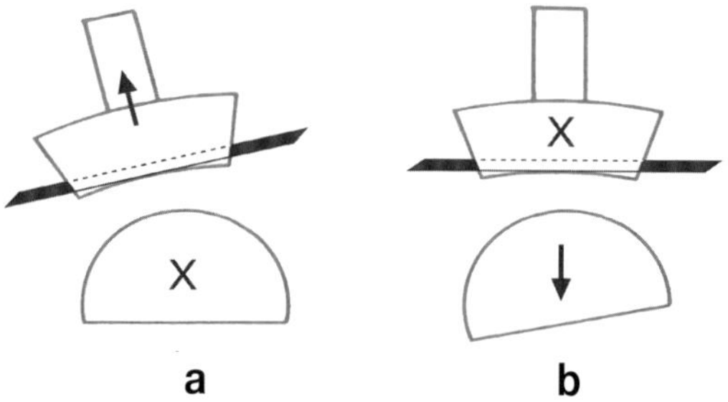

The line of drive lies at a right angle to the Treatment Plane through the concave joint partner.

If the traction-manipulation is applied to the concave joint partner (*Figure 5.6a*) the line of drive follows the orientation of the moving concave joint partner, for example, when treating the finger, elbow, and knee joints, and most cervical and thoracic segments treated from a cranial orientation. The line of drive direction changes if the orientation of the concave joint partner changes.

If the traction-manipulation is applied to the convex joint partner (*Figure 5.6b*), the line of drive follows the orientation of the fixed concave joint partner, for example, when treating the wrist, shoulder, and ankle joints, and lumbar segments when treated from a caudal orientation. In this case, the direction of the thrust remains the same even if the convex joint partner changes position.

Apply the manipulative thrust

Timing	Quickness	Amplitude	Force	Grade

A manipulative thrust is a high-velocity, low-amplitude impulse applied spontaneously at the instant the practitioner senses that the joint relaxes and is ready to go. It takes place as if by reflex.

Timing

In order for a manipulative thrust to be applied successfully, the contractile tissues surrounding the joint must be fully relaxed while taking up the slack and at the moment of the thrust. Relaxation is facilitated in the seconds immediately preceding the manipulation with a variety of techniques, including reflex facilitation and inhibition techniques (e.g., hold-relax/direct action; contraction of antagonists/reciprocal inhibition), breathing maneuvers, and precise positioning.

Some patients with significant pain or tension find relaxation difficult, especially when being handled, prodded, tested and moved by a manual therapist. Slow mobilizations and joint movements can aggravate their pain and increase their muscle guarding response. If such patients can relax even for a second, a skilled manipulator can apply a thrust in that instant of opportunity to provide the patient with relief. Skilled practitioners sometimes distract the patient's attention with a verbal comment or suggestion, and in that moment of distraction find a split-second of opportunity to apply a manipulative thrust.

Quickness

Quickness is the most important element of the manipulation.

The practitioner must already be in position with correct contact pressures and line of drive, so that the moment the joint reaches its manipulative window the practitioner can instantly react with the thrust. There is no time for the practitioner to think at this point. Practitioners who think about the thrust as a step-by-step movement will not develop sufficient speed to be successful.

It is quickness that distinguishes a manipulation from a mobilization. The thrust occurs so quickly it is not possible for the patient to interrupt it. The patient has no chance to provide feedback about pain as the thrust is applied. Patient feedback can only occur during premanipulative procedures. The therapist must be certain of the indications for the thrust prior to initiating the thrust.

Techniques without fixation must be *extremely* quick to produce a local effect. Slower movements have a more general effect and can impact neighboring joints with unwanted movement. Speed is particularly important with cervical and lumbar manipulations applied without fixation. For example, if a traction-manipulation intended for the upper cervical spine is performed too slowly, it may instead produce unwanted movement in the lower cervical spine or even into the thoracic region, especially if the movement is large.

Some practitioners skilled in mobilization techniques have difficulty breaking the "slow mobilization habit" and never develop the quickness to become a skilled manipulator. In order to produce a quick movement, a manipulative thrust is typically generated by isolated muscles in the practitioner‘s arm or shoulder (as push or pull) rather than by the practitioner‘s body. This is in contrast to mobilization techniques in which slow movements are produced by movement of the practitioner‘s entire body. It is important that practitioners learn to isolate these muscles to generate the small, explosive, spontaneous impulse required for an effective thrust.

The beneficial neurological reflex effects of manipulation depend in large part upon the quickness of the maneuver. Practitioners who are unable to generate the necessary speed for a successful manipulative thrust, must depend upon slower mobilization techniques for patient treatment which rely more on mechanical tissue change for their effect.

Amplitude

Amplitude is the second-most important element of the manipulation.

The amplitude (length) of movement that is produced in a manipulative thrust is so small, there may be no perceptible movement in the joint. The movement is no more than a quick impulse applied after the slack is tightened to the restricted first stop. An extremely small movement amplitude is essential to prevent damage to the joint tissues and surrounding structures with a rapid thrust.

The impulse of the thrust stops as quickly as it starts, like a contained explosion. When learning manipulation, it is useful to think the words "Go" and "Stop" at the same time (i.e., say, "GoStop" as a single word) upon initiating the thrust.[1]

Force

In a manipulative thrust, the practitioner uses the least possible force necessary to achieve the desired effect. The more skilled a practitioner becomes with palpation, tightening the slack, sensing end-feel, timing, positioning and movement coordination, the less force is needed.

The exact force required for an effective manipulative thrust is impossible to ascertain with certainty. Various joints, variations in individual anatomy and different types and stages of joint pathology, characteristically require more or less thrusting force. A joint in a child may only require a force of 5 Newtons, whereas a large joint in an adult may require a force of 40 or 50 Newtons. Therapeutic manipulation for hypomobility requires relatively more force than manipulations used as a trial treatment or to differentiate an acutely fixated hypermobile joint from a longer standing hypomobility. The best guideline for practitioners is to use as much force as necessary and as little force as possible.

There is no shortcut for learning how to determine the optimal force for a particular manipulation. Only time and experience can teach this, with hands-on guidance from an experienced clinical instructor.

Grade

The traction thrust is applied precisely when the slack has been slowly taken up and *tightened* at the start of the pathological Grade III range, called the restricted first stop. Manipulation is not applied at the end of a prolonged stretch-mobilization.

A common misconception among manual therapists, is that a manipulation is a continuation of a stretch-mobilization.

---

1 In Norwegian, the word "ballotere" describes a movement that is stopped suddenly by an antagonist muscle. A manipulative thrust is a "ballotere" movement that stops *immediately* after it starts. There is no equivalent word in the English language, so we created one: "GoStop".

A practitioner's ability to apply an effective traction thrust requires the ability to detect and instantaneously react at the moment the movement approaches the marked resistance of the restricted first stop.

A common error of student practitioners is to thrust "at a run" through the IITZ range into the Grade III range. In practice, the thrust is a continuation of a slow translatoric movement from the Slack Zone (IISZ) which begins to tighten the tissue through the Transition Zone (IITZ). The quick thrust is initiated the instant the practitioner senses marked resistance at the start of the restricted first stop.

Prior to application of any manipulative thrust, the practitioner should have confirmed that the patient can safely tolerate a manipulation by applying a Grade III pre-manipulative stretch-test and feeling the precise location of the first stop where the thrust will be applied.

Manipulative thrust treatment progression

Pre-manipulative procedures

The joint must have an end-feel suitable for manipulation. In cases where the joint end-feel is too restricted or when associated soft tissue restrictions interfere with a manipulative maneuver, it may be necessary to prepare the joint with other treatments. The joint can be loosened over a period of time in the days preceding the manipulation with the application of stretch mobilization, soft tissue treatment (e.g., muscle stretching, functional massage), acupuncture or acupressure, therapeutic exercise, or other modalities (e.g., heat, cold, electrotherapy).

Progression of manipulative treatments

When the application of a manipulative thrust results in normalization of joint function along with decreased symptoms, treatment should be stopped for that day.

It can take more than one manipulative thrust to achieve success. If the first attempt is unsuccessful and reassessment reveals no improvement, the practitioner can try again with variations in technique (e.g., with better patient relaxation, changes in timing, positioning, direction of force, etc.) or a different technique. If a second attempt at manipulation is unsuccessful, or if the patient's condition is worsened, reevaluation is necessary and may indicate a change in treatment.

Some patients benefit from a series of manipulation treatments over time. As long as reassessment confirms that the patient improves with each treatment, there is no harm in repeating the same manipulation in subsequent treatment sessions. Periodic treatment with manipulation is often useful in cases when self-treatment measures (e.g., home exercise) are not adequate to maintain joint function. Periodic manipulation treatments over time are also helpful in chronic cases (e.g., ankylosing spondylitis) to help maintain joint function.

If there is no change after three treatments with manipulation it makes little sense to continue. At this point the practitioner must determine whether another form of treatment is indicated. In some cases the patient might benefit from manipulation delivered by a specialist with more advanced manipulative skill. Unfortunately, patient referrals to colleagues with specialty training is discouraged in some clinical settings, to the detriment of quality patient care.

Post-manipulative procedures

Appropriate after-manipulation care and patient instruction follows the same OMT guidelines as for other manual therapy techniques. Following manipulation, additional treatment or special management of the condition may be necessary. Some joint conditions benefit from a period of rest after the manipulation, especially in the cervical spine. Other conditions benefit from therapeutic exercise (e.g., Medical Training Therapy) in the area where the manipulation was applied.

Avoiding negative outcomes with manual treatment

How much treatment is enough?

One of the most frequently asked questions, and also hardest to answer is, "How much treatment is enough?" The easiest answer is, "As much as necessary and as little as possible." The answer is accurate but rarely satisfies students. We therefore provide the following general guidelines which are both conservative and safe. With experience, the nuances of clinical decision-making will become more apparent and you will find answers to these difficult questions.

Reassessment of the patient's chief complaints and dominant physical signs is important at the beginning and end of each treatment session as well as during the treatment session.

» When reassessment reveals increased range of motion or decreased pain, then treatment may continue as before, perhaps with increased intensity.

» When reassessment reveals a *marked* improvement in range of motion, we advise student practitioners to stop treatment for that day and continue the treatment on a subsequent day. We make this recommendation because student practitioners often overtreat the patient in the mistaken belief that "more is better."

» When reassessment during a treatment session indicates that function is not normalizing or that symptoms are not decreasing, the therapist must be alert to the need for further evaluation to determine a more appropriate technique, positioning, direction of force, or treatment intensity.

Treatment should not result in discomfort or pain which persists beyond the day of treatment.

■ Risks of rotation mobilization

We do not teach rotation joint mobilization or manipulation around an axis because such techniques can produce significant compressive forces with adverse effects.

The safest way to increase joint rotation range is to use a Grade III stretch-traction mobilization in conjunction with specific three-dimensional positioning. The specific joint is positioned near the point of its restricted rotation, at which point a Grade III traction mobilization is applied at a right angle to the treatment plane. If this procedure does not completely restore the rotation movement, treatment is progressed to a linear stretch-glide mobilization at the end-range of the restricted rotation with a simultaneous Grade I traction force to protect the joint.

The skilled application of three-dimensional stretch-traction mobilization or specific stretch-glide mobilizations is safer and, in skilled hands, just as effective as rotation mobilization. (See *Afterword: Recommendation to abandon rotatory joint techniques.*)

■ Risks of joint compression

Some practitioners believe that passive manual joint compression can stimulate cartilage nutrition and regeneration and use it for that purpose, particularly in certain extremity joints. We do not teach joint compression techniques because they can too easily aggravate a joint condition.

Little is known about the physiological effects of manual joint compression treatment. Critical to the maintenance of articular cartilage is its fluid supply of nutrients by diffusion. This fluid nutrient transfer is facilitated by *changes in joint loading* which create pressure changes. Therefore, it has been hypothesized that compression may be a useful joint mobilization technique. Following the same logic, our intermittent traction approach may also provide the necessary pressure changes, thus facilitating articular cartilage nutrition.

Rolling, gliding, and compression are physiological stresses joints experience with normal movement. In fact, these stresses are *necessary* for the maintenance of articular cartilage. When there is an imbalance of rolling, gliding and compression, joints begin to show the effects of wear and tear, marking the onset of degenerative joint disease (DJD). For example, too much compression may occur with excessive running or jumping activities which can lead to DJD. On the other hand, not enough stress to the joint, as with prolonged immobilization in a cast or bed rest, can also lead to DJD.

If joint compression occurs during a patient's treatment program, the amount of load-bearing is increased gradually and monitored closely to avoid pain. Therapists use standard protocols for graduated return to full weight-bearing in the lower extremity joints. The progression usually begins with toe-touch weight-bearing using two crutches and progresses to one crutch, then a cane, and eventually full weight-bearing. Another common progression starts with active assisted movement, then active movement, and finally resisted movement. These progressions represent a kind of "graduated" compression therapy which the patient controls based on their tolerance to the activity. Premature load-bearing treatment can lead to joint swelling and additional injury to the patient.

Many daily activities produce joint compression and can aggravate a patients symptoms. For example, sidelying induces significant compression in the hip joint. Management of this patient would include instruction in how to position pillows during sidelying sleep.

Traction and glide mobilizations are safer than joint compression techniques, and may very well provide the needed pressure changes to facilitate articular maintenance. However, gliding techniques also have a compression effect, especially at the end range of motion, and can also produce pain. If glide mobilizations produce pain, reduce the force and add traction. If pain persists with this treatment, discontinue the technique.

6 Supplemental OMT treatment

Mobilization is often more effective when supplemented with other therapeutic procedures and modalities. The sequencing of these adjunctive procedures can influence the outcome of manual mobilization techniques. For example, a stretch mobilization preceded by heat application can produce greater mobility gains, and specific home exercise following a stretch mobilization can better preserve mobility gains.

While you study the following treatment guidelines, remember that clinical experience, not theory, is the most important criteria upon which treatment decisions are made.

OMT Treatment

A. For symptom control

1. *Immobilization*
2. *Thermo-Hydro-Electro (T-H-E) therapy*
3. *Joint mobilization* (see Chapter 5)
    a. Non-thrust Grade I - IISZ: Pain-relief mobilization
4. *Special procedures*

B. To increase mobility

1. *Soft tissue mobilization*
    a. Passive soft tissue mobilization
    b. Active soft tissue mobilization
2. *Joint mobilization* (see Chapter 5)
    a. Non-thrust Grade I - II: Relaxation mobilization
    b. Non-thrust Grade III: Stretch mobilization
    c. Thrust Grade III: Manipulation
3. *Neural tissue mobilization*
4. *Specialized exercise*

C. To limit movement

1. *Specialized exercise*
2. *Increasing movement in adjacent joints*

D. Supportive devices

E. To inform, instruct, and train

Treatment for symptom control

Symptom control treatments can be useful for both hypermobile and hypomobile joint conditions and in the presence of nerve root findings. Use symptom control techniques when:

» severe pain or other symptoms (for example, an empty end-feel) interfere with biomechanical assessment of the joint.

» treatment with movement is contraindicated or cannot be tolerated.

» inflammatory processes, disc pathology, or increased muscle reactivity around a symptomatic joint decrease gliding movement and restrict functional movement without structural soft tissue shortening (e.g., in the presence of normal muscle length or a normal or even a lax joint capsule).

In cases where nerve root irritation or the status of the intervertebral disc interferes with assessment of the biomechanical status of the joint (for example, due to severe pain or spasm), or when the nature of the condition does not allow for biomechanically based treatment, direct treatment toward symptom relief.

Immobilization

With some clinical conditions, immobilization is appropriate and necessary for a prescribed time. Selecting the correct general or specific immobilization method as well as *timing when and how long* to immobilize is important to the success of treatment. Acutely severe, painful and inflammatory conditions, instabilities, and recent post-surgeries may benefit from a prescribed duration of immobilization. General bed rest may be the only alternative with certain painful, inflammatory conditions, especially in the weight-bearing joints. Specific immobilization methods such as the use of casts, splints, braces, and taping can be used to protect a joint while the patient continues to function.

Thermo-Hydro-Electro (T-H-E) therapy

The judicious use of various forms of cold, heat, water, or electrotherapy can be an effective means to modulate pain, enhance relaxation, and reduce swelling. Integrated with manual therapy, modalities are used in preparation for mobilization and afterwards to prevent or limit treatment-related soreness. As with all treatments, selecting the correct technique, and determining when and how long to use it, is critical.

■ Pain-relief mobilization (Grade I-II SZ)

See *"Pain relief mobilization"* in *Chapter 5: Joint Mobilization.*

■ Special procedures to relieve pain

Acupuncture, acupressure, and various forms of soft tissue mobilization have long been used for pain relief through reflex pain modification, inhibition of muscle spasm, and the reduction of swelling. These are safe treatments even in the presence of serious musculoskeletal dysfunction.

■ Treatment to increase mobility

Soft tissue mobilization can facilitate Grade III stretch mobilization by loosening tight soft tissues that limit joint movement. In practice, treatment often begins with soft tissue treatments such as functional/ pumping massage and muscle stretching to increase soft tissue mobility. In some cases, particularly with chronic disorders, both periarticular tissues and muscles are restricted near the same point in the range. In such cases it is necessary to alternate Grade III stretch joint mobilization with soft tissue mobilization or muscle stretching and to take care not to move joints beyond their natural or actual range of movement during the soft tissue procedures.

■ Soft tissue mobilization

Whether or not a particular technique is viewed as soft tissue mobilization depends on the viewpoint of the clinician. Soft tissue treatments can affect many structures including joints, nerves and blood vessels. What distinguishes the soft tissue treatment from other forms of treatment is that the clinician uses soft tissue assessment to monitor change. The intention is to change soft tissues. Assessment is made by monitoring soft tissues. The clinician continuously monitors tissue response and instantaneously modifies treatment.

Good manual soft tissue technique requires sensitivity to constantly fluctuating patient responses. The clinician must recognize these subtle changes and immediately and continuously modify the treatment.

Just as joint movements are classified as either translations (i.e., joint play accessory movements) or rotations (i.e. physiological bone movements), so are soft tissue movements.

Accessory soft tissue movements (muscle play) cannot be performed actively. Friction massage, a passive lateral movement of muscle, is one example of muscle play.

Physiological soft tissue movements can be performed actively or passively. Traditional muscle stretching, and the lengthening and shortening movements that occur with muscle contraction and relaxation, are examples of physiological soft tissue movements. Treatment using physiological soft tissue movements generally utilize limb movement (e.g., combined functional movements) to alter soft tissue tension.

Some forms of soft tissue mobilization such as functional/pumping massage are most effective when the underlying joints are allowed to move as well. We often encourage and guide underlying joint movement by using a coupled movement pattern during soft tissue mobilization.

Soft tissue mobilization techniques can be broadly classified according to the amount of patient participation as either passive or active. The level and type of patient participation is an important clinical decision. Patient participation can vary from none at all, to the patient supplying most of the mobilizing force. Patient participation depends on many factors, including the chronicity and painfulness of the problem as well as the patient's willingness and ability to move.

■ Passive soft tissue mobilization

During passive soft tissue mobilization (STM) the patient does nothing but relax while the therapist provides the movement and force. Passive STM is appropriate for treatment of many acute soft tissue injuries where the objective is early movement with minimal tissue elongation or stretching. This approach may not be effective if the patient has difficulty relaxing while they are passively moved. There are many forms of passive STM, including classical massage, functional massage (Evjenth), and friction massage (Cyriax).

■ Active soft tissue mobilization

Contract-relax followed by passive physiological lengthening of soft tissues (muscle stretching).

Following a muscle contraction there is a brief period of relaxation when the muscle can be more easily stretched. During the relaxation phase, the practitioner stretches the soft tissues by moving muscle attachments maximally apart and holding them there. This kind of passive stretching can be uncomfortable and even painful in the stretched tissues, but should not increase the patients primary symptoms. The patient must be able to relax despite discomfort.

Contract-relax followed by passive accessory mobilization of soft tissues.

Following a muscle contraction there is a brief period of relaxation when the muscle can be more easily mobilized. During the relaxation phase, the muscle can be passively moved in a variety of ways depending on how the muscle responds. The practitioner times the soft tissue mobilization to take full advantage of the relaxation period. This technique is useful for passive manipulation of a muscle in cases where the muscle will not easily relax.

Contract with simultaneous mobilization of soft tissues.

The practitioner uses resistance to guide the patient's movement in order to actively elongate specific muscles. Simultaneously, the practitioner passively manipulates the antagonistic muscle. An example is manipulation of the hamstring muscles while simultaneously resisting knee extension (quadriceps activation). This technique takes advantage of the neurological phenomena called "reciprocal inhibition" and can be quite strong. This is useful when patients have difficulty relaxing while they are passively moved. It is also useful for more forceful or vigorous stretching. Patients seem to tolerate this technique well, perhaps because they control much of the force.

■ Passive muscle stretching

Integrate passive muscle stretching with active soft tissue relaxation techniques whenever possible. Before stretching, test muscle length, nerve mobility, end-feel, and the underlying joints to make sure stretching is indicated and safe.

Passive stretching principles

- » To test muscle length, position muscle attachments maximally apart, taking into consideration both primary and secondary muscle functions.
- » Determine that shortened muscles, and not a joint stop, are limiting movement.
- » Examine underlying joints to insure they can withstand the stresses imposed on them during stretching. Stretching muscles over joints that are unstable, inflamed, or have decreased joint play can result in their injury.

When stretching muscles, observe the following principles:

- » Warm the muscle prior to stretching, with exercise or passive heat applications, to facilitate relaxation.
- » Precede stretching with an isometric contraction of the muscle to be stretched to obtain maximal relaxation.
- » If the muscle crosses more than one joint, apply the stretch movement through the least painful, most stable, and largest joint.
- » It is generally more effective, and comfortable for the patient, to stretch using a lower force sustained for a longer time (60 seconds or more) than greater force for shorter time. Applying stretching force for a longer time is more likely to result in plastic deformation of soft tissues rather than the more temporary elastic changes.

■ Joint mobilization to increase mobility

See *"Stretch mobilization"* in *Chapter 5: Joint mobilization.*

Preparation for stretch mobilization

Soft tissue dysfunction can alter joint movement and decrease the effectiveness of joint stretch-mobilizations. That is why treatment often begins with procedures to decrease pain and muscle spasm or increase soft tissue mobility. These adjunct procedures may also make the joint mobilization easier to perform and produce a longer lasting effect.

Treatment to improve circulation and thereby elevate soft tissue temperatures is useful preparation for Grade III stretch mobilizations. Warming tissues surrounding the joint prior to Grade III mobilizations makes them easier to stretch. Effective warming can be achieved by surface heat application or deep heat application (e.g., ultrasound, diathermy). However, the most effective way to "warm-up" tissues is with exercise.

The most effective way to improve circulation and "warm-up" soft tissues is with exercise.

It is reported that cooling tissues after stretch mobilization treatment helps preserve mobility gains for a longer period of time. We do not recommend cold application prior to or during stretch technique, since cooled tissues can be more easily injured from overstretching.

Reflex inhibition for stretch mobilization

Stretch mobilization is more effective and better controlled when joint stretching is carefully timed to occur during periods of maximum muscle relaxation. Reflex inhibition relaxation techniques such as PNF contract-relax and hold-relax techniques (i.e., active relaxation, post-isometric relaxation) and contraction of antagonists (i.e., reciprocal inhibition) can be very effective.

■ Neural tissue mobilization

In cases where overt or suspected nerve involvement is accompanied by severe symptoms, treatment often begins before the physical evaluation is complete. Less critical biomechanical joint assessments and physical examination maneuvers that could risk further injury, may need to be deferred until the patient can tolerate them safely.

In certain clinical situations when joint and soft tissue mobilization techniques have not succeeded in alleviating neural symptoms, neural tissue mobilization may be indicated. There are specific techniques for mobilizing nerves in relation to their perineural tissue which, when appropriately applied, can be effective.

Neural tissue mobilization is sometimes used to prevent soft tissue adhesions in the presence of a peripheral neuropathy, for example, with carpal tunnel syndrome.

Entrapment syndromes associated with paraesthesias, can sometimes be helped by stretching the structures that are compromising the neuro-vascular tissues. For example, stretching the flexor and pronator muscles of the forearm may relieve paraesthesias in the hand. Stretching exercises for the scaleni and pectoralis minor, mobilization of the first rib, and posture exercise may relieve neurovascular symptoms associated with thoracic outlet syndrome. While these stretching maneuvers are directed primarily to muscle tissues, the maneuvers also mobilize the symptomatic neural tissues.

■ Specialized exercise to increase mobility

The therapeutic application of exercise is the cornerstone of physical therapy. Almost all physical therapy patients can benefit from exercise as part of their treatment program. Exercise should begin as early as possible during the course of care and each patient should have a home exercise program.

Exercise should be specifically tailored for the individual. Just as for mobilization, there is no uniform regimen of exercise applicable to all patients. We do not recommend the routine issue of preprinted exercise protocols based on medical diagnosis rather than examination findings. For exercise to effectively complement mobilization, it should be administered by the same clinician providing the mobilization treatment and not delegated to another practitioner as an afterthought.

In weight-bearing lower extremity joints, it may be necessary to modify exercises to reduce joint compression loads. For example, walking on a treadmill produces lower ground force reactions in the legs compared with walking on the ground. Reduced joint loading can also be accomplished with an exercise bike, water exercise, a Pilates shuttle, or whole-body traction used in conjunction with treadmill or leg press equipment.

In patients with both hypomobility and hypermobility in adjacent joints, the patient may need stabilization training to protect the hypermobile area during mobilization exercise for the hypomobile area.

There are times when it may not be advisable to increase range of movement in a hypomobile joint, whether by exercise or by manual mobilization. For example, in some advanced degenerative joint conditions, increased mobility may aggravate the condition and result in instability or decreased function.

Automobilization (self-mobilization) exercise can be useful for patients with joint hypomobility to maintain or increase mobility. However, automobilization cannot take the place of skilled manual mobilization performed by a therapist. Very few patients can control specific joint movements with the same precision as the skilled hands of a therapist.

Treatment to limit movement

Hypermobility treatment is a long-term process and requires persistence and patience from both patient and therapist. The goal is to limit or minimize joint movement in the excessively mobile directions. This is accomplished in four ways, often concurrently:

1. Specialized exercises
2. Increasing movement in kinetically related (i.e., adjacent) stiff joints
3. Taping, orthoses, and other supportive and controlling applications
4. Instruction in body mechanics and ergonomics.

Hypermobile joints are often misdiagnosed as hypomobile and therefore mismanaged by practitioners unskilled in passive movement testing. Misdiagnosis can occur when a hypermobile joint, especially a significant hypermobility (Class 5), gets "stuck" outside of its normal resting position (i.e., in a positional fault), for example, with the scaphoid and lunate bones in the wrist. The skilled application of traction and gliding test maneuvers sometimes releases the joint and clearly reveals the underlying hypermobility.

Grade III stretch mobilization is contraindicated for hypermobile joints. However, in the case of a fixated positional fault, the underlying hypermobility may only become apparent after the application of a Grade III stretch-glide mobilization or manipulative thrust.

The nature of the end-feel determines whether an unusually large movement range is a normal anatomical variation and should not be treated, or whether it is a pathological hypermobility that might benefit from treatment.

■ Specialized exercises for hypermobility

A patient with a hypermobile joint must learn how to limit and control the excessive movements with specialized muscle training. The patient must change the habitual motor behaviors that stretch the joint in a hypermobile direction. This usually involves a long-term movement reeducation program emphasizing coordination and kinesthetic retraining in a variety of functional activities until the patient can demonstrate safe behaviors in timing, recruitment, and intensity of muscle activity around the hypermobile joint.

Slight hypermobilities (Class 4), while often asymptomatic, may still be at risk for overstretching injuries during activities that place the joint at end ranges of motion and can progress to a symptomatic (Class 5) hypermobility. For this reason, specialized muscle training and ergonomic instruction may be important whether or not the hypermobility is symptomatic.

■ Increasing movement in adjacent joints

Increasing movement in kinetically related joints will decrease movement forces through the hypermobile joint during functional activities and will increase the opportunity for a hypermobile segment to heal and stabilize. Movement in the joints proximal and distal to a hypermobile joint can be enhanced with joint and soft tissue mobilization, automobilization, and other specialized exercises.

Limited movement in one joint can increase joint stresses elsewhere and may eventually lead to symptomatic hypermobility in a kinetically related joint. For example, a stiff ankle joint can lead to increased stress and eventual hypermobility in the metatarsal and tarsal joints. It is therefore important to mobilize adjacent joints displaying limited mobility as soon as possible, even if they are asymptomatic.

■ Supportive devices

Supportive devices such as braces, splints, orthotics and taping, can help protect symptomatic joints during an acute phase, limit specific movements, reduce joint loading, and help retrain movement to facilitate healthy movement patterns. Supports that specifically limit movement in some directions and allow movement in other directions can protect a joint from excessive movement and at the same time guide and train healthy movement patterns. For example, foot orthotics that support normal foot alignment can relieve stress to painful structures and at the same time improve gait patterns and proprioception. A three-point knee brace designed to unload the medial or lateral compartment can still allow full functional knee flexion.

Supportive devices can also be useful long after treatment is completed to reduce joint loads and limit movement in vulnerable joints during work activities and sports.

In more serious cases a rigid support that limits all movement may be necessary. In these cases, a strengthening program may be helpful to counteract the deconditioning that often accompanies rigid immobilization.

To inform, instruct, and train

It is important that the patient be motivated to take responsibility for their own health. Patient education takes time, but often saves time in the end as it leads to active participation by the patient and clearer communication between patient and health care provider. Many disturbances of the locomotor system are chronic, recurrent conditions which require self-management by the patient both at home and at work. Our manual therapy system stresses the role of the patient in reestablishing and maintaining normal mobility, in preventing recurrence, and in improving arthro-neuro-muscular health.

Patients need instruction in what postures and movements to avoid and in developing new and more healthful ways of moving and working. Medical Training Therapy[1] (MTT) is a form of exercise that applies the principles of Kaltenborn OMT. MTT programs emphasize coordination, kinesthetic retraining, strength, mobility, and endurance until the patient can demonstrate consistent and safe behaviors in timing, recruitment, and intensity of muscle activity during a variety of functional activities. MTT can be provided on an individual basis or in groups. Training is medicine. Exercise is the only modality that can have a positive effect on every organ system in the body. Ideally, patients will continue their training even after discharge from formal treatment, preferably at a facility with qualified MTT instructors.

1 Medical Training Therapy (MTT) is called "Medical Exercise Therapy (MET)" in some countries.

In addition to both supervised and at-home exercise, we instruct patients in activities of daily living (ADL), body mechanics, and ergonomics. Instruction should also be given in methods for pain relief, for example traction, ice, heat or taping. Home instruction is especially important if the patient's activities exacerbate neurological symptoms. Patients can be taught how to monitor their neurological signs and use them as a guide to determine safe activity levels.

With proper OMT management and education, the patient will often complete their course of care in a healthier state than they were before the episode that brought them to treatment.

TECHNIQUE

7 Manual technique principles

One cannot learn orthopedic manipulative therapy from books and classroom teaching alone. The speed, timing, coordination and feel required to master manual joint mobilization can take many years of daily practice. Students must take the time to observe the intricacies and effectiveness of treatment delivered by a master clinician and must work to develop their own manual skills in a supervised clinical setting with real patients.

A passive joint movement is guided and controlled not only with the therapist's hands, but also through the therapist's body. The therapist's body moves around an axis of motion in the targeted tissue or joint. This requires that the therapist have a thorough understanding of axes of movement and the physical coordination and capacity to accurately perform the movement.

A common error of student practitioners is to stand still and use only the hands and arms to move the patient. This creates an axis of movement between themselves and the patient and reduces or distorts movement at the targeted segment or tissue. Since accurate palpation of movement quantity and quality depends not only on the sensitivity of the therapist's palpating hands but also on the specificity with which a movement is produced, students of manual therapy must practice and perfect their own body movements before they can accurately evaluate and effectively treat with specific manual therapy techniques.

The application of manual joint techniques requires that the practitioner possess a certain degree of strength and fitness, especially for the treatment of the spine and larger joints such as the knee and hip. The physical loads experienced by a practitioner during the application of a manual joint mobilization maneuver must be within the safe limits of the therapist's functional capacity.

Proper equipment is essential to reduce risk of work-related injury to the therapist. High-low adjustable treatment tables are a standard requirement in all manual therapy treatment settings. Proper treatment table height reduces a therapist's reach distances, minimizes awkward working postures, and allows the therapist to position their body for best leverage and physical control of the manual treatment procedure. Skillful use of fixation belts, wedges, and other patient positioning devices can both maximize the treatment effect and at the same time reduce the physical loads experienced by the practitioner.

The techniques outlined in this basic text are guidelines only. Skilled practitioners will adapt and modify techniques as the patient's condition and treatment goals dictate.

Symbols

The photographs describing the techniques presented in this text incorporate symbols that indicate which joint partner should be stabilized or fixated, and in which direction the corresponding joint partner should be moved.

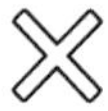 = Fixation or stabilization

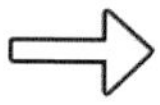 = Direction of linear movement (testing and treatment)

■ Applying manual techniques

■ Objective

The difference between a joint testing technique and a joint treatment technique is not always obvious. Joint play testing techniques can also be applied in the resting position as gentle Grade I and II traction mobilizations for pain relief or relaxation. Grade III stretch-mobilization techniques can also be used for symptom localization and end-feel testing.

With changes in grip, fixation, and positioning, many joint mobilizations can be adapted for use as a test, as a treatment for pain relief and relaxation, or as a stretch-mobilization. In addition, with changes in joint position the effect of the test or treatment can be much more specific. In the following chapters, we suggest the best application for each technique in its title:

» **Test:** Indicates that the technique is usually used for testing only. We illustrate linear, translatoric tests with straight arrows. We also indicate whether the objective of the test is for "mobility and symptom screening" or to "evaluate range and quality of movement, including end-feel."

» **Test and Mobilization:** Indicates that the technique can be used for testing joint play (Grade II), for testing end-feel (Grade III), and also for stretch-mobilizations (Grade III). Both test and mobilization procedures usually use the same grip. "Test and Mobilization" traction techniques in the resting position can also be applied for pain relief (Grade I and IISZ) or muscle relaxation (Grade I through IITZ).

» **Mobilization:** Indicates that the technique is adapted with alternate grips or stronger fixation (for example, with straps) for more effective stretch-mobilizations (Grade III).

» **Manipulation**: Indicates that the technique is suitable for the safe practice of manipulative thrust by students, in addition to its applications for patient treatment.

■ Starting position

Therapist position

It is important the practitioner employ sound ergonomics principles to protect themselves from the rigors of long hours of manual therapy practice.

» Stand as close to the patient as possible to minimize reach distance.

» Maintain a solid base of support with a wide stance, flexed hips and knees, and a natural lumbar lordosis.

» Adjust the height of the treatment table to ensure efficient and effective body mechanics.

The therapist should be relaxed, and insure that the patient is also relaxed.

Patient position

Manual techniques should be applied in a sequence that is efficient and requires a minimum of patient repositioning.

First, place the patient's body in a position of comfort to encourage relaxation and minimize muscle tension, then position the specific joint(s) to be mobilized.

» **If the patient is sitting** the feet should be supported if possible. Foot support contributes to the stability of the patient's body necessary for proper positioning during evaluation and treatment.

» **If the patient is prone** it is usually necessary to place an appropriately sized pillow under the patient's stomach (even if the patient has a protruding abdomen) to position the lumbar spine in a comfortable position. A pillow may also be necessary under the thorax to maintain a resting position there. In some cases it is necessary to lower the head piece of the treatment table in order to achieve adequate muscle relaxation.

The head piece of a manual therapy treatment table should have an opening for the patient's nose and mouth so they need not rotate their necks in order to breathe. Cervical rotation can compromise vascular flow, impinge nerve roots, and may increase tension in the shoulder girdle and entire spinal musculature.

» **If the patient is sidelying** the hip and knee joints should be flexed to provide stability. In sidelying, the patient's position should approximate the normal spinal curvatures observed in standing. In many cases, especially in females with a broad pelvis, it is necessary to place a pillow under the patient's waist, between the knees, or under the upper limb both for comfort and to control joint position.

» **If the patient is supine** the patient's head should be supported directly by the table or by a pillow, and the patient's legs should be slightly abducted and relaxed. For comfort and relaxation, it may be necessary to place a pillow under the patient's knees, to have the patient in a hooklying position, or to place a positioning pillow under the lumbar area.

For most evaluation and basic mobilization techniques, position the patient so that the involved joints are in the resting position or in the momentary resting position. In these positions the muscles surrounding the involved joint usually also relax. However, repeated trials may be necessary to find the best starting position, for example, the momentary resting position for pre-positioned pain-relieving, three-dimensional traction.

The therapist must often modify some other positions to accommodate the characteristics and flexibility of individual patients.

Joint position

For best effect and to avoid pain, the joint must be carefully positioned prior to the application of a test or treatment procedure. A uniaxial joint can be positioned within one plane of movement; a biaxial joint in two planes; and a triaxial joint in three planes.

If the intent of the technique is pain relief or relaxation, treatment begins in the momentary resting position. As the condition tolerates, the joint is positioned nearer to the true resting position.

If the intent of the technique is stretching, the joint can be positioned three-dimensionally anywhere within the available range-of-motion. Treatment begins in the resting position and progresses toward the restriction outside the resting position. The closer the joint position to the limit of movement, the more effective – and risky – the technique.

For the Grade III stretch-mobilizations illustrated in this book which are outside the resting position, the targeted joint has been positioned at a theoretical limit of joint motion.

If the intent of the technique is manipulation, the thrust must be initiated from the joint's momentary resting position.

Joint positioning cannot be based solely on established norms or typical movement patterns, as actual patient joint characteristics can vary widely.

■ Hand placement and fixation/stabilization

During most basic joint test and mobilization techniques, the therapist moves one hand with the patient's distal joint partner while keeping the other hand stable for palpation, stabilization or fixation. Both the moving hand and the palpating/stabilizing hand monitor the quality and quantity of movement.

Grip

Grips for testing maneuvers and gentle Grade I and II mobilizations differ from grips for longer duration stretch-mobilizations. Grips for testing and gentle mid-range mobilizations use a smaller contact surface, sometimes using only the fingers for grip. Grips for longer duration stretch-mobilizations use the broader contact surfaces of the hand along with more efficient therapist body mechanics and stronger fixation. In larger joints the grip may be reinforced with straps or with the therapist's body.

The less contact pressure used the better. Lighter grip pressures enhance sensitivity of the therapist's hands for palpation and sensory feedback. Only a small degree of linear movement is available in any individual joint, so excessive contact pressure can reduce movement, mask feedback about movement quality, distort the movement, and even elicit muscle guarding in the patient.

Grips are continuously modified and adjusted for patient comfort. The grip must be comfortable for the patient. A broad grip with greater surface contact area is usually better tolerated by patients than a "pointy" grip with smaller surface contact area. Subtle adjustments in grip positioning to avoid tender bony prominences can make a big difference in patient comfort. It may be necessary to push aside sensitive soft tissue structures such as nerves, muscles, or tendons.

A well-placed grip close to the joint space of two adjacent joint partners, can simultaneously produce a Grade I traction sufficient to neutralize or decompress the joint and thus facilitate a glide-test or glide-mobilization procedure.

A skilled manual therapist can perform stabilizing/fixating and moving/mobilizing functions equally well with either hand, from either side of the patient. The techniques in this book are accompanied by photographs (figures) that show a technique after it has been performed, i.e., in the terminal position. To perform the same technique on the opposite side of that shown in the picture, the therapist simply stands on the opposite side of the patient and switches the stabilizing and moving hands. Students should practice testing and mobilization techniques on both sides to train both hands for both functions.

Therapist's stable hand

With many mobilization techniques, the therapist keeps one hand stable while the other moves. The stable hand provides fixation and is usually positioned just proximal to the joint space. The fingers of the stable hand are also used to palpate the joint space. It is much easier to palpate movement in a joint if the palpating finger is stable rather than moving.

During most specific passive joint function tests and some mobilizations the therapist palpates with one finger of the stable hand. Most therapists use the index finger as the palpating finger, but individual practitioners may find another finger more sensitive or more comfortable to use. The palpating finger is positioned at the targeted joint space with contact to both joint partners. (In the photographs in this text, the stable hand or fixation is marked with an "X").

When testing end-feel, the contact pressure is increased slightly in the stable hand (and if necessary also the forearm of the stable hand) to *fixate* one joint partner. *Stabilize* neighboring joints by increasing the contact area of the grip. With adequate fixation, an end-range test technique can also be used as a specific Grade III mobilization.

Fixation is an essential component of specific Grade III stretch mobilization techniques, which are performed slowly and sustained for longer periods of time. Fixation can also be supplemented with wedges, belts, and other external fixating devices. External fixation devices are usually not necessary for specific movement testing because these tests use small movements with little force.

Therapist's moving hand

With smaller joints, the mobilizing hand grips the joint partner to be moved as close to the joint space as possible.

The moving hand performs the test or treatment procedure. With larger joints, the therapist's hands and body may move together to apply the movement while fixation is provided by the table, a wedge, or a strap. The moving hand and fingers should be placed as specifically as possible, close to the joint space, so that the movement occurs specifically at the targeted joint.

■ Procedure

Therapist safety and treatment effectiveness are enhanced with the application of ergonomic principles.

» Diligent use of body mechanics will help protect the therapist's body from the rigors of long hours of manual therapy practice, for example, by absorbing movement forces through the legs rather than through the back.

» The therapist should position their body close to the patient, facing the treatment direction to the extent possible.

» When treating larger joints, the therapist should stand with feet apart to maintain a solid base of support.

» When necessary, the therapist should use gravity and body weight to supplement treatment forces.

» We encourage the use of ergonomic devices and treatment accessories such as adjustable treatment tables, fixation belts, sand bags, wedges, and patient positioning aids should be incorporated to improve treatment outcomes and therapist safety.

Student manual therapists must practice and perfect their own body movements before they can accurately evaluate and effectively treat using specific manual therapy techniques.

Mobilization procedure

Mobilization techniques are applied slowly so that the patient may interrupt treatment at any time. For best effect, the speed and rhythm of the test movement or mobilization is varied to control pain and encourage relaxation.

A common error of student manual therapists is to stand still and use only the hands and arms to mobilize a joint. Movement should be produced and controlled not only through hand movement but also through body movement.

» **For joint play testing including end-feel** (Grade I - III), move slowly and ease into the Grade III range.

» **For pain relief** (Grade I - IISZ), use oscillations or slow, repetitive, intermittent traction movements, staying well short of the Transition Zone.

» **For relaxation** (Grade I - IITZ), apply slow intermittent traction mobilizations, staying well short of the first stop.

» **For stretching** (Grade III non-thrust), apply linear traction or glide movements even more slowly and sustain each stretch for 30 - 40 seconds or more. For lasting effect, repeat the stretch in a cyclic manner for a 10 - 15 minute session or to patient tolerance. Note that home exercise is usually necessary to maintain mobility gains.

When possible, the patient can be encouraged to assist a "passive" movement actively. This lessens the effort exerted by the therapist to produce and control a particular movement, but can only be used if the patient can assist without creating muscular tension at the joint targeted for evaluation or treatment.

Manipulation procedure

A common misconception among manual therapists is that manipulation is a "continuation" of a stretch-mobilization or a further movement at the end of a prolonged mobilization. Manipulation is fundamentally different from mobilization. A manipulative thrust is always quick, is never under the patient's control, is always initiated from the momentary resting position, and primarily impacts intra-articular restrictions. A manipulative thrust is applied so quickly, a patient cannot voluntarily interrupt the movement. A joint mobilization is always slow, can be initiated from any joint position (not only the momentary resting position), is especially effective for stretching specific extra-articular and peri-articular tissues, and is always under the patient's control.

In order to produce a manipulative thrust that is sufficiently quick in speed and short in amplitude, the therapist must apply the movement primarily with the hands and arms. One's body cannot move as quickly as one's arms. This is in contrast to the slow movements of non-thrust mobilization techniques in which movements are often controlled with slow movements of the therapist's body.

A pre-manipulative stretch test is required prior to practice of manipulative thrusts in classroom practice settings.

■ Notes

CHAPTER 8

FINGERS

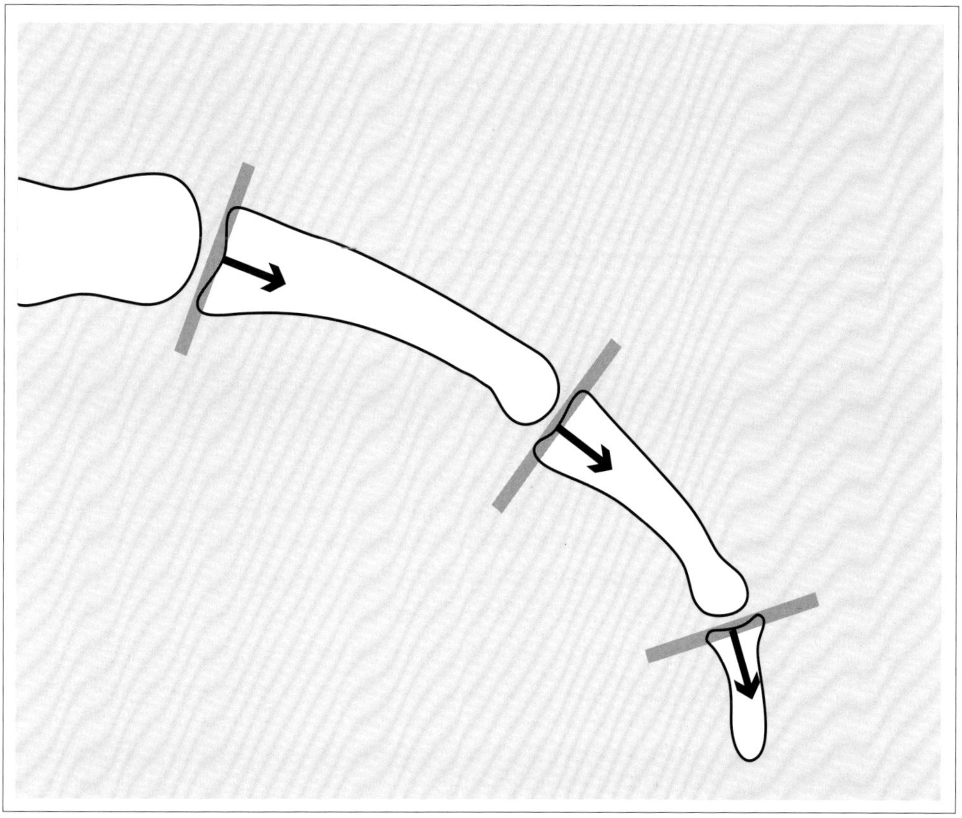

8 Fingers

■ Functional anatomy and movement

■ Finger joints

(artt. interphalangeales manus distalis et proximalis, abbrev. DIP, PIP)

The finger joints are anatomically and mechanically simple uniaxial hinge joints (ginglymus, modified sellar). Each phalanx has a head or distal end with a convex surface, a body, and a base or proximal end with a concave surface. The trochlea of the head of the phalanx has a sulcus. The eminence on the base of the phalanx fits into the guiding sulcus provided by the head.

Bony palpation

- Finger bones
- DIP and PIP joint spaces
- One sesamoid bone on IP I

Ligaments

- Collateral ligaments
- Palmar ligaments

Bone movement and axes

- Flexion - extension: around a transverse (radial-ulnar) axis through the head of the phalanx

End feel

- Firm

Joint movement (gliding)

- Concave Rule

Treatment plane

- On the concave joint surface at the base of the phalanx

Zero position

- The longitudinal axis through the metacarpal and corresponding phalangeal bone forms a straight line

Resting position

- Slight flexion in all joints

Close-packed position

- DIPs, PIPs and MCP I: maximal extension

Capsular pattern

- Restricted in all directions with slightly more limitation into flexion

■ "Knuckle" joints II-V

(artt. metacarpophalangeales, abbreviated MCP)

The "knuckle" joints of the 2nd through 5th digits are anatomically and mechanically simple biaxial joints (ellipsoid, modified ovoid). The convex surface of the head, on the distal part of the metacarpal bone, fits into the concave surface of the base of the proximal phalanx. When the hand is fisted, the MCP joints lie approximately one centimeter distal to the knuckles. There are also guiding sulci on the heads of the metacarpals; when the fingers are individually flexed, each finger tip moves towards the middle of the hand.

Bony palpation

- Proximal phalanges II-V
- Metacarpal bones II-V
- Joint spaces of MCP joints II-V
- One sesamoid bone on MCP II and MCP V

Ligaments

- Collateral ligaments
- Palmar ligaments

Bone movement and axes

- Flexion - extension: around a transverse (radial-ulnar) axis through the head of the metacarpal bone
- Radial flexion - ulnar flexion: around a sagittal (dorsal-palmar) axis through the head of the metacarpal bone. Alternate terminology: Abduction and adduction of the fingers is defined as movement away from and toward the third digit. Movement of the middle finger around the dorsal-palmar axis is called radial and ulnar deviation.
- Passive rotation: around a longitudinal axis through the phalanx

End feel

- Firm

Joint movement (gliding)

- Concave Rule

Treatment plane

- On the concave joint surface at the base of the proximal phalanx

Zero position

- The longitudinal axis through the metacarpal and corresponding phalangeal bone forms a straight line

Resting position

- Slight flexion and ulnar flexion

Close-packed position

- Maximal flexion

Capsular pattern

- Restricted in all directions with slightly more limitation into flexion

■ Metacarpal-phalangeal joint of the thumb

(art. metacarpophalangealis I, abbreviated MCP I)

The metacarpal-phalangeal joint of the thumb is an anatomically and mechanically simple uniaxial joint (ginglymus, modified sellar) with a very lax capsule.

Bony palpation

- Proximal phalanx I
- Joint space of MCP I
- Two sesamoid bones of MCP I

Ligaments

- Collateral ligaments

Bone movement and axes

- Flexion - extension: around a transverse (radial-ulnar) axis through the head of metacarpal I

End feel

- Firm

Joint movement (gliding)

- Concave Rule: The concave surface is on the proximal end of the phalangeal bone; the convex surface is on the distal end of the metacarpal bone.

Treatment plane

- On the concave joint surface at the base of phalanx I

Zero position

- The longitudinal axis through the metacarpal and corresponding phalangeal bone forms a straight line.

Resting position

- Slight flexion

Close-packed position

- Maximal extension

Capsular pattern

- Restricted in all directions with slightly more limitation into flexion

■ Finger examination scheme

(Refer to Chapters 3 and 4 for more information on examination)

Tests of function

1. Active and passive movements, including stability tests and end-feel

Flexion	*DIP*	45°- 60°
	PIP	100°
	MCP I-V	90°
Extension from zero	*MCP II-V*	10°- 30°
Abduction	*MCP II-V*	total of 90°

2. Translatoric joint play movements, including end-feel

Traction - compression	(Figure 1a)
Gliding	
Palmar	(Figure 2a)
Dorsal	(Figure 2d)
Radial	(Figure 3a)
Ulnar	(Figure 3c)

3. Resisted movements

	ACTS AT:
Flexion	
Flexor digitorum superficialis	PIP
Flexor digitorum profundus	DIP
Lumbricals	MCP
Flexor pollicis brevis	MCP
Flexor pollicis longus	IP
Extension	
Lumbricals	DIP, PIP
Extensor digitorum	DIP, PIP
Extensor digiti minimi	DIP, PIP
Extensor indicis	DIP, PIP
Extensor pollicis brevis	MCP
Extensor pollicis longus	IP
Abduction	
Dorsal interossei	MCP
Abductor digiti minimi	MCP
Adduction	
Palmar interossei	MCP

4. Passive soft tissue movements

Physiological
Accessory

5. Additional tests

Trial treatment

Traction	(Figure 1b)

Fingers

Finger techniques

The following techniques can also be applied to the thumb MCP and IP joints.

Figure 1a,b	Traction for pain and hypomobility
Figure 1c,d	Traction for restricted flexion and extension
Figure 2a,b,c	Palmar glide for restricted flexion
Figure 2d,e,f	Dorsal glide for restricted extension
Figure 3a,b	Radial glide for restricted flexion and extension
Figure 3c,d	Ulnar glide for restricted flexion and extension

Finger traction
for pain and hypomobility

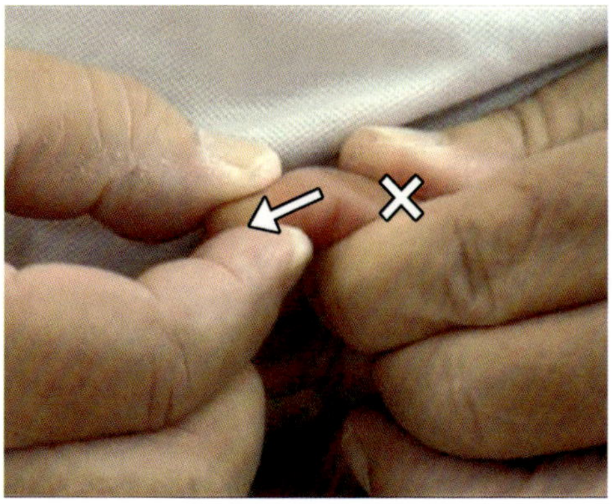

Figure 1a – test and mobilization in resting position

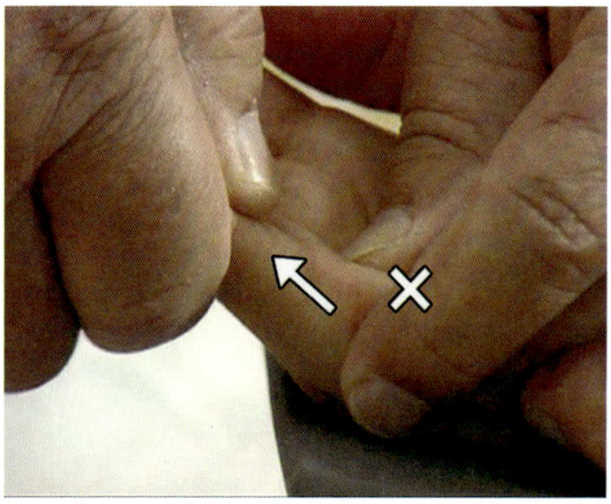

Figure 1b – mobilization in resting position

■ Figure 1a: Test and mobilization in resting position

Objective

- To evaluate the quantity and quality of traction joint play in a DIP, PIP, or MCP joint, including end-feel.
- To decrease pain or increase range-of-motion in a DIP, PIP, or MCP joint.

Starting position

- The patient's palm faces down.
- Position the joint in its resting position.

Hand placement and fixation

- **Therapist's stable hand (left):** Hold the patient's hand and finger in your hand; fixate the patient's hand against your body; grip with your fingers just proximal to the targeted joint space.
- **Therapist's moving hand (right):** Hold the patient's finger in your hand; grip with your fingers just distal to the targeted joint space.

Procedure

- Apply a Grade I, II, or III distal traction movement to the distal phalanx.
- Suitable for early training in manipulative thrust techniques.

■ Figure 1b: Alternate mobilization technique in resting position

- Traction the MCP joint with the dorsal side of the patient's hand resting on a wedge: fixate the patient's metacarpal bone against the wedge with your hand; grip with your fingers or thenar eminence just proximal to the patient's MCP joint space; apply a Grade III distal traction movement.
- Suitable for early training in manipulative thrust techniques.

Fingers

Finger traction
for restricted flexion and extension

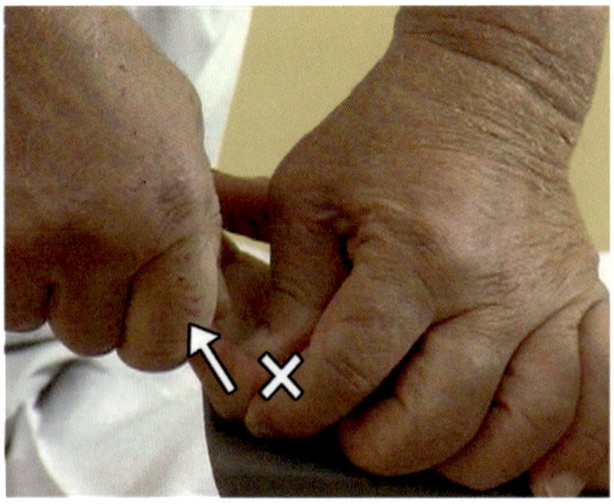

Figure 1c
MCP traction-mobilization in flexion

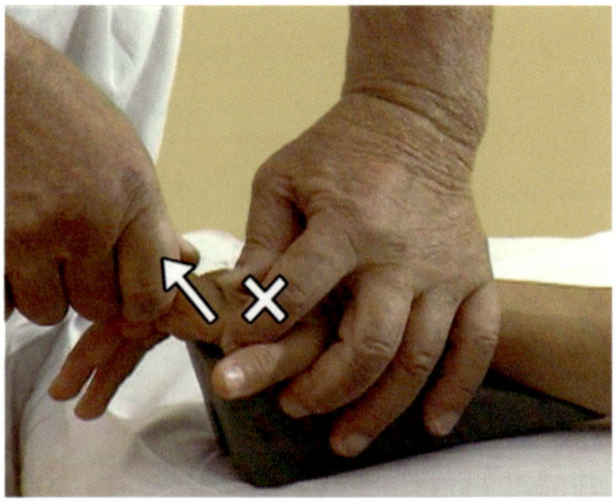

Figure 1d
MCP traction-mobilization in extension

■ Figure 1c: Flexion progression

Objective

- To increase flexion range-of-motion in a DIP, PIP, or MCP joint.

Starting position

- The dorsal side of the patient's hand rests on a wedge.
- Position the joint close to its end range-of-motion in flexion.

Hand placement and fixation

- **Therapist's stable hand (left):** Fixate the patient's proximal joint partner against the wedge with your hand; grip with your fingers or thenar eminence just proximal to the targeted joint space.
- **Therapist's moving hand (right):** Hold the patient's finger in your hand; grip with your fingers just distal to the targeted joint space.

Procedure

- Apply a Grade III distal traction movement to the distal phalanx.

■ Figure 1d: Extension progression for the MCP joint

- The patient's palm rests on a wedge with the MCP joint positioned near to its end range-of-motion in extension. Apply a Grade III distal traction movement to the distal phalanx.

Finger palmar glide
for restricted flexion

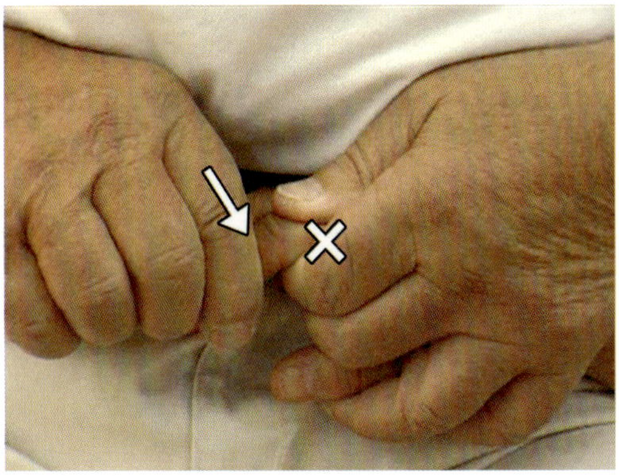

Figure 2a – test and mobilization in resting position

■ Figure 2a: Test and mobilization in resting position

Objective

- To evaluate the quantity and quality of palmar glide joint play in a DIP, PIP, or MCP joint, including end-feel.
- To increase flexion range-of-motion in a DIP, PIP, or MCP joint (Concave Rule).

Starting position

- The patient's palm faces down.
- Position the joint in its resting position.

Hand placement and fixation

- **Therapist's stable hand (left):** Hold the patient's hand and finger in your hand; fixate the patient's hand against your body; grip with your fingers just proximal to the targeted joint space.
- **Therapist's moving hand (right):** Hold the patient's finger in your hand; grip with your fingers just distal to the targeted joint space.

Procedure

- Apply a Grade II or III palmar glide movement to the distal phalanx.

Finger palmar glide

for restricted flexion (cont'd)

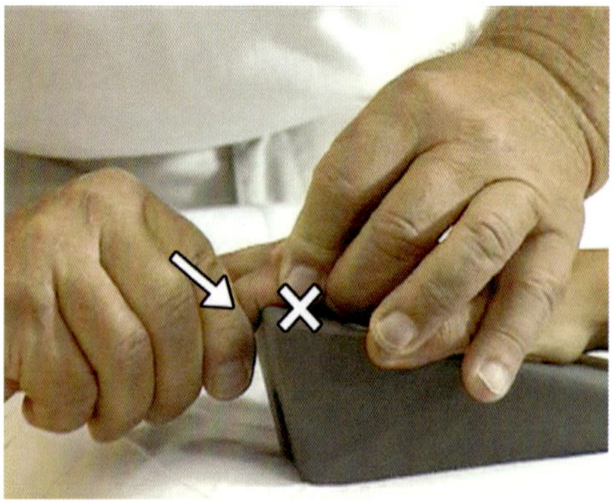

Figure 2b – mobilization in resting position

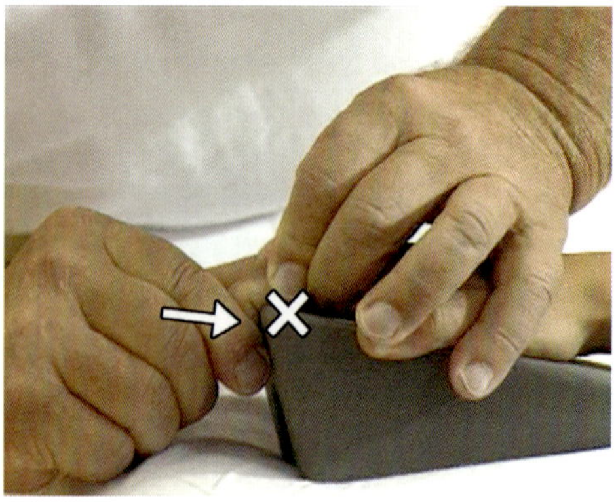

Figure 2c – mobilization in flexion

■ Figure 2b: Alternate mobilization technique in resting position

Objective

- To increase flexion range-of-motion in a DIP, PIP, or MCP joint (Concave Rule).

Starting position

- The patient's palm rests on a wedge.
- Position the joint in its resting position.

Hand placement and fixation

- **Therapist's stable hand (left):** Fixate the patient's proximal joint partner against the wedge with your hand; grip with your fingers or thenar eminence just proximal to the targeted joint space.
- **Therapist's moving hand (right):** Hold the patient's finger in your hand; grip with your fingers just distal to the targeted joint space.

Procedure

- Apply a Grade III palmar glide movement to the distal phalanx.

■ Figure 2c: Flexion progression

- Apply a Grade III palmar glide movement with the targeted finger joint positioned close to its end range-of-motion in flexion.

Finger dorsal glide
for restricted extension

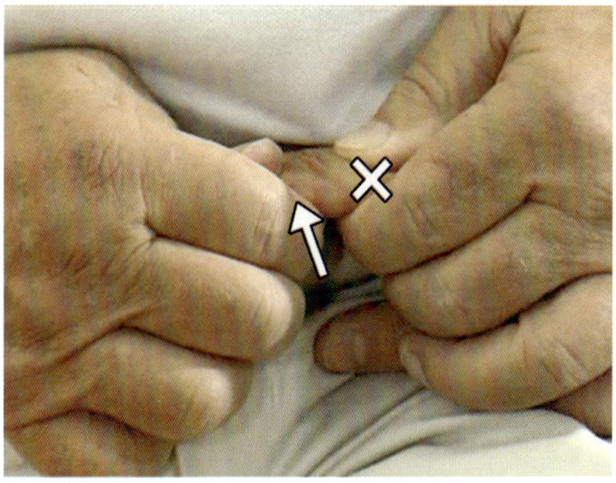

Figure 2d – test and mobilization in resting position

■ Figure 2d: Test and mobilization in resting position

Objective

- To evaluate the quantity and quality of dorsal glide joint play in a DIP, PIP, or MCP joint, including end-feel.
- To increase extension range-of-motion in a DIP, PIP, or MCP joint (Concave Rule).

Starting position

- The patient's palm faces down.
- Position the joint in its resting position.

Hand placement and fixation

- **Therapist's stable hand (left):** Hold the patient's hand and finger in your hand; fixate the patient’s hand against your body; grip with your fingers just proximal to the targeted joint space.
- **Therapist's moving hand (right):** Hold the patient's finger in your hand; grip with your fingers just distal to the targeted joint space.

Procedure

- Apply a Grade II or III dorsal glide movement to the distal phalanx.

Finger dorsal glide
for restricted extension (cont'd)

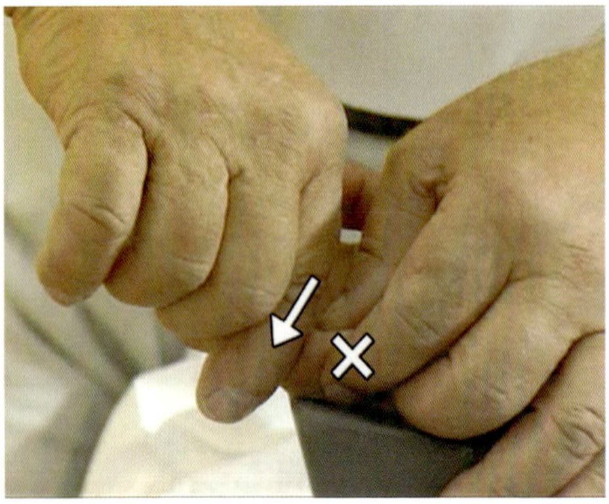

Figure 2e – mobilization in resting position

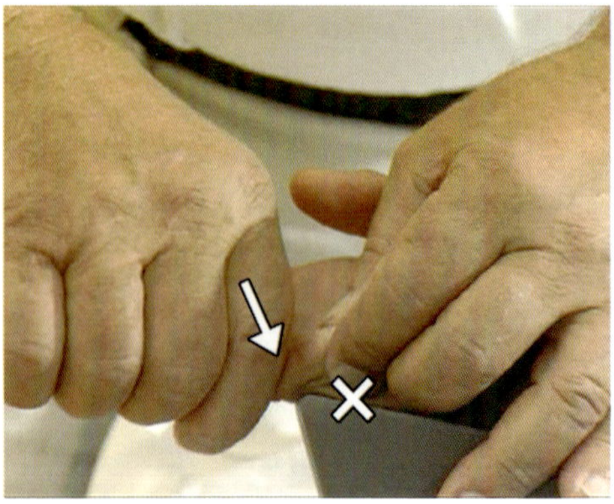

Figure 2f – mobilization in extension

■ Figure 2e: Mobilization in resting position

Objective

- To increase extension range-of-motion in a DIP, PIP, or MCP joint (Concave Rule).

Starting position

- The dorsal side of the patient's hand rests on a wedge.
- Position the joint in its resting position.

Hand placement and fixation

- **Therapist's stable hand (left):** Fixate the patient's proximal joint partner against the wedge with your hand; grip with your fingers or thenar eminence just proximal to the targeted joint space.
- **Therapist's moving hand (right):** Hold the patient's finger in your hand; grip with your fingers just distal to the targeted joint space.

Procedure

- Apply a Grade III dorsal glide movement to the distal phalanx.

■ Figure 2f: Extension progression

- Apply a Grade III dorsal glide movement with the targeted finger joint positioned close to its end range-of-motion in extension.

Finger radial glide

for restricted flexion and extension

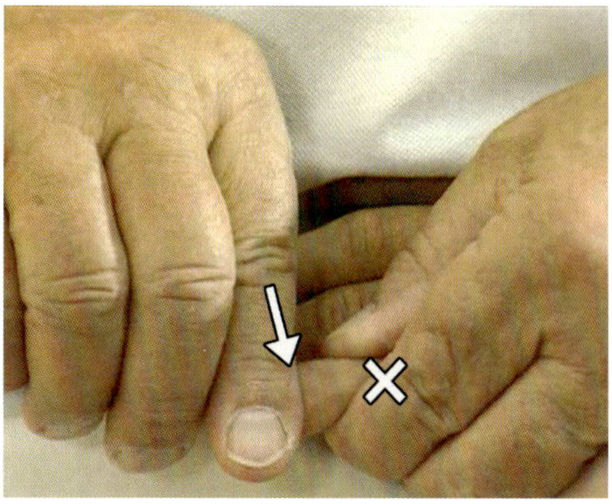

Figure 3a – test and mobilization in resting position

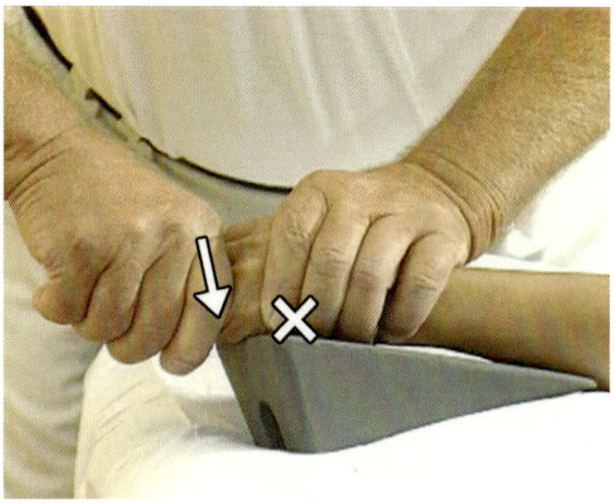

Figure 3b – mobilization in resting position

■ Figure 3a: Test and mobilization in resting position

Objective

- To evaluate the quantity and quality of radial glide joint play in a DIP, PIP, or MCP joint, including end-feel.
- To increase flexion and extension range-of-motion in a DIP, PIP, or MCP joint (Concave Rule).

Starting position

- The patient's palm faces the therapist.
- Position the joint in its resting position.

Hand placement and fixation

- **Therapist's stable hand (left):** Hold the patient's hand and finger in your hand; fixate the patient's hand against your body; grip with your fingers just proximal to the targeted joint space.
- **Therapist's moving hand (right):** Hold the patient's finger in your hand; grip with your fingers just distal to the targeted joint space.

Procedure

- Apply a Grade II or III radial glide movement to the distal phalanx.

■ Figure 3b: Alternate mobilization technique in resting position

- Apply a Grade III radial glide movement to the MCP joint with the radial side of the patient's hand resting on a wedge. Fixate the patient's metacarpal bone against the wedge with your hand; grip just proximal to the patient's MCP joint spaces.
- This technique can be used to increase radial glide joint play (Concave Rule) both in the resting position and approaching the end range-of-motion into flexion, extension, and MCP radial flexion.

Finger ulnar glide

for restricted flexion and extension

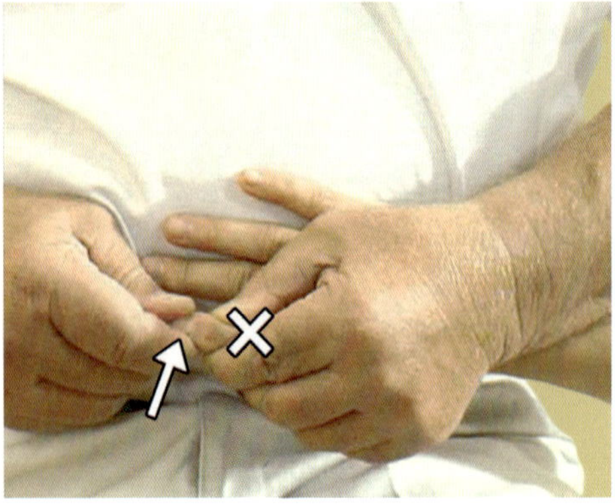

Figure 3c – test and mobilization in resting position

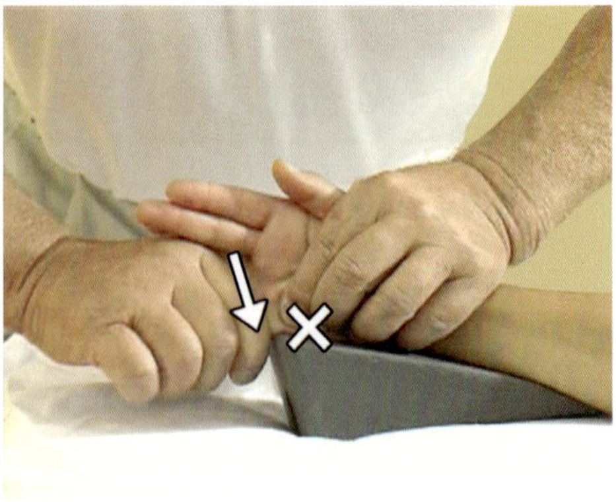

Figure 3d – mobilization in resting position

■ Figure 3c: Test and mobilization in resting position

Objective

- To evaluate the quantity and quality of ulnar glide joint play in a DIP, PIP, or MCP joint, including end-feel.
- To increase flexion and extension range-of-motion in a DIP, PIP, or MCP joint (Concave Rule).

Starting position

- The patient's palm faces the therapist.
- Position the joint in its resting position.

Hand placement and fixation

- **Therapist's stable hand (left):** Hold the patient's hand and finger in your hand; fixate the patient's hand against your body; grip with your fingers just proximal to the targeted joint space.
- **Therapist's moving hand (right):** Hold the patient's finger in your hand; grip with your fingers just distal to the targeted joint space.

Procedure

- Apply a Grade II or III ulnar glide movement to the distal phalanx.

■ Figure 3d: Alternate mobilization technique in resting position

- Apply a Grade III ulnar glide movement in an MCP joint with the ulnar side of the patient's hand resting on a wedge; fixate the patient's metacarpal bone against the wedge with your hand; grip just proximal to the patient's MCP joint spaces.
- This technique can be used to increase ulnar glide joint play (Concave Rule) both in the resting position and near the end range-of-motion into flexion, extension, or MCP ulnar flexion.

CHAPTER 9

METACARPALS

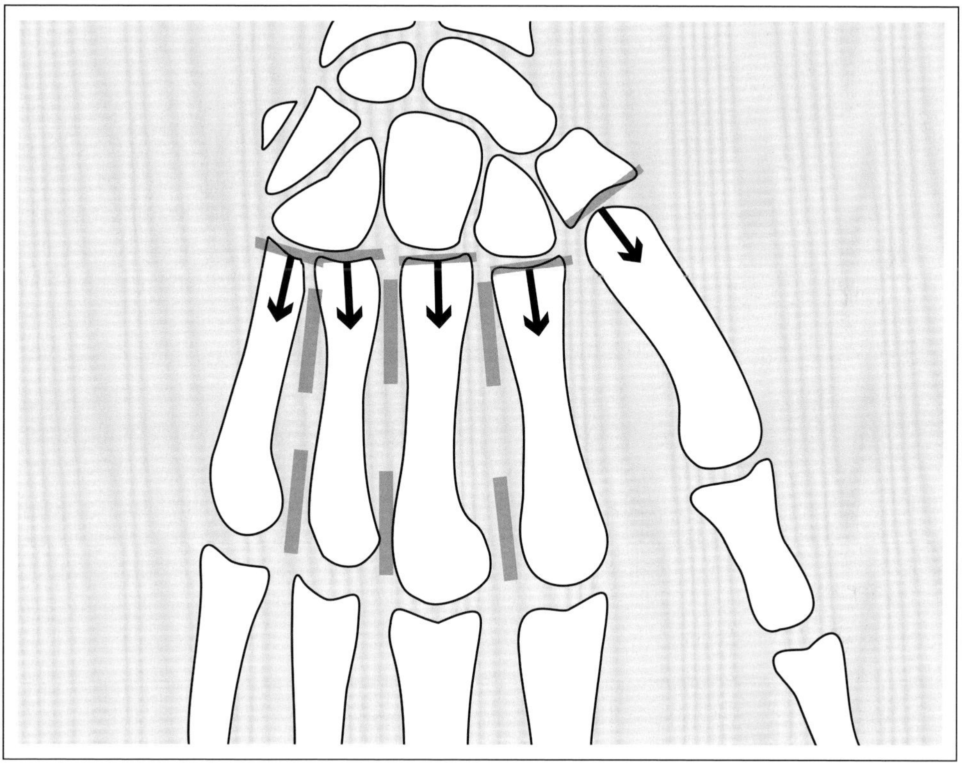

9 Metacarpals

■ Functional anatomy and movement

When there is movement restriction in the hand, first treat the metacarpals and later progress to treatment of the fingers.

■ Hand proper
(metacarpus)

The hand proper is made up of five metacarpal bones corresponding to the five digits. Each metacarpal has a head or distal end with a convex surface, a body, and a base or proximal end with a concave surface. The heads of the metacarpals have no joints in relation to each other, but are joined together by the deep transverse metacarpal ligaments.

The joints between the bases of the second through fifth metacarpals and the adjacent row of carpal bones (*artt. carpometacarpales*; abbreviated CM), and the joints between the bases of the metacarpal bones (*artt. intermetacarpales*; abbreviated IM) are plane or nearly flat. However, these joints individually are anatomically simple and mechanically compound plane amphiarthroses (Figure 13). All of these "plane" joints have a small curvature, but this need not be taken into consideration during treatment, since only traction and dorsal-palmar gliding techniques are used.

The intermetacarpal joints of the hand share one complex cavity with the carpometacarpal joints I-V. Therefore, all these joints together are often called the "big carpometacarpal joint." This complex joint cavity does not communicate with the first carpometacarpal or pisiform joints.

The dorsal convex arch of the hand proper changes shape with all finger movements.

Bony palpation

- Metacarpals II-V
- Distal row of carpals (trapezoid, capitate, hamate)
- Carpometacarpal joint space II-V

Ligaments

- Dorsal interosseous ligaments
- Palmar metacarpal ligaments
- Dorsal and palmar carpometacarpal ligaments

Bone movement and axes

There is relatively more movement in the ulnar metacarpal joints than in the radial metacarpal joints. For example, the metacarpal V - hamate articulation, a saddle joint, is capable of flexion-extension, radial-ulnar flexion, and also opposition.

Intermetacarpal joints:

- There are no defined axes for the small movements that occur in these joints. As the curve of the transverse metacarpal arch increases, the metacarpals move in a palmar direction with relation to metacarpal III.
- As the curve of the transverse metacarpal arch decreases, the metacarpals move in a dorsal direction with relation to metacarpal III

Carpometacarpal joints:

- Flexion - extension: around a transverse (radial-ulnar) axis through the carpal bones
- Radial - ulnar flexion: around a sagittal (dorsal-palmar) axis through the carpal bones

End feel

- Firm

Joint movement (gliding)

- Concave Rule

Treatment plane

- Distal and proximal intermetacarpal II-V treatment plane lies between and perpendicular to the metacarpal bones
- Carpometacarpal treatment plane lies on the concave joint surface at the base of the metacarpal

Zero position

- *CM joints II-V:* not described

Resting position

- *CM joints II-V:* not described

Close-packed position

- Unknown

Capsular pattern

- *CM joints II-V:* limited equally in all directions

First ("little") carpometacarpal joint

(art. carpometacarpalis pollicis)

The first carpometacarpal joint between the first metacarpal bone and trapezium, is an anatomically and mechanically simple biaxial joint (sellaris, unmodified sellar). It must be treated as a saddle joint, but because there is a lax capsule it is functionally a triaxial ball and socket joint (sphaeroidea).

Bony palpation

- Base of metacarpal I
- Trapezium
- Carpometacarpal I joint space

Ligaments

- Strengthen the capsule on all sides

Bone movement and axes

The joint surface of the trapezium is not parallel to the joint surfaces of the other distal carpal bones because the trapezium is rotated 90° towards the palm. Therefore, when describing movements of the first carpometacarpal joint it must be remembered that the axes are also rotated 90°.

- Palmar abduction - adduction: The base of the first metacarpal bone moves with its convex surface around a radial-ulnar axis through its base.
- Flexion - extension: The base of the first metacarpal bone moves with its concave surface around a dorsal-palmar axis through the trapezium.
- Rotation: The axis passes longitudinally through the metacarpal bone. Rotation can only be performed passively.
- Opposition - reposition: Opposition occurs when the abducted thumb is flexed; reposition occurs when the adducted thumb is extended.

End feel

- Firm

Joint movement (gliding)

- Flexion - extension: Concave Rule
- Abduction - adduction: Convex Rule

Treatment plane

- Flexion - extension: on the concave joint surface at the base of the metacarpal.
- Abduction - adduction: on the concave joint surface of the trapezium

Zero position

- MC I bone midway between maximal abduction-adduction and flexion-extension from zero.

Resting position

- MC I bone midway between abduction-adduction and flexion-extension

Close-packed position

- Maximal opposition

Capsular pattern

- Abduction-extension

Metacarpal examination scheme

(Refer to Chapters 3 and 4 for more information on examination)

Tests of function

1. Active and passive movements, including stability tests and end-feel

CM I	Flexion - extension	50° total
	Abduction - adduction	40° total
CM II-V	Flexion - extension	little movement
	Abduction - adduction	
CM V	Opposition	

2. Translatoric joint play, including end-feel

CM I	Traction - compression	(Figure 7a)
	Gliding	
	Ulnar	(Figure 7c)
	Radial	(Figure 7e)
	Palmar	(Figure 7g)
	Dorsal	(Figure 7i)
CM II-V	Traction - compression	(Figure 6a)
	Gliding	
	Palmar	
	Dorsal	
IMC II-V	Gliding	(Figure 5a)

3. Resisted movements

			ACTS AT:
CM I	Flexion:	*Flexor pollicis longus*	IP, MCP
		Flexor pollicis brevis	IP
	Extension:	*Extensor pollicis longus*	IP, MCP
		Extensor pollicis brevis	IP
	Abduction:	*Abductor pollicis longus*	
		Abductor pollicis brevis	
	Adduction:	*Adductor pollicis*	
	Opposition:	*Opponens pollicis,*	
		Flexor pollicis brevis	
CM V	Opposition:	*Opponens digiti minimi*	

4. Passive soft tissue movements
   Physiological
   Accessory

5. Additional tests

Trial treatment

CM I	Traction	(Figure 7b)
CM II-V	Traction	(Figure 6b)

Metacarpal techniques

Metacarpal arch

Figure 4a,b	For hypomobility

Proximal intermetacarpals

Figure 5a,b	Palmar glide for hypomobility

Carpometacarpal joints II - V

Figure 6a,b	Traction for pain and hypomobility

Thumb carpometacarpal joint

Figure 7a,b	Traction for pain and hypomobility
Figure 7c,d	Ulnar glide for restricted flexion
Figure 7e,f	Radial glide for restricted extension
Figure 7g,h	Palmar glide for restricted adduction
Figure 7i,j	Dorsal glide for restricted abduction

Recommended mobilization sequence for the hand

1. Carpometacarpal traction (Figure 6)
2. Proximal metacarpal glide (Figure 5)
3. Metacarpal arch mobilization (Figure 4)

Metacarpal arch
for hypomobility

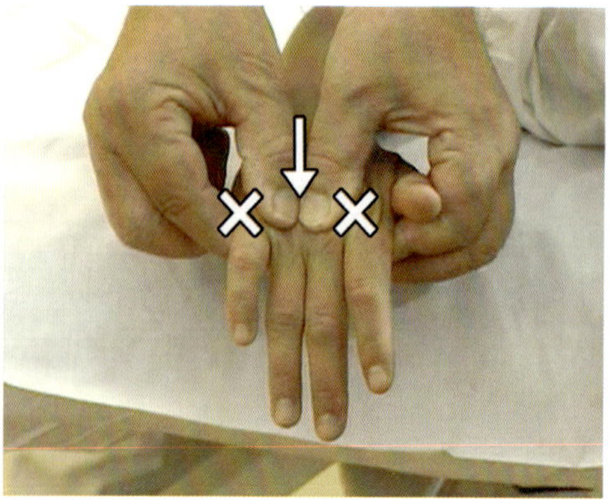

Figure 4a – test and mobilization

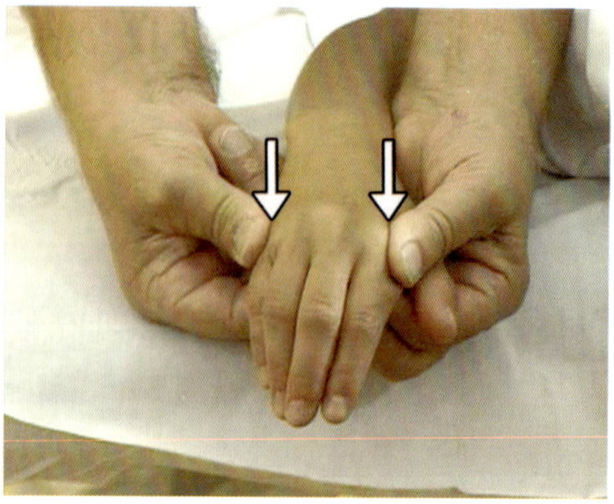

Figure 4b – test and mobilization

■ Figure 4a: Test and mobilization, dorsal-concave arch

Objective

- To evaluate the quantity and quality of metacarpal arch mobility, including end-feel.
- To increase metacarpal arch mobility; to stretch the distal syndesmosis. See *Figure 5b* for an alternate stretch for the distal syndesmosis.

Starting position

- The patient's palm rests on the treatment surface.

Hand placement and fixation

- Grip the patient's hand with your fingers on the palmar side of the patient's hand to provide fixation; place your thumbs together on the dorsal side of metacarpal III to apply the movement.

Procedure

- Apply a Grade II or III downward pressure with your thumbs to reverse the patient's metacarpal arch (dorsal concave).

■ Figure 4b: Test and mobilization, dorsal-convex arch

- Fixate metacarpal III with your fingers on the palmar surface of the hand; mobilize with your thumbs pressing down on metacarpals II and IV/V.

Proximal intermetacarpal palmar glide
for hypomobility

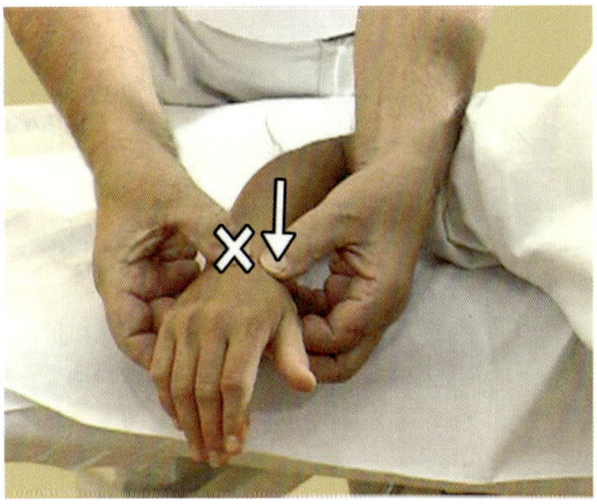

Figure 5a – test and mobilization in resting position

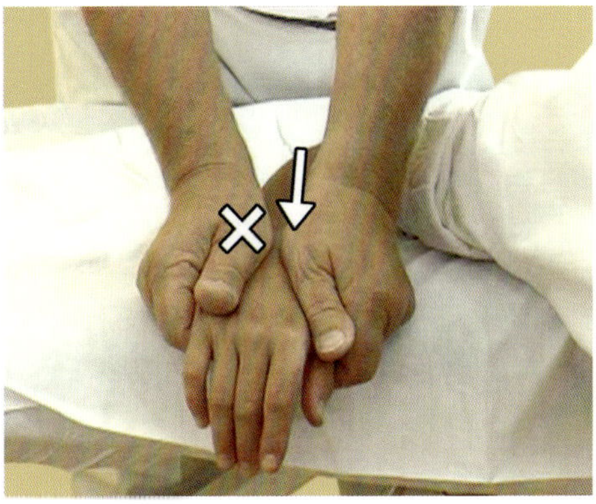

Figure 5b – mobilization in resting position

■ Figure 5a: Test and mobilization in resting position

Objective

- To evaluate the quantity and quality of metacarpal palmar glide joint play, including end-feel.
- To increase intermetacarpal mobility.

Starting position

- The patient's palm faces down.

Hand placement and fixation

- **Therapist's stable hand (right):** Hold the patient's hand from the ulnar side; grip your thumb and fingers around the base of the patient's metacarpal (metacarpal III shown).
- **Therapist's moving hand (left):** Hold the patient's hand from the radial side; grip with your thumb and fingers around the base of the adjacent metacarpal (metacarpal II shown).

Procedure

- Press your left hand downward to apply a Grade II or III palmar glide movement.

■ Figure 5b: Mobilization in resting position

- Grip for fixation and mobilization with your thenar eminences and thumbs. Apply a Grade III palmar glide movement.

■ Alternate technique (not shown)

- Apply a Grade II or III dorsal glide movement to increase intermetacarpal mobility with the dorsal side of the patient's hand facing down.

Metacarpals

Carpometacarpal traction
for pain and hypomobility

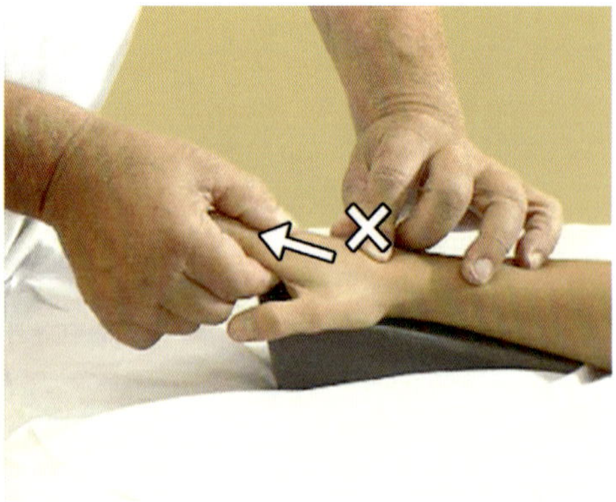

Figure 6a – test and mobilization in resting position

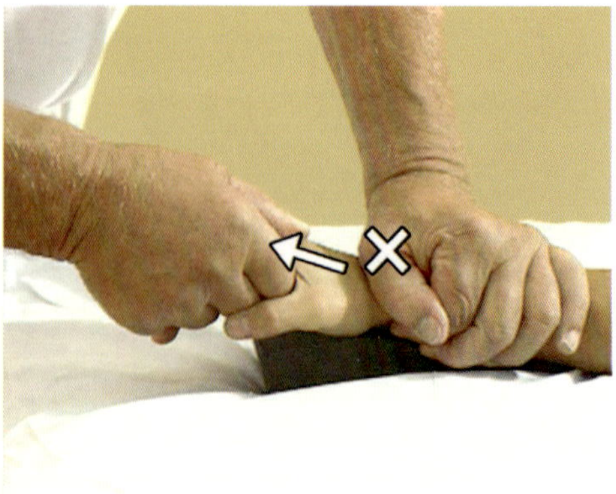

Figure 6b – mobilization in resting position

■ Figure 6a: Test and mobilization in resting position

Objective

- To evaluate the quantity and quality of traction joint play in a carpometacarpal joint, including end-feel.
- To decrease pain or increase range-of-motion in the carpometacarpal joints.

Starting position

- The patient's hand rests on the wedge with their palm facing down.
- Position the joint in its resting position.

Hand placement and fixation

- **Therapist's stable hand (left):** Grip around the targeted carpal bone just proximal to the joint space (trapezoid shown).
- **Therapist's moving hand (right):** Grip the patient's targeted metacarpal bone just distal to the joint space (metacarpal II shown).

Procedure

- Apply a Grade I, II or III traction movement to the metacarpal bone.
- For testing and mobilization, the joint space can be palpated with the thumb or finger of your fixating hand.
- Suitable for early training in manipulative thrust techniques.

■ Figure 6b: Mobilization in resting position

- Apply a Grade III traction movement to increase carpometacarpal mobility. Use your left thenar eminence to fixate the patient's carpal bone against the treatment surface or wedge.
- Suitable for early training in manipulative thrust techniques.

Thumb carpometacarpal traction

for pain and hypomobility

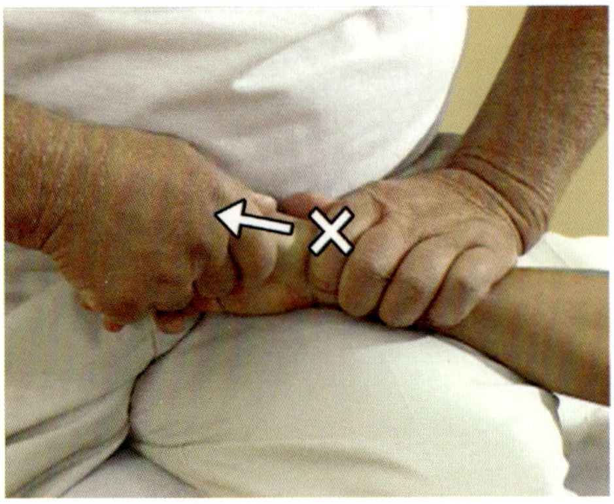

Figure 7a – test and mobilization in resting position

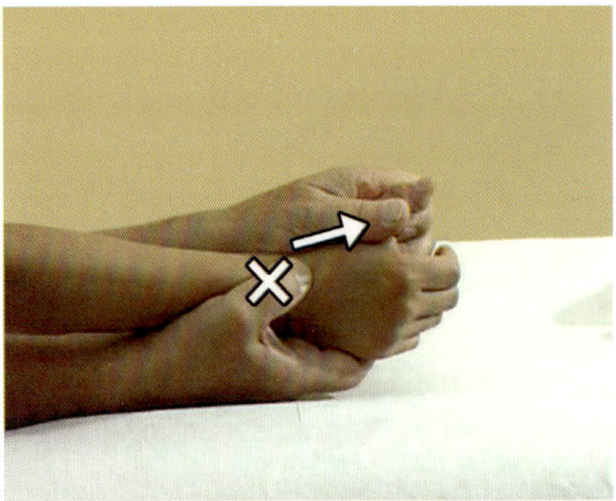

Figure 7b – mobilization in resting position

■ Figure 7a: Test and mobilization in resting position

Objective

- To evaluate the quantity and quality of distal traction joint play in the carpometacarpal I joint, including end-feel.
- To decrease pain or increase range-of-motion in a carpometacarpal joint.

Starting position

- The ulnar side of the patient's hand faces down.
- Position the joint in its resting position.

Hand placement and fixation

- **Therapist's stable hand (left):** Hold the patient's distal forearm with your hand; grip around the trapezium just proximal to the joint space; fixate the patient's hand against your body.
- **Therapist's moving hand (right):** Grip the patient's metacarpal I just distal to the joint space.

Procedure

- Apply a Grade I, II, or III distal traction movement to metacarpal I.
- Suitable for early training in manipulative thrust techniques.

■ Figure 7b: Mobilization in resting position

- Use your thenar eminence and finger tips to grip around the ulnar side of the patient's hand, to fixate the trapezium. Your left hand grips around the 1st metacarpal.
- Suitable for early training in manipulative thrust techniques.

■ Flexion and extension progression (not shown)

- Position the carpometacarpal I joint near the end range-of-motion into flexion or extension.

Thumb carpometacarpal ulnar glide
for restricted flexion

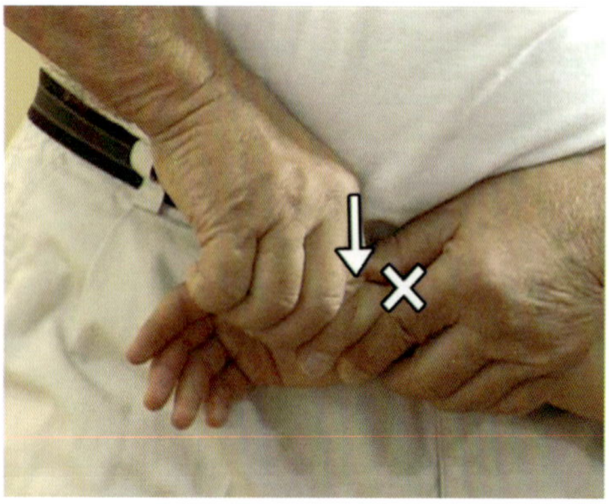
Figure 7c – test and mobilization in resting position

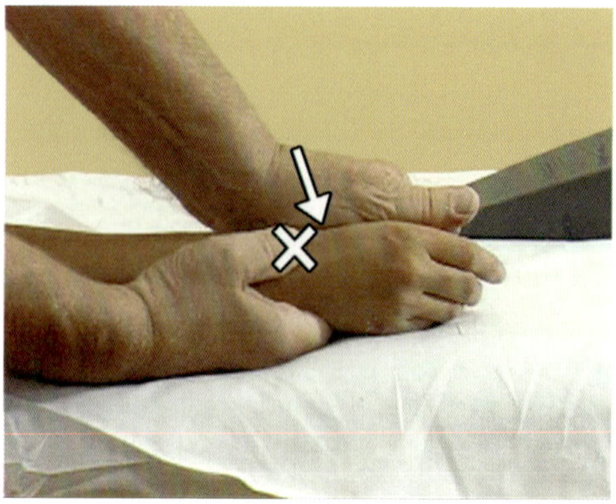
Figure 7d – mobilization in resting position

■ Figure 7c: Test and mobilization in resting position

Objective

- To evaluate the quantity and quality of ulnar glide joint play in the carpometacarpal I joint, including end-feel.
- To increase thumb flexion range-of-motion in the carpometacarpal I joint (Concave Rule).

Starting position

- The ulnar side of the patient's hand faces down.
- Position the joint in its resting position.

Hand placement and fixation

- **Therapist's stable hand (left):** Hold the patient's distal forearm with your hand; grip around the trapezium just proximal to the joint space; fixate the patient's hand against your body.
- **Therapist's moving hand (right):** Grip the patient's metacarpal I just distal to the joint space.

Procedure

- Apply a Grade II or III ulnar glide movement to metacarpal I.

■ Figure 7d: Mobilization in resting position

- Apply a Grade III ulnar glide movement to increase thumb flexion. The ulnar side of the patient's hand rests on the treatment surface; use your right thenar eminence and finger tips to grip around the ulnar side of the patient's hand, to fixate the trapezium; your left hand grips around 1st metacarpal.

■ Flexion progression (not shown)

- Position the carpometacarpal I joint near the end range-of-motion into flexion.

Thumb carpometacarpal radial glide

for restricted extension

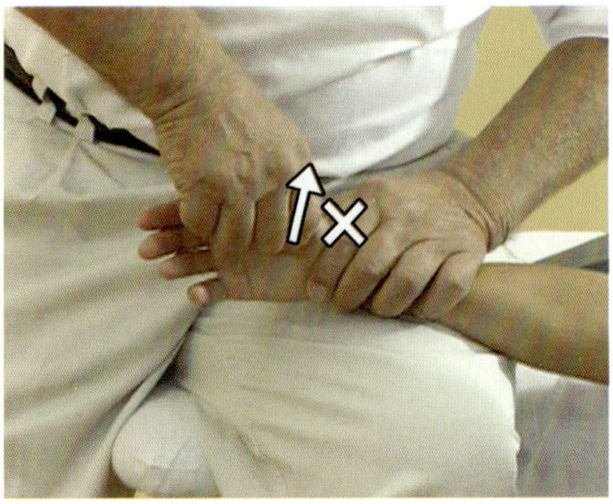

Figure 7e – test and mobilization in resting position

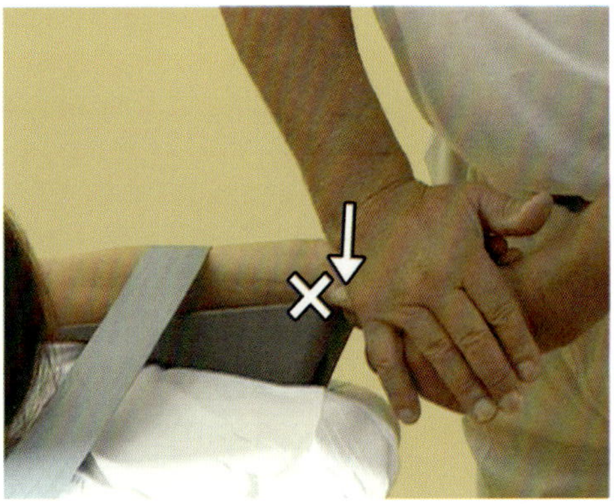

Figure 7f – mobilization in resting position

■ Figure 7e: Test and mobilization in resting position

Objective

- To evaluate the quantity and quality of radial glide joint play in the carpometacarpal I joint, including end-feel.
- To increase thumb extension range-of-motion (Concave Rule).

Starting position

- The ulnar side of the patient's hand faces down.
- Position the joint in its resting position.

Hand placement and fixation

- **Therapist's stable hand (left):** Hold the patient's distal forearm with your hand; grip around the trapezium just proximal to the joint space; fixate the patient's hand against your body.
- **Therapist's moving hand (right):** Grip the patient's metacarpal I just distal to the joint space.

Procedure

- Apply a Grade II or III radial glide movement to metacarpal I.

■ Figure 7f: Mobilization in resting position

- Apply a Grade III radial glide movement to increase thumb extension. The patient lies supine; the radial side of the patient's carpus and the distal forearm (with a strap) rests on the wedge with the patient's hand extended over the edge. Grip around metacarpal I with your left thumb and fingers; reinforce your grip with your right hand and lean your body through your extended arm.

■ Extension progression (not shown)

- Position the carpometacarpal I joint near its end range-of-motion into extension.

Thumb carpometacarpal palmar glide
for restricted adduction

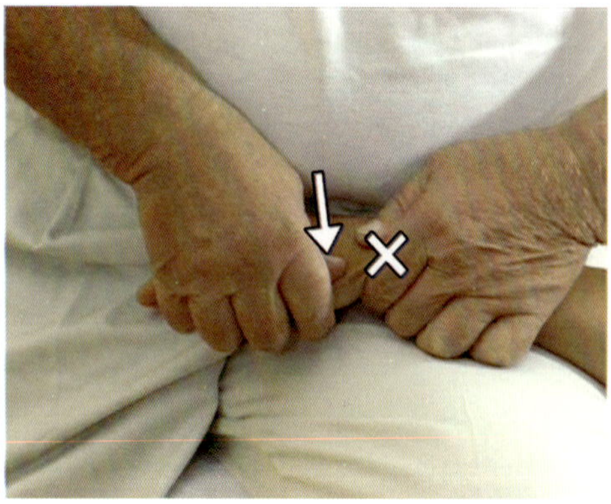

Figure 7g – test and mobilization in resting position

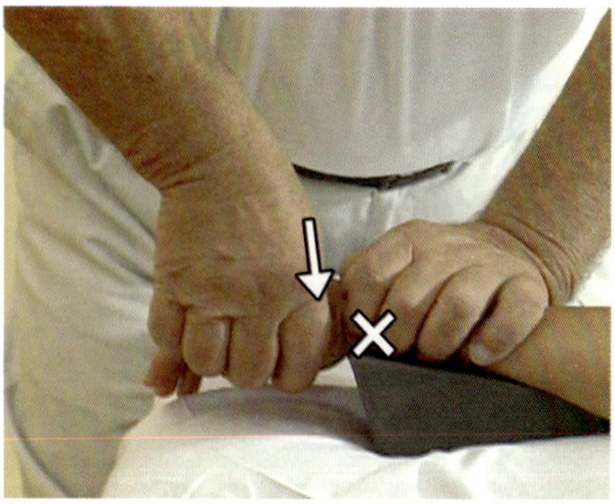

Figure 7h – mobilization in resting position

■ Figure 7g: Test and mobilization in resting position

Objective

- To evaluate the quantity and quality of palmar glide joint play in the carpometacarpal I joint, including end-feel.
- To increase thumb adduction range-of-motion (Convex Rule).

Starting position

- The palmar side of the patient's hand faces down.
- Position the joint in its resting position.

Hand placement and fixation

- **Therapist's stable hand (left):** Hold the patient's distal forearm with your hand; grip around the trapezium just proximal to the joint space; fixate the patient's hand against your body.
- **Therapist's moving hand (right):** Grip the patient's metacarpal I just distal to the joint space.

Procedure

- Apply a Grade II or III palmar glide movement to metacarpal I.

■ Figure 7h: Mobilization in resting position

- Apply a Grade III palmar glide movement to increase thumb adduction. The palmar side of the patient's hand, including the trapezium, rests on the treatment wedge; grip around metacarpal I with your left thumb and fingers. You may reinforce your grip with your right hand and lean your body through your extended arm.

■ Adduction progression (not shown)

- Position the carpometacarpal I joint near the end range-of-motion into adduction. Note that in cases of extreme hypomobility the joint may remain in an abducted position.

Thumb carpometacarpal dorsal glide
for restricted abduction

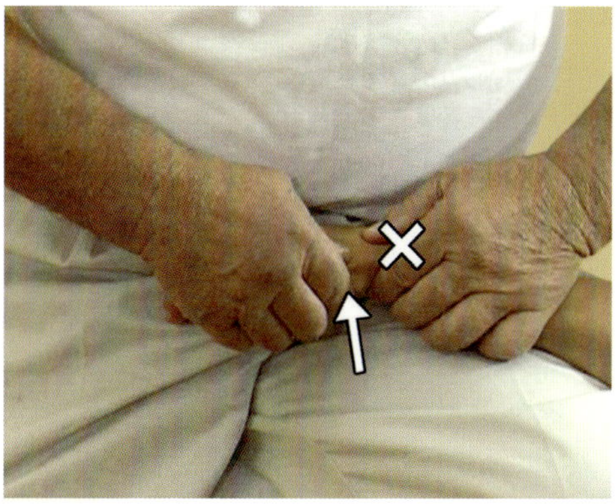

Figure 7i – test and mobilization in resting position

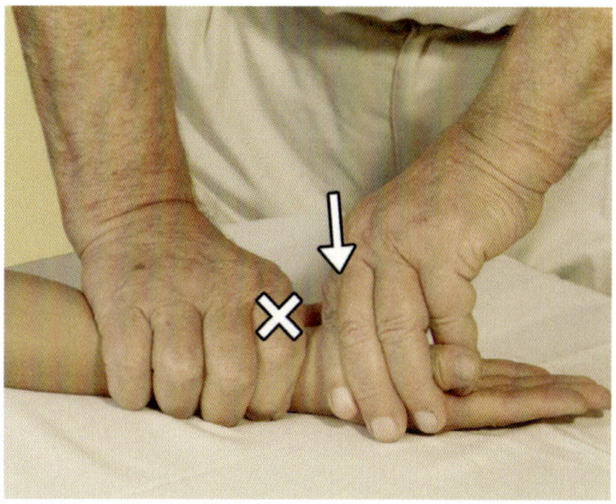

Figure 7j – mobilization in resting position

■ Figure 7i: Test and mobilization in resting position

Objective

- To evaluate the quantity and quality of dorsal glide joint play in the carpometacarpal I joint, including end-feel.
- To increase thumb abduction range-of-motion (Convex Rule).

Starting position

- The palmar side of the patient's hand faces down.
- Position the joint in its resting position.

Hand placement and fixation

- **Therapist's stable hand (left):** Hold the patient's distal forearm with your hand; grip around the trapezium just proximal to the joint space; fixate the patient's hand against your body.
- **Therapist's moving hand (right):** Grip the patient's metacarpal I just distal to the joint space.

Procedure

- Apply a Grade II or III dorsal glide movement to metacarpal I.

■ Figure 7j: Mobilization in resting position

- Apply a Grade III dorsal glide movement to increase thumb abduction. The dorsal side of the patient's hands rests on the treatment surface; grip around metacarpal I with your left hand; place your metacarpal II-phalangeal joint just distal to the joint space; lean your body through your extended arm.

■ Abduction progression (not shown)

- Position the carpometacarpal I joint near its end range-of-motion into abduction.

Notes

Metacarpals

CHAPTER 10

WRIST

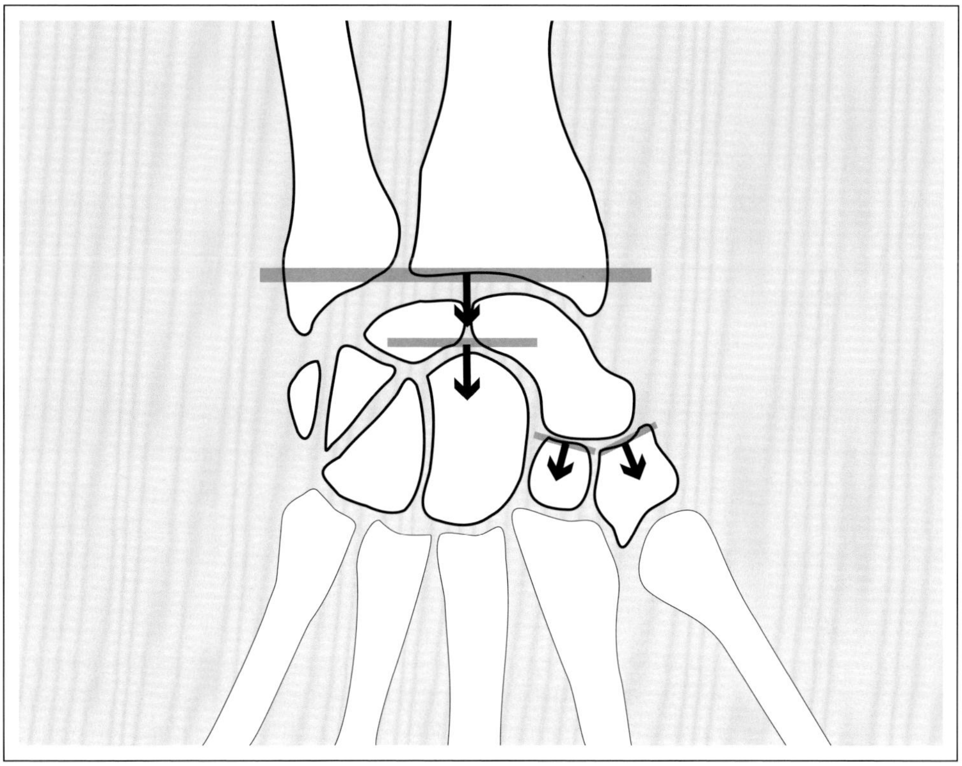

Wrist

10 Wrist

(carpus)

Functional anatomy and movement

The wrist joint complex consists of eight carpal bones arranged in two rows, the distal radius and ulna, and an articular disc (see *Figure 13*).

The proximal or first row of carpal bones are, starting from the radial side:

- scaphoid (navicular = os scaphoideum)
- lunate (semi-lunate = os lunatum)
- triquetral (cuneiform = os triquetral)
- pisiform (os pisiforme).

In the second or distal row, starting from the radial side

- trapezium (multangulum majus = os trapezium)
- trapezoid (multangulum minus = os trapezoideum)
- capitate (magnum = os capitatum); and hamate (unciform = os hamatum).

An articular disc binds the distal end of the radius and ulna together and its lower surface forms part of the radiocarpal joint. The articular disc takes part in all movements of the radiocarpal joint in addition to forearm pronation and supination.

The wrist is divided into three joints,

Radiocarpal joint

(art. radiocarpalis)

The radiocarpal joint, the "true" wrist joint, is an anatomically and mechanically simple biaxial joint (ellipsoid, modified ovoid). The convex surface is made up of the scaphoid, lunate and triquetral and their interosseous ligaments, which are often calcified. Therefore, these three bones act as one joint surface. The scaphoid and radial part of the lunate articulates with the radius, and the triquetral and ulnar part of the lunate articulates with the articular disc. A concave surface is formed by the radius and the articular disc.

■ Midcarpal joint

(art. mediocarpalis)

The midcarpal joint is an anatomically simple and mechanically compound joint between the bones of the proximal and distal rows of carpals. The scaphoid has a convex surface distally and articulates with the two trapezii, which together can be considered as having a concave surface. On the ulnar side, the scaphoid, lunate and triquetral form a concave surface which articulates with the convex surface formed by the capitate and hamate.

■ Pisiform joint

(art. ossis pisiformis)

The pisiform joint is an anatomically simple and mechanically compound plane gliding joint. The pisiform is a sesamoid bone in the tendon of the flexor carpi ulnaris. Proximal gliding is prevented by the pisohamate and pisometacarpal ligaments. The abductor digiti minimi arises from the pisiform bone. Therefore, the pisiform will be fixated during contraction of both the abductor digiti minimi and flexor carpi ulnaris.

Bony palpation

- Scaphoid, lunate, triquetral, pisiform, radius
- Ulna and articular disc
- Joint spaces between radial-carpal and ulnar-carpal joints
- Intercarpal joints of proximal carpal row
- Trapezium, trapezoid, capitate, hamate with its hook
- Joint spaces between the proximal and distal row of carpals
- Intercarpal joints of distal carpal row

Ligaments

- Intercarpal ligaments: dorsal, palmar and interosseous
- Radiocarpal ligament: deep
- Collateral ligaments: radial and ulnar
- Ulnocarpal ligament: palmar
- Radiocarpal ligaments: dorsal and palmar
- Pisohamate and pisometacarpal ligaments

Bone movement and axes

- **Dorsal flexion** (extension) and **palmar flexion** (flexion): Movement begins in the radiocarpal joint around a transverse axis running through the lunate, and continues in the intercarpal joint around a transverse axis running through the capitate. Approximately half the range of wrist extension and flexion takes place in the intercarpal joint and the other half in the radiocarpal joint.

  During *dorsal flexion,* the proximal part of the capitate moves in a palmar direction in relation to lunate; the same occurs with lunate in relation to the radius. The proximal part of the scaphoid also moves in a palmar direction in relation to the radius; the distal part of the scaphoid appears to move in a palmar direction in relation to the trapezii because these bones glide dorsally on the scaphoid. During *palmar flexion* these movements are reversed.

- **Ulnar flexion** (ulnar deviation, adduction): Movement takes place primarily in the radiocarpal joint around a dorsal-palmar axis through the head of the capitate. The proximal row of carpals glide in a radial direction in relation to the radius. Laxity in the ligaments on the radial side of the joint allows this gliding to take place.
- **Radial flexion** (radial deviation, abduction): The primary movement also takes place around the above mentioned axis and the proximal carpal row glides in an ulnar direction in relation to the radius. However, due to tightening of ligaments, radial flexion (ulnar gliding) is less than ulnar flexion (radial gliding). Full radial flexion requires that the two trapezii glide onto the dorsal side of the scaphoid. This approximates the trapezii and the radius; the movement is similar to that occurring with extension of the wrist.

End feel

- Firm

Joint movement (gliding)

- Convex Rule for all wrist joints with the following exception:
- Concave Rule for trapezium/trapezoid-scaphoid joint

Treatment plane

- On the concave surface of the targeted wrist joint

Zero position

- The longitudinal axes through the radius and the third metacarpal bone form a straight line.

Resting position

- Slight palmar flexion and slight ulnar flexion (midway between maximal radial and ulnar flexion)

Close-packed position

- Wrist in maximal extension

Capsular pattern

- Restricted equally in all directions

Wrist examination scheme

(Refer to Chapters 3 and 4 for more information on examination)

Tests of function

1. **Active and passive movements, including stability tests and end-feel**

Palmar flexion	90°
Extension	80°
Radial flexion	20°
Ulnar flexion	30°

2. **Translatoric joint play movements, including end-feel**

Traction - compression	(Figure 8a)
Gliding	
Palmar	(Figure 9a)
Dorsal	(Figure 10a)
Radial	(Figure 11a)
Ulnar	(Figure 12a)
Carpal bones	(Figures 14a)

3. **Resisted movements**

	OTHER FUNCTIONS
Palmar flexion	
Flexor carpi radialis	Radial flexion
Flexor carpi ulnaris	Ulnar flexion
Palmaris longus	
Extension	
Extensor carpi radialis longus	Radial flexion
Extensor carpi radialis brevis	
Extensor carpi ulnaris	Ulnar flexion
Radial flexion	
Flexor carpi radialis	Palmar flexion
Extensor carpi radialis	Extension
Ulnar flexion	
Flexor carpi ulnaris	Palmar flexion
Extensor carpi ulnaris	Extension

4. **Passive soft tissue movements**
   - Physiological
   - Accessory

5. **Additional tests**

Trial treatment

Traction	(Figure 8b)

Wrist techniques

General techniques

Figure 8a,b	Traction for pain and hypomobility
Figure 8c,d	Traction for restricted palmar and dorsal flexion
Figure 9a,b	Palmar glide for restricted dorsal flexion
Figure 10a,b	Dorsal glide for restricted palmar flexion
Figure 11a,b	Radial glide for restricted ulnar flexion
Figure 12a,b	Ulnar glide for restricted radial flexion

Specific techniques

Figure 13	Wrist glide tests recommended sequence
Figure 14a	Wrist palmar and dorsal glide test

Capitate-lunate

Figure 14b,c	Palmar glide for restricted dorsal flexion
Figure 14d,e	Dorsal glide for restricted palmar flexion

Lunate-radius

(not shown)	Palmar glide for restricted dorsal flexion
(not shown)	Dorsal glide for restricted palmar flexion

Scaphoid-radius

Figure 15a,b	Palmar glide for restricted dorsal flexion
(not shown)	Dorsal glide for restricted palmar flexion

Trapezii-scaphoid

(not shown)	Palmar glide for restricted palmar flexion
Figure 15c,d	Dorsal glide for restricted dorsal flexion

Triquetral-ulna

Figure 16a,b	Palmar glide for restricted dorsal flexion

Wrist traction
for pain and hypomobility

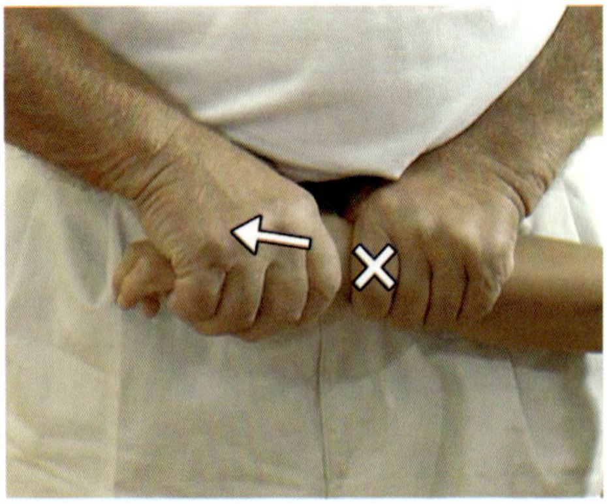

Figure 8a – test and mobilization in resting position

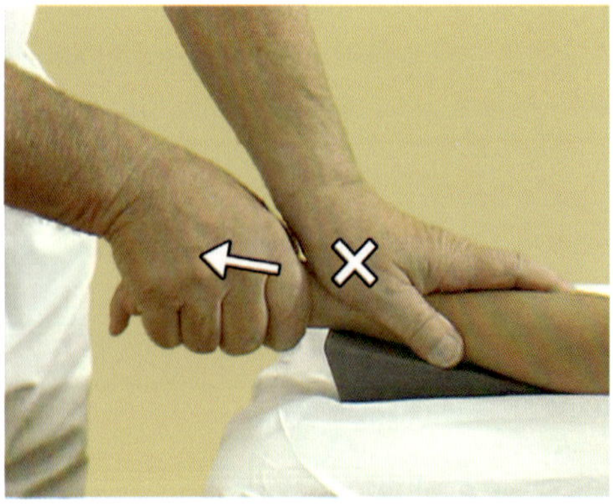

Figure 8b – mobilization in resting position

■ Figure 8a: Test and mobilization in resting position

Objective

- To evaluate the quantity and quality of traction joint play in the wrist, including end-feel.
- To decrease pain or increase range-of-motion in the wrist joints.

Starting position

- The patient's palm faces down.
- Position the joint in its resting position.

Hand placement and fixation

- **Therapist's stable hand (left):** Grip the patient's forearm just proximal to the wrist joint; fixate the patient's forearm against your body.
- **Therapist's moving hand (right):** Grip the patient's hand just distal to the wrist joint.

Procedure

- Apply a Grade I, II or III distal traction movement to the distal joint partners.
- Modify your grip to apply more specific traction between the radius and proximal row of carpals, or between the proximal and distal row of carpals.
- Suitable for early training in manipulative thrust techniques.

■ Figure 8b: Mobilization in resting position

- Stabilize the patient's forearm on a wedge. Fixate the patient's anterior distal forearm against the wedge with your hand. Grip with your thenar eminence just proximal to the targeted wrist joints.
- Suitable for early training in manipulative thrust techniques.

Wrist traction
for restricted palmar and dorsal flexion

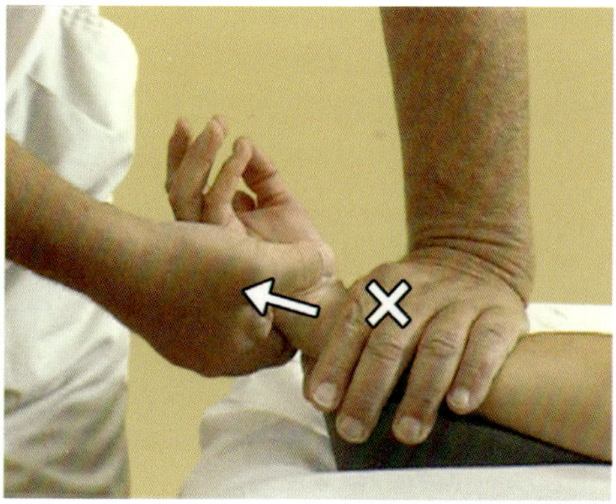

Figure 8c – mobilization in palmar flexion

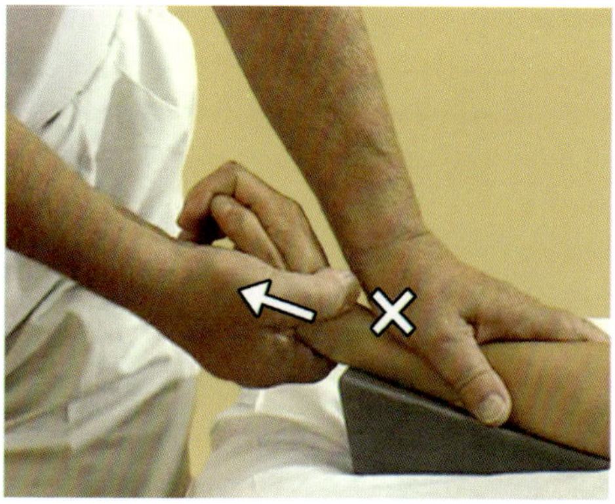

Figure 8d – mobilization in dorsal flexion

■ Figure 8c: Palmar progression

Objective

- To increase wrist palmar flexion range-of-motion.

Starting position

- The posterior side of the patient's distal forearm rests on the wedge.
- Position the joint near the end range-of-motion into palmar flexion.

Hand placement and fixation

- **Therapist's stable hand (left):** Fixate the patient's distal forearm against the wedge, including, if necessary, the proximal row of carpals; grip the patient's distal forearm just proximal to the targeted wrist joints.
- **Therapist's moving hand (right):** Grip the patient's hand just distal to the targeted wrist joints.

Procedure

- Apply a Grade III distal traction movement to the distal joint partners.
- Modify your grip to apply more specific traction between the radius and proximal row of carpals, or between the proximal and distal row of carpals.

■ Figure 8d: Dorsal progression

- Apply a Grade III distal traction movement to the wrist positioned near to its end range-of-motion into dorsal flexion.
- The anterior side of the patient's distal forearm rests on the wedge.

Wrist palmar glide

for restricted dorsal flexion

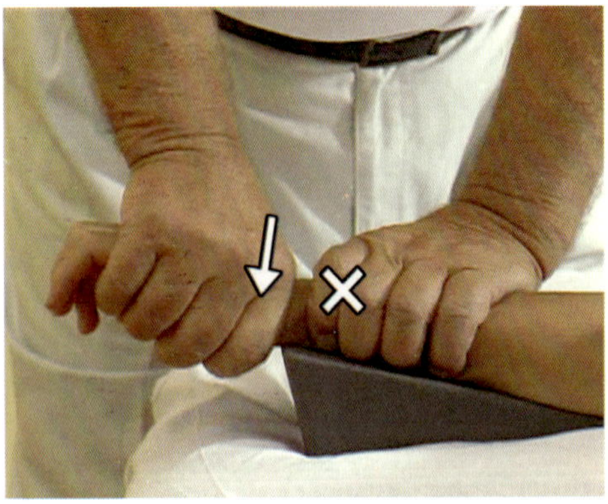

Figure 9a – test and mobilization in resting position

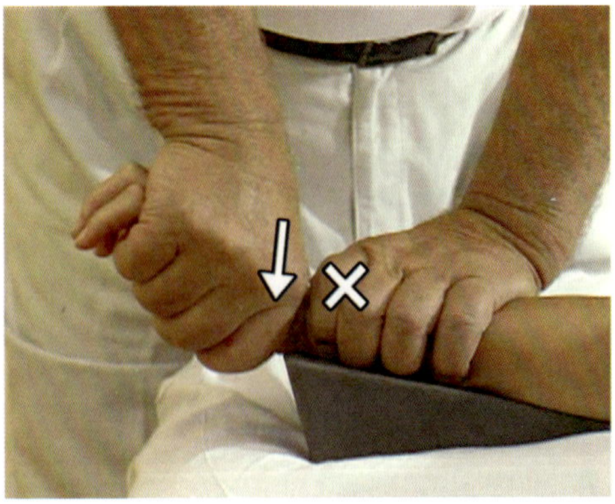

Figure 9b – mobilization in dorsal flexion

■ Figure 9a: Test and mobilization in resting position

Objective

- To evaluate the quantity and quality of palmar glide joint play in the wrist joints.
- To increase wrist dorsal flexion range-of-motion (Convex Rule).

Starting position

- The anterior side of the patient's distal forearm rests on the wedge.
- Position the joint in its resting position.

Hand placement and fixation

- **Therapist's stable hand (left):** Fixate the patient's distal forearm against the wedge, including, if necessary, the proximal row of carpals; grip the patient's distal forearm just proximal to the targeted wrist joints.
- **Therapist's moving hand (right):** Hold the patient's hand in your hand; grip just distal to the targeted joint spaces.

Procedure

- Apply a Grade II or III palmar glide movement to the distal joint partners.
- Modify your grip to apply more specific mobilization between the radius and proximal row of carpals, or between the proximal and distal row of carpals.

■ Figure 9b: Dorsal progression

- Apply a Grade III palmar glide movement with the targeted wrist joints positioned close to their end range-of-motion into dorsal flexion (Convex Rule).

Wrist dorsal glide
for restricted palmar flexion

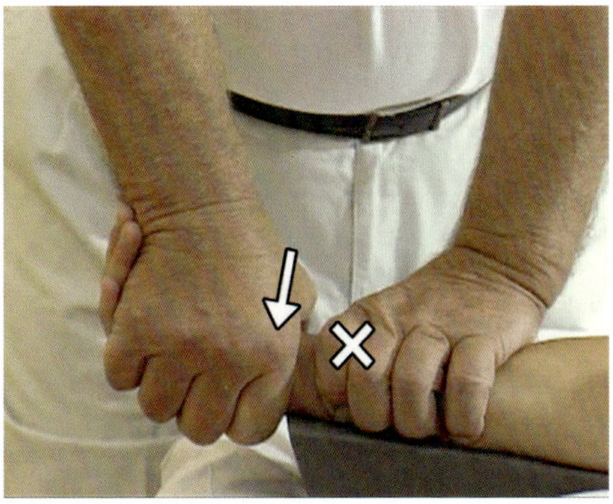
Figure 10a – test and mobilization in resting position

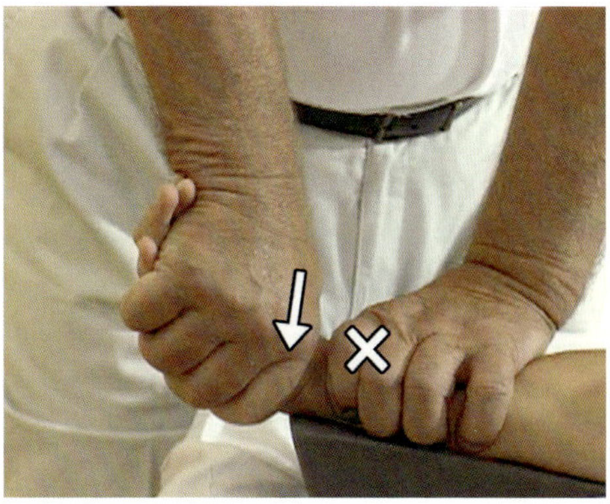
Figure 10b – mobilization in palmar flexion

■ Figure 10a: Test and mobilization in resting position

Objective

- To evaluate the quantity and quality of dorsal glide joint play in the wrist joints.
- To increase wrist palmar flexion range-of-motion (Convex Rule).

Starting position

- The posterior side of the patient's distal forearm rests on the wedge.
- Position the joint in its resting position.

Hand placement and fixation

- **Therapist's stable hand (left):** Fixate the patient's distal forearm against the wedge, including, if necessary, the proximal row of carpals; grip the patient's distal forearm just proximal to the targeted wrist joints.
- **Therapist's moving hand (right):** Hold the patient's hand in your hand; grip just distal to the targeted joints.

Procedure

- Apply a Grade II or III dorsal glide movement to the distal joint partners.
- Modify your grip to apply more specific mobilization between the radius and proximal row of carpals, or between the proximal and distal row of carpals.

■ Figure 10b: Palmar progression

- Apply a Grade III dorsal glide movement with the targeted wrist joints positioned close to their end range-of-motion into palmar flexion (Convex Rule).

Wrist radial glide

for restricted ulnar flexion

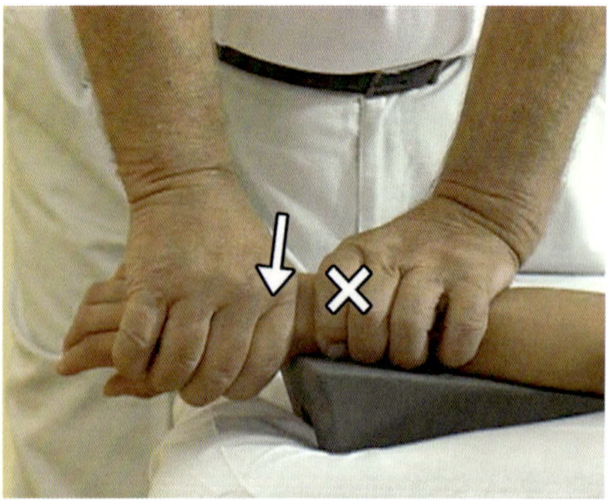

Figure 11a – test and mobilization in resting position

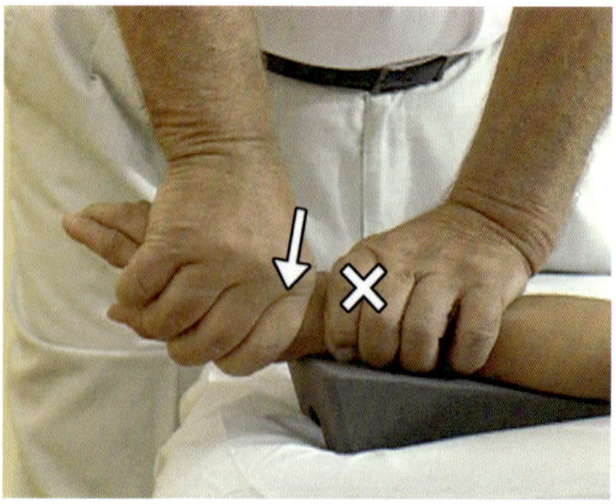

Figure 11b – mobilization in ulnar flexion

Wrist

■ Figure 11a: Test and mobilization in resting position

Objective

- To evaluate the quantity and quality of radial glide joint play in the wrist joints.
- To increase ulnar flexion range-of-motion (Convex Rule).

Starting position

- The radial side of the patient's distal forearm rests on the wedge.
- Position the joint in its resting position.

Hand placement and fixation

- **Therapist's stable hand (left):** Fixate the patient's distal forearm against the wedge, including, if necessary, the proximal row of carpals; grip the patient's distal forearm just proximal to the targeted wrist joints.
- **Therapist's moving hand (right):** Hold the patient's hand in your hand; grip just distal to the targeted joint spaces.

Procedure

- Apply a Grade II or III radial glide movement to the distal joint partners.

■ Figure 11b: Ulnar progression

- Apply a Grade III radial glide movement with the targeted wrist joints positioned close to their end range-of-motion into ulnar flexion (Convex Rule).

Wrist ulnar glide
for restricted radial flexion

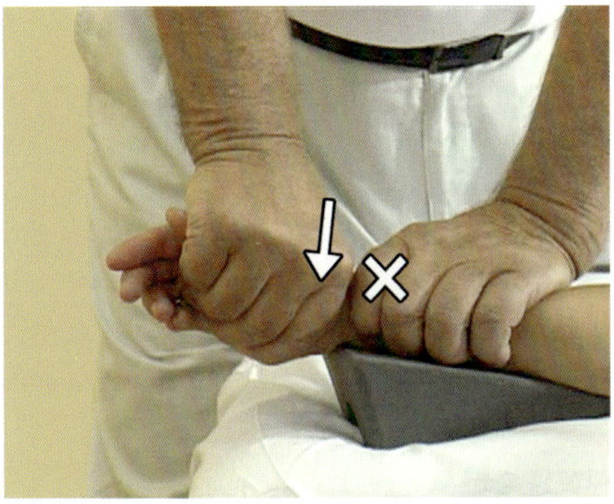

Figure 12a – test and mobilization in resting position

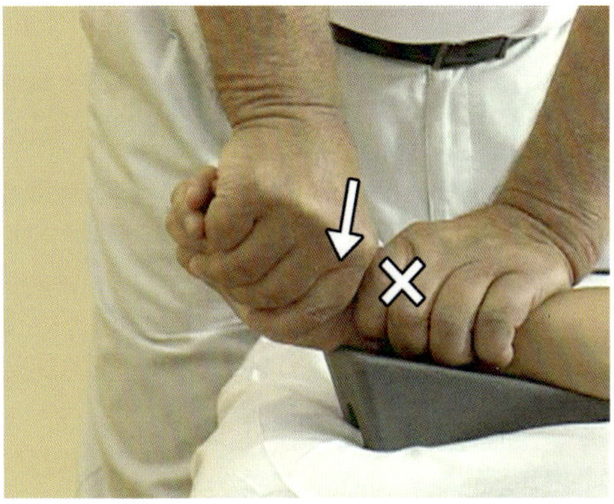

Figure 12b – mobilization in radial flexion

Wrist

■ Figure 12a: Test and mobilization in resting position

Objective

- To evaluate the quantity and quality of ulnar glide joint play in the wrist joints.
- To increase radial flexion range-of-motion (Convex Rule).

Starting position

- The ulnar side of the patient's distal forearm rests on the wedge.
- Position the joint in its resting position.

Hand placement and fixation

- **Therapist's stable hand (left):** Fixate the patient's distal forearm against the wedge, including, if necessary, the proximal row of carpals; grip the patient's distal forearm just proximal to the targeted wrist joints.
- **Therapist's moving hand (right):** Hold the patient's hand in your hand; grip just distal to the targeted joint spaces.

Procedure

- Apply a Grade II or III ulnar glide movement to the distal joint partners.

■ Figure 12b: Radial progression

- Apply a Grade III ulnar glide movement with the targeted wrist joints positioned close to their end range-of-motion into radial flexion (Convex Rule).

Wrist glide tests
Recommended sequence

■ **Figure 13: Recommended glide test sequence for the wrist**

Use one hand for fixation and the other hand for movement.

Movements around the capitate ......(Figure 14a)

Fixate capitate and move:

1. Trapezoid
2. Scaphoid
3. Lunate

Fixate capitate and move:

4. Hamate ....(adapt from Figure 14a, 15a or 16a)

Movements on the radial side of the wrist

Fixate scaphoid and move:

5. The two trapezii ....(Figure 15c)

Movements of the radiocarpal joint

Fixate radius and move:

6. Scaphoid ....(Figure 15a)
7. Lunate ....(adapt from Figure 14a, 15a or 16a)

Fixate ulna, including the disc, and move:

8. Triquetral ....(Figure 16a)

Movements on the ulnar side of the wrist

Fixate triquetral and move:

9. Hamate ....(adapt from Figure 14a, 15a or 16a)
10. Pisiform (position the patient's hand in palmar flexion)

Movements between triquetral-lunate, lunate-scaphoid and between the two trapezii can also be tested.

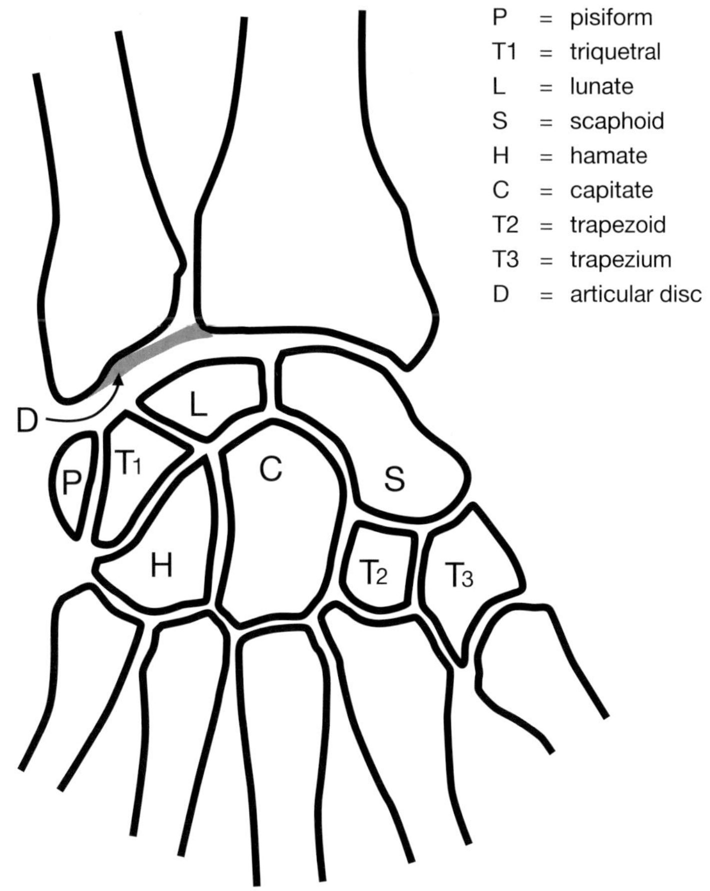

Figure 13
Dorsal aspect of the right wrist

Wrist

Wrist palmar and dorsal glide

Test

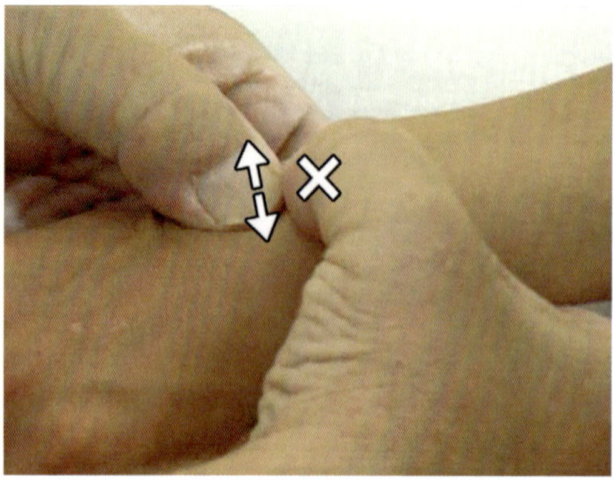

Figure 14a – specific wrist joint tests

Wrist

■ Figure 14a: Test with proximal fixation in resting position

Objective

- To evaluate the quantity and quality of palmar and dorsal glide joint play in specific wrist joints, including end-feel.

Starting position

- The patient rests the palmar side of their forearm on the treatment surface.
- Position the joint in its resting position.

Fixation

- **Therapist's stable hand (right):** Grip the proximal joint partner with your fingers; fixate your hand against the treatment surface.
- **Therapist's moving hand (left):** Hold the patient's fingers in your hand; grip with your fingers just distal to the targeted joint space.

Procedure

- Apply a palmar or dorsal glide movement; use simultaneous Grade I traction to facilitate the movement.

■ Distal or lateral fixation in resting position (not shown)

- All joints between the eight carpal bones can be similarly tested using proximal, distal, or lateral fixation: fixate one carpal bone and move an adjacent carpal bone in a dorsal or palmar direction.

Capitate-lunate palmar glide
for restricted dorsal flexion

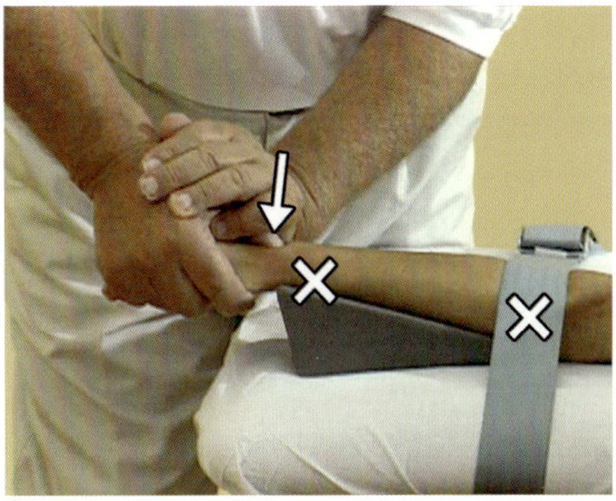

Figure 14b – mobilization in resting position

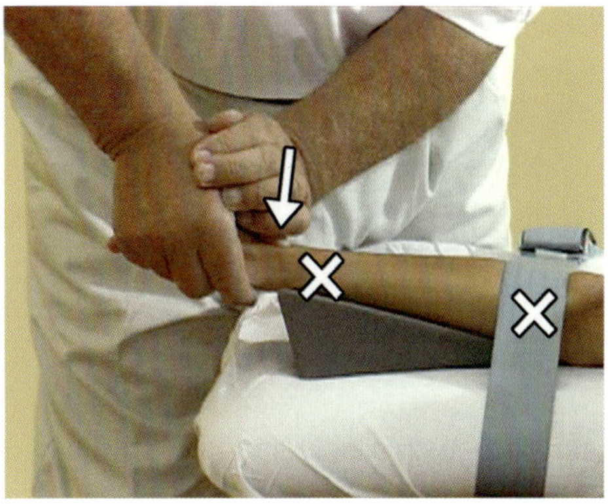

Figure 14c – mobilization in dorsal flexion

■ Figure 14b: Mobilization in resting position

Objective

- To increase wrist dorsal flexion range-of-motion (Convex Rule).

Starting position

- The anterior side of the patient's distal forearm, including the lunate, rests on the wedge.
- Position the joint in its resting position.

Hand placement and fixation

- **Fixation:** The lunate is fixated by the wedge; a belt fixates the proximal forearm.
- **Therapist's moving hands:** Support the patient's hand and thumb in your right hand with your thumb on the capitate; use your left hand to supplement your grip.

Procedure

- Apply a Grade III palmar glide movement to the capitate.

■ Figure 14c: Dorsal flexion progression

- Apply a Grade III palmar glide joint play movement to the capitate near the end range-of-motion into wrist dorsal flexion (Convex Rule)

■ Lunate-radius mobilization (not shown)

- Fixate the radius; apply a Grade III palmar glide movement to the lunate (Convex Rule).

Capitate-lunate dorsal glide
for restricted palmar flexion

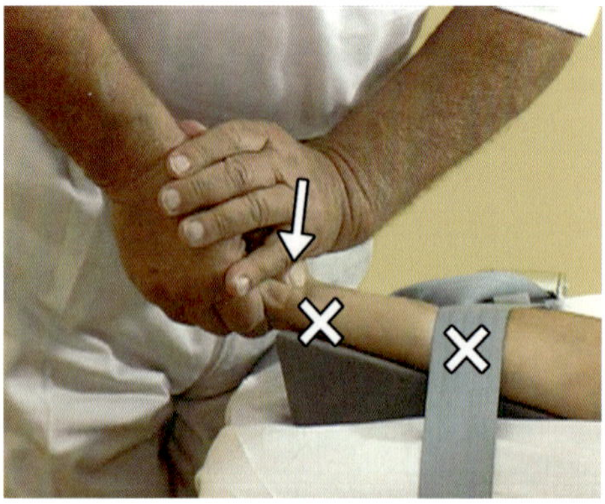

Figure 14d – mobilization in resting position

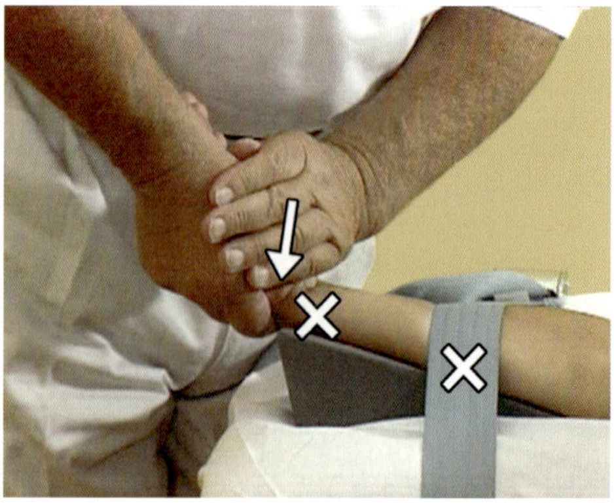

Figure 14e – mobilization in palmar flexion

■ Figure 14d: Mobilization in resting position

Objective

- To increase wrist palmar flexion range-of-motion (Convex Rule).

Starting position

- The posterior side of the patient's distal forearm, including the lunate, rests on the wedge.
- Position the joint in its resting position.

Hand placement and fixation

- **Fixation:** The lunate is fixated by the wedge; a belt fixates the proximal forearm.
- **Therapist's moving hands:** Support the patient's hand and thumb in your right hand with your thumb on the capitate; use your left hand to supplement your grip.

Procedure

- Apply a Grade III dorsal glide movement to the capitate.

■ Figure 14e: Palmar flexion progression

- Apply a Grade III dorsal glide joint play movement near the end range-of-motion into wrist palmar flexion (Convex Rule).

■ Radius-lunate mobilization (not shown)

- Fixate the radius; apply a Grade III dorsal glide movement to the lunate (Convex Rule).

Scaphoid-radius palmar glide
for restricted dorsal flexion

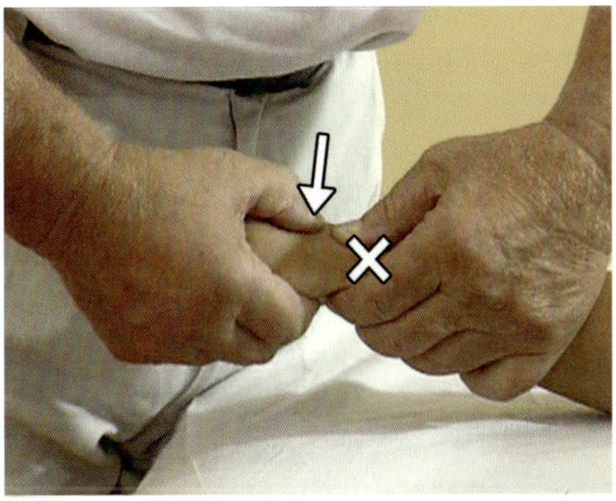

Figure 15a – test and mobilization in resting position

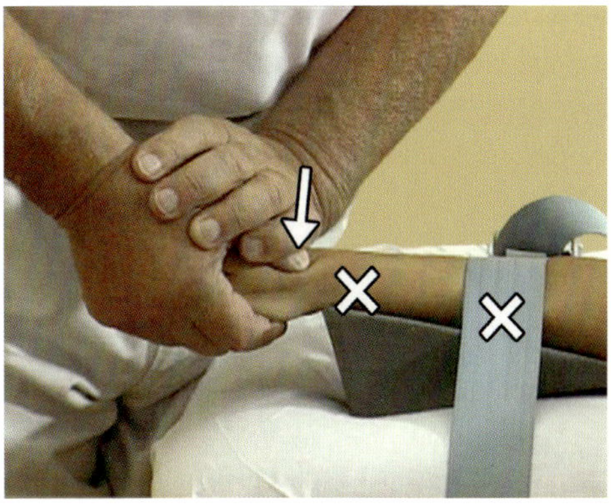

Figure 15b – mobilization in resting position

Wrist

■ Figure 15a: Test and mobilization in resting position

Objective

- To evaluate the quantity and quality of scaphoid palmar glide joint play in relation to the radius, including end-feel.
- To increase wrist dorsal and radial flexion range-of-motion (Convex Rule).

Starting position

- The anterior side of the patient's forearm faces down.
- Position the joint in its resting position.

Hand placement and fixation

- **Therapist's stable hand (left):** Hold the patient's distal forearm; grip with your fingers just proximal to the scaphoid-radius joint space.
- **Therapist's moving hand (right):** Support the patient's hand in your hand; grip with your thumb and index finger surrounding the scaphoid.

Procedure

- Apply a Grade II or III palmar glide movement to the scaphoid.

■ Figure 15b: Mobilization in resting position

- The anterior side of the patient's distal forearm rests on the wedge; the distal radius is fixated by the wedge; a belt fixates the proximal forearm; support the patient's hand and thumb in your right hand with your thumb on the scaphoid; use your left hand to supplement your grip; apply a Grade III palmar glide movement to the scaphoid.

  For progression, position the hand near the end range-of-motion into wrist dorsal flexion.

■ Trapezii-scaphoid palmar glide for restricted palmar flexion (not shown)

- Fixate the scaphoid; apply a Grade III palmar glide movement to the trapezii (Concave Rule).

Trapezii-scaphoid dorsal glide
for restricted dorsal flexion

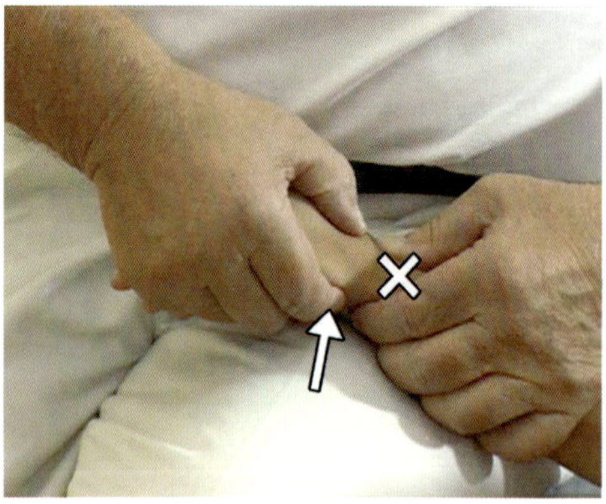

Figure 15c – test and mobilization in resting position

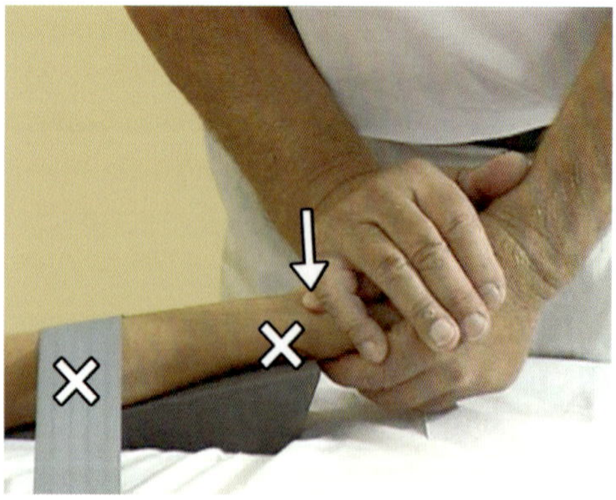

Figure 15d – mobilization in resting position

■ Figure 15c: Test and mobilization in resting position

Objective

- To evaluate the quantity and quality of dorsal glide joint play of the trapezii in relation to the scaphoid, including end-feel.
- To increase wrist dorsal flexion (Concave Rule).

Starting position

- The anterior side of the patient's forearm faces down.
- Position the joint in its resting position.

Hand placement and fixation

- **Therapist's stable hand (left):** Hold the patient's distal forearm against your body; grip with your fingers surrounding the scaphoid.
- **Therapist's moving hand (right):** Support the patient's hand in your hand; grip with your thumb and index finger surrounding the trapezii.

Procedure

- Apply a Grade II or III dorsal glide movement to the trapezii.

■ Figure 15d: Mobilization in resting position

- The posterior side of the patient's distal forearm rests on the wedge; the distal radius, including the scaphoid, is fixated by the wedge; a belt fixates the proximal forearm; support the patient's hand and thumb in your left hand with your thumb on the trapezii; use your right hand to supplement your grip; apply a Grade III dorsal glide movement to the trapezii.

■ Scaphoid-radius dorsal glide for restricted palmar flexion (not shown)

- Fixate the radius; apply a Grade III dorsal glide movement to the scaphoid (Convex Rule).

Triquetral-ulna palmar glide

for restricted dorsal flexion

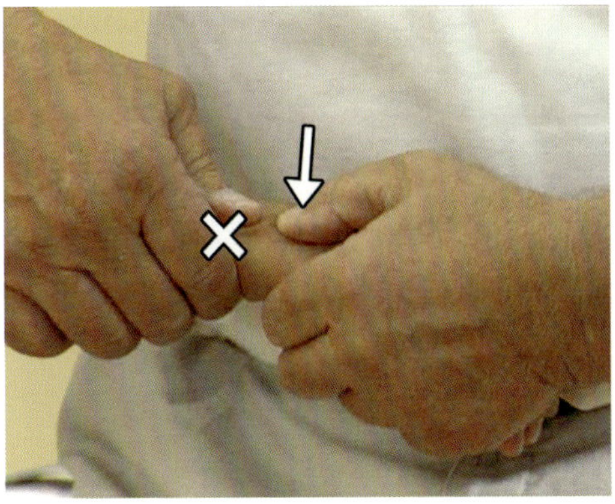

Figure 16a – test and mobilization in resting position

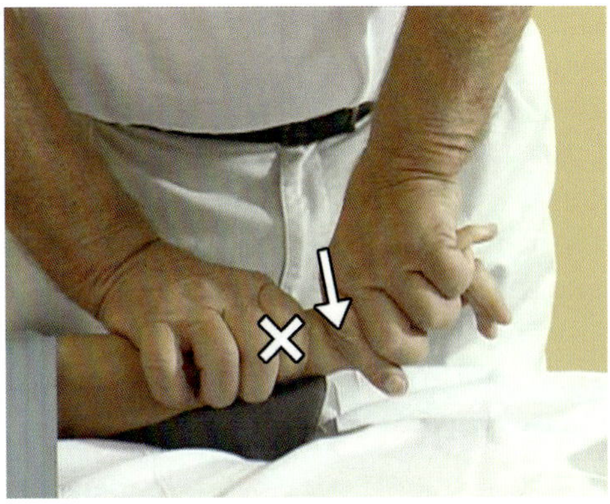

Figure 16b – mobilization in resting position

■ Figure 16a: Test and mobilization in resting position

Objective

- To evaluate the quantity and quality of palmar glide joint play of the triquetral in relation to the ulna, including end-feel.
- To release a fixated articular disc between triquetral and ulna. The fixated articular disc can restrict forearm pronation, supination, and all wrist movements.
- To increase wrist dorsal flexion (Convex Rule).

Starting position

- The palmar side of the patient's hand faces down.
- Position the joint in its resting position.

Hand placement and fixation

- **Therapist's stable hand (right):** Hold the patient's distal forearm against your body; grip with your fingers around the head of the ulna.
- **Therapist's moving hand (left):** Support the patient's hand in your hand; grip with your thumb and index finger surrounding the triquetral.

Procedure

- Apply a Grade II or III palmar glide movement to the triquetral.

■ Figure 16b: Mobilization in resting position

- The anterior side of the patient's distal forearm rests on the wedge; the distal ulna is fixated by the wedge; a belt fixates the proximal forearm; support the patient's hand in your right hand with your MCP II joint on the triquetral; apply a Grade III palmar glide joint play movement of the triquetral.

■ Hamate-triquetral palmar glide (not shown)

- Fixate the triquetral; apply a Grade III palmar glide movement to the hamate.

■ Hamate-triquetral dorsal glide (not shown)

- Supinate the patient's forearm and fixate the triquetral; apply a Grade III dorsal glide movement to the hamate.

■ Notes

Wrist

CHAPTER 11

FOREARM

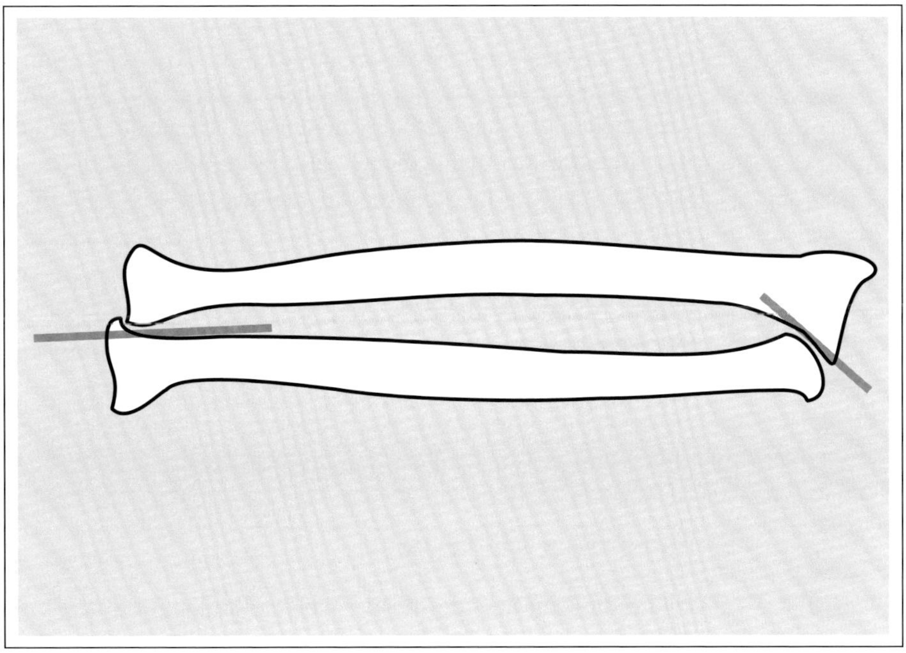

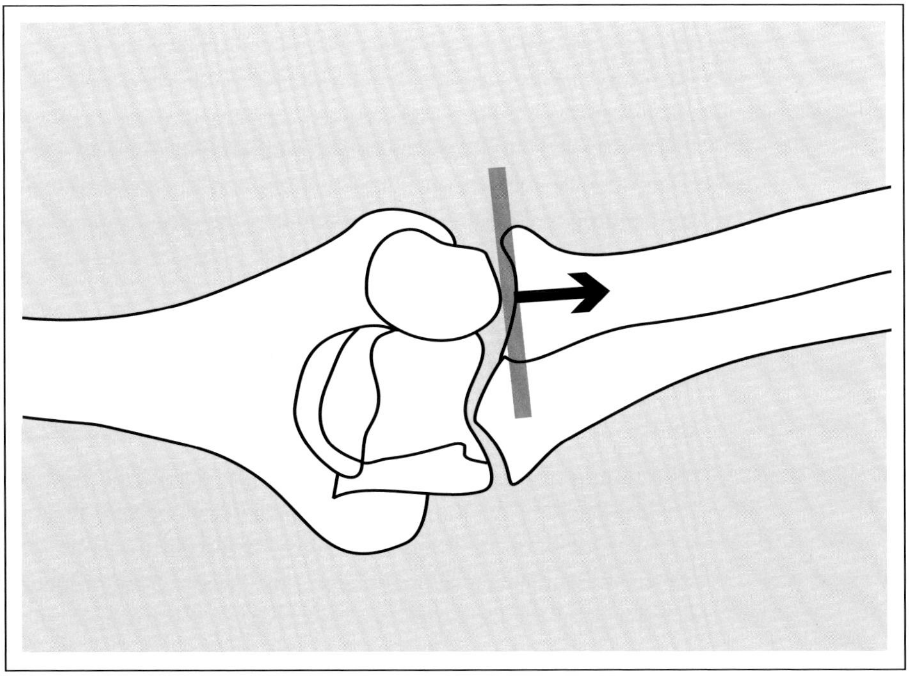

11 Forearm

Functional anatomy and movement

The forearm (antebrachium) consists of the radius and ulna with the antebrachial interosseous membrane. The distal broad part of the radius has the main contact with the carpus while the proximal, thickened part of the ulna has the main connection with the upper arm.

Distal radio-ulnar joint
(art. radio-ulnaris distalis)

The distal radio-ulnar joint is an anatomically and mechanically simple biaxial joint (trochoid, modified ovoid). The head of the ulna moves in the notch on the distal end of the radius.

Radio-ulnar syndesmosis

The radio-ulnar syndesmosis involves the length of the ulna and radius with the antebrachial interosseous membrane lying between their sharp interosseous borders.

Proximal radio-ulnar joint
(art. radio-ulnaris proximalis)

The proximal radio-ulnar joint is anatomically part of the elbow joint; it is a biaxial pivot joint (trochoid, modified ovoid). The head of the radius moves in the radial notch of the ulna.

Humeroradial joint
(art. humeroradialis)

The humeroradial joint is anatomically part of the elbow, but functionally also part of the forearm, and therefore is described here.

The humeroradial joint is a triaxial joint (spheroid, unmodified ovoid). During flexion-extension, the shallow concave facet on the radius moves on the convex surface of the capitulum of the humerus. Movements also take place at this joint during pronation and supination of the forearm.

Bony palpation

- Proximal radius (radial head)
- Radial tuberosity
- Distal radius and styloid process
- Distal ulna and styloid process
- Distal radio-ulnar joint space
- Proximal radio-ulnar joint space
- Humeroradial joint space

Ligaments

- Annular ligament: The annular ligament is cone-shaped, narrows distally and is only attached to the ulna which allows free movement of the head of the radius.
- Radial collateral ligament

Bone movement and axes

- Pronation - supination: The radius rotates around the ulna and produces torsion of the forearm; the axis of movement lies obliquely in the forearm passing through the radial and ulnar heads.
- Abduction (passive): The radius glides distally in relation to the ulna.
- Adduction (passive): The radius glides proximally in relation to the ulna.

End feel

- Pronation: hard end-feel. Pronation stops when the radius comes in contact with the ulna (bone to bone) producing a hard end-feel.
- Supination: firm end-feel. Supination is limited by soft tissues being stretched, especially ligaments, which results in a firm end-feel.

Joint movement (gliding)

- Distal radio-ulnar joint: Concave Rule
- Proximal radio-ulnar joint: Convex Rule
- Radius-humerus: Concave Rule

Treatment plane

- Distal radio-ulnar joint: on the concave joint surface of the radius
- Proximal radio-ulnar joint: on the concave joint surface of the ulna
- Humeroradial joint: on the concave joint surface of the radius

Zero position

- Distal and proximal radio-ulnar joints: upper arm parallel to the trunk with the elbow at a right angle, wrist in the Zero Position, and hand in the sagittal plane
- Humeroradial joint: arm and forearm in the frontal plane with the forearm fully supinated and the elbow extended

Resting position

All joints in the forearm cannot be placed in the resting position simultaneously.

- Distal radio-ulnar joint: The forearm is supinated approximately 10°.
- Proximal radio-ulnar joint: Forearm supination is approximately 35° and elbow flexion approximately 70°.
- Humeroradial joint: The forearm is fully supinated and the elbow fully extended.

Close-packed position

- Distal and proximal radio-ulnar joints: maximal pronation or supination
- Humeroradial joint: 90° elbow flexion

Capsular pattern

- Pronation and supination are restricted equally; occurs usually only when there is marked limitation of flexion and extension of the elbow joint.

■ Forearm examination scheme

(Refer to Chapters 3 and 4 for more information on examination)

Tests of function

1. Active and passive movements, including stability tests and end-feel

Pronation	80°
Supination	90°

2. Translatoric joint play movements

Traction - compression	(adapt techniques from Figure 17)
Gliding	
Distal radio-ulnar joint	
Ventral	(Figure 17a)
Dorsal	(Figure 18a)
Proximal radio-ulnar joint	
Ventral	(Figure 19a)
Dorsal	(Figure 19d)
Humeroradial joint	
Bilateral	(Figure 20)
Dorsal	(Figure 21a)

3. Resisted movements

	OTHER FUNCTIONS
Pronation	
Pronator teres	Flexion
Pronator quadratus	
Brachioradialis	Flexion; functions from supinated to zero starting position
Supination	
Supinator	Flexion
Biceps brachii	Flexion
Brachioradialis	Flexion; functions from pronated to zero starting position

4. Passive soft tissue movements

Physiological

Accessory

5. Additional tests

Trial treatment

Distal radio-ulnar joint	
Anterior-posterior gliding	(Figure 17b,18b)
Proximal radio-ulnar joint	
Anterior-posterior gliding	(Figure 19b, 19e)
Radius-humerus	
Posterior gliding	(Figure 21b)
Traction	(Figure 22)

■ Forearm techniques

Distal radio-ulnar joint

Figure 17a	Anterior glide for hypomobility
Figure 17b,c	Anterior glide for restricted pronation
Figure 18a,b	Posterior glide for hypomobility
Figure 18b,c	Posterior glide for restricted supination

Proximal radio-ulnar joint

Figure 19a,b,c	Anterior glide for restricted supination
Figure 19d,e,f	Posterior glide for restricted pronation

Humeroradial joint

Figure 20	Test
Figure 21a,b	Posterior glide for restricted extension
(not shown)	Anterior glide for restricted flexion
Figure 22	Distal traction for elbow and forearm hypomobility
Figure 23	Approximation for elbow and forearm hypomobility

Distal radio-ulnar joint anterior glide
for hypomobility

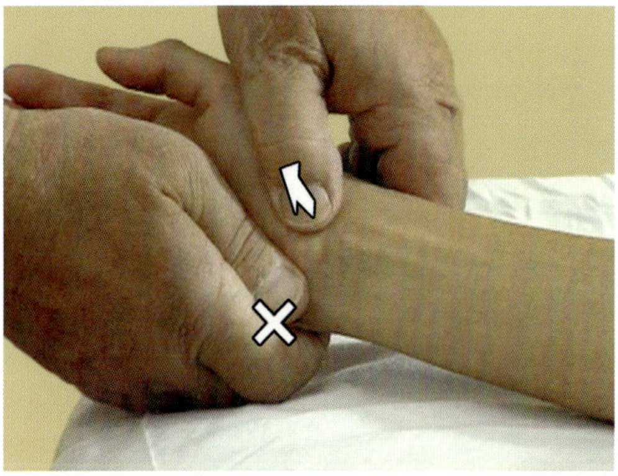

Figure 17a – test and mobilization in resting position

■ Figure 17a: Test and mobilization in resting position

Objective

- To evaluate the quantity and quality of anterior glide joint play in the radio-ulnar joint, including end-feel.
- To increase forearm pronation (Concave Rule).

Starting position

- The posterior side of the patient's forearm rests on the treatment surface, the elbow slightly flexed.
- Position the joint in its resting position.

Hand placement and fixation

- **Therapist's stable hand (right):** Hold the patient's hand from the ulnar side; grip around the patient's distal ulna near the joint space.
- **Therapist's moving hand (left):** Hold the patient's hand from the radial side; grip around the patient's distal radius near the joint space.

Procedure

- Apply a Grade II or III anterior glide movement to the radius.

Note

- Passive pronation, which is greater with the elbow flexed than extended, implicates a shortened supinator.

Distal radio-ulnar joint anterior glide

for restricted pronation

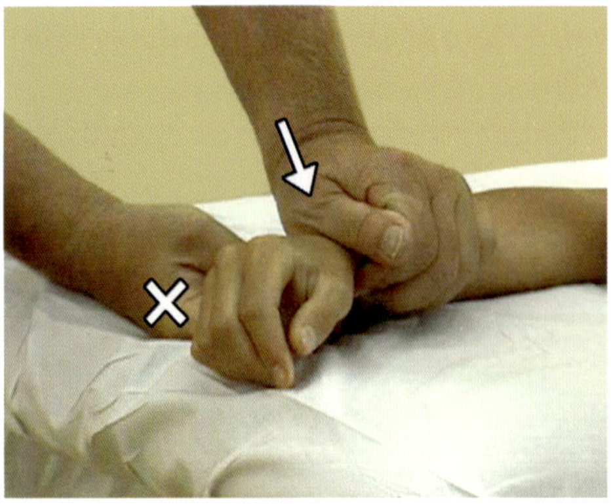

Figure 17b – mobilization in resting position

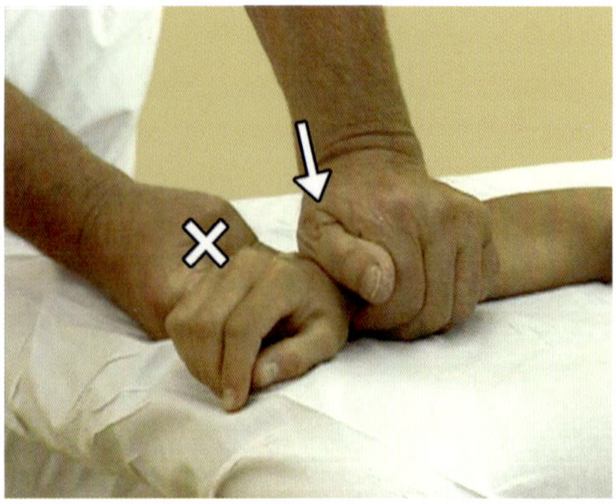

Figure 17c – mobilization in pronation

■ Figure 17b: Mobilization in resting position

Objective

- To increase forearm pronation (Concave Rule).

Starting position

- The ulnar side of the patient's forearm rests on the treatment surface, the elbow slightly flexed.
- Position the joint in its resting position.

Hand placement and fixation

- **Therapist's stable hand (right):** Grip with your thumb and fingers around the patient's ulnar head; rest your forearm on the treatment surface.
- **Therapist's moving hand (left):** Hold the patient's distal forearm from the radial side; grip around the distal radius with your thenar eminence close to the joint space; position your forearm in line with the treatment plane.

Procedure

- Press your left hand downward to apply a Grade III anterior glide movement.

■ Figure 17c: Pronation progression

- Apply a Grade III anterior glide movement with the forearm positioned near its end range-of-motion into pronation.

Distal radio-ulnar joint posterior glide
for hypomobility

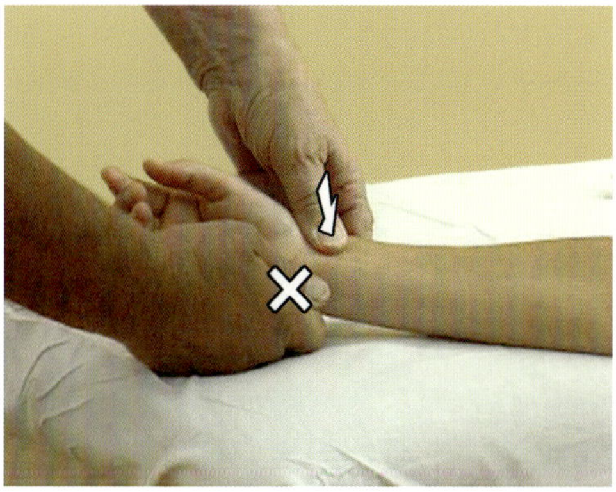

Figure 18a – test and mobilization in resting position

■ Figure 18a: Test and mobilization in resting position

Objective

- To evaluate the quantity and quality of posterior glide movement in the radio-ulnar joint, including end-feel.
- To increase forearm supination (Concave Rule).

Starting position

- The posterior side of the patient's forearm rests on the treatment surface, the elbow slightly flexed.
- Position the joint in its resting position. Note that in positions of greater shoulder abduction, the patient's hand moves into the horizontal plane making it difficult to perform these procedures in the resting position.

Hand placement and fixation

- **Therapist's stable hand (right):** Hold the patient's hand and distal forearm from the ulnar side; grip around the patient's distal ulna near the joint space.
- **Therapist's moving hand (left):** Hold the patient's hand and distal forearm from the radial side; grip around the patient's distal radius near the joint space.

Procedure

- Apply a Grade II or III posterior glide movement to the radius.

Note

- Passive supination, which is greater with the elbow flexed than extended, implicates a shortened pronator teres.

Distal radio-ulnar joint posterior glide
for restricted supination

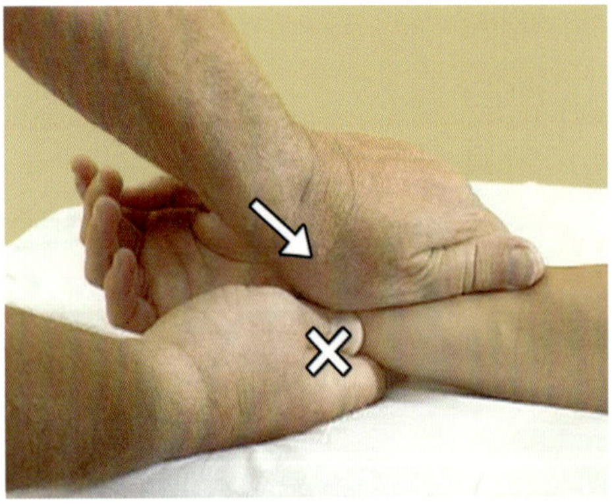

Figure 18b – mobilization in resting position

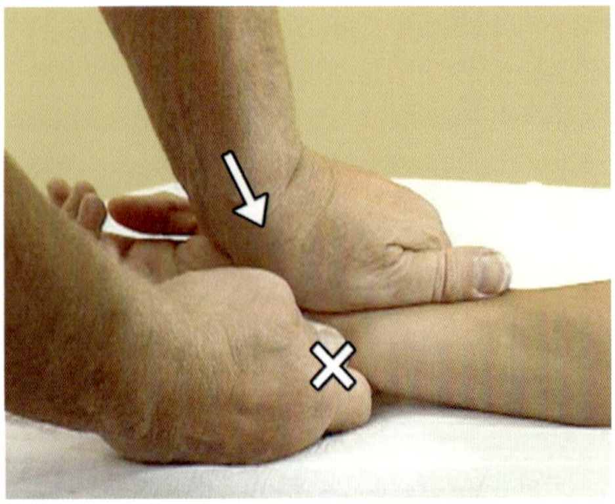

Figure 18c – mobilization in supination

■ Figure 18b: Mobilization in resting position

Objective

- To increase forearm supination (Concave Rule).

Starting position

- The ulnar side of the patient's forearm rests on the treatment surface, the elbow slightly flexed.
- Position the joint in its resting position.

Hand placement and fixation

- **Therapist's stable hand (right):** Grip with your thumb and fingers around the patient's ulnar head; rest your hand on the treatment surface.
- **Therapist's moving hand (left):** Hold the patient's distal forearm from the radial side; grip around the distal radius with your thenar eminence close to the joint space; position your forearm in line with the treatment plane.

Procedure

- Apply a Grade III posterior glide movement to the radius by pressing your left hand in a posterior direction.

■ Figure 18c: Supination progression

- Apply a Grade III posterior glide movement to the radius with the forearm positioned near its end range-of-motion into supination.

Proximal radio-ulnar joint anterior glide
for restricted supination

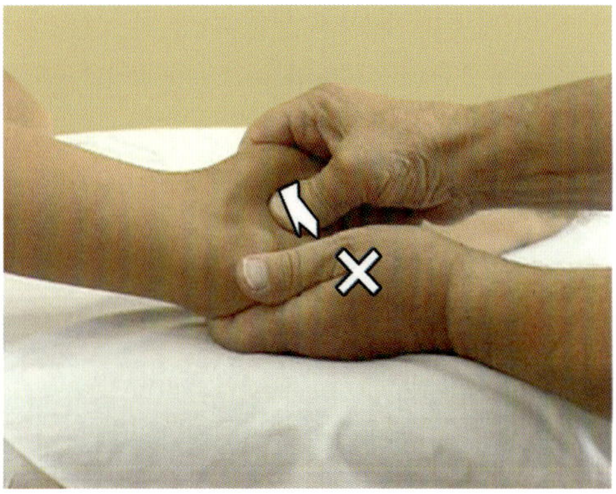

Figure 19a – test and mobilization in resting position

■ Figure 19a: Test and mobilization in resting position

Objective

- To evaluate the quantity and quality of anterior glide joint play in the proximal radio-ulnar joint, including end-feel.
- To increase forearm supination (Convex Rule).

Starting position

- The ulnar side of the patient's forearm rests on the treatment surface, the elbow flexed, shoulder in abduction.
- Position the joint in its resting position.

Hand placement and fixation

- **Therapist's stable hand (left):** Hold the patient's proximal forearm from the ulnar side; grip around the patient's proximal ulna.
- **Therapist's moving hand (right):** Hold the patient's proximal forearm from the radial side; grip around the patient's proximal radius near the joint space.

Procedure

- Apply a Grade II or III anterior glide movement to the radius.

Proximal radio-ulnar joint anterior glide
for restricted supination (cont'd)

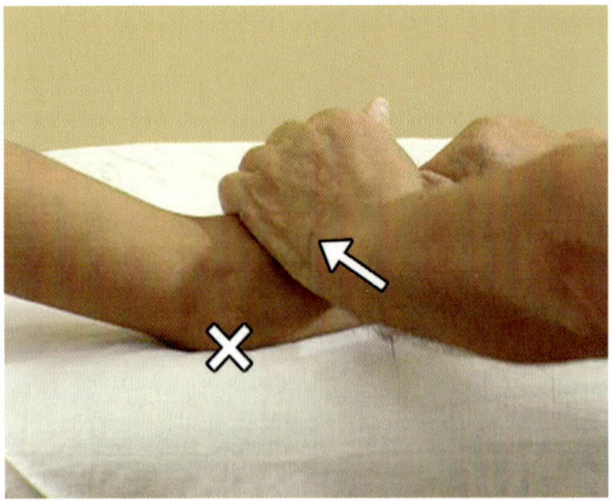

Figure 19b – mobilization in resting position

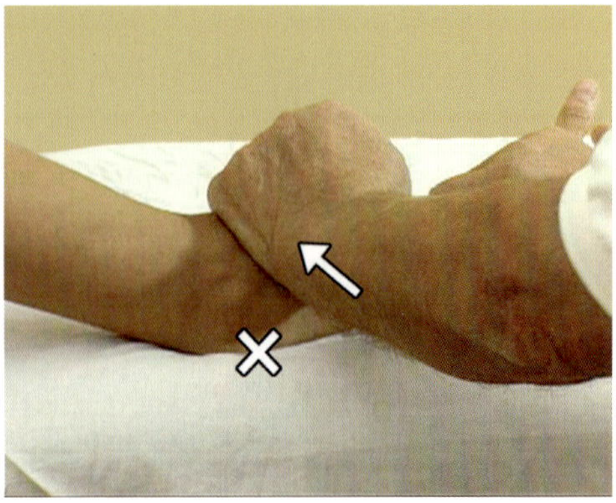

Figure 19c – mobilization in supination

■ Figure 19b: Mobilization in resting position

Objective

- To increase forearm supination (Convex Rule).

Starting position

- The ulnar side of the patient's forearm rests on the treatment surface, the elbow flexed, shoulder in abduction.
- Position the joint in its resting position.

Hand placement and fixation

- **Therapist's stable hand (right):** Hold the patient's forearm from the ulnar or radial side; fixate the patient's forearm against the treatment surface.
- **Therapist's moving hand (left):** Hold the patient's proximal radius with your hand and fingers, with your hypothenar eminence near the joint space; position your forearm in line with the treatment plane.

Procedure

- Apply a Grade III anterior glide movement to the proximal radius. To keep your movement in the treatment plane, you must keep your forearm close to the treatment surface. If you lift your forearm and press downward you will compress the proximal radio-ulnar joint.

■ Figure 19c: Supination progression

- Position the forearm near the end range-of-motion into supination.

Proximal radio-ulnar joint posterior glide

for restricted pronation

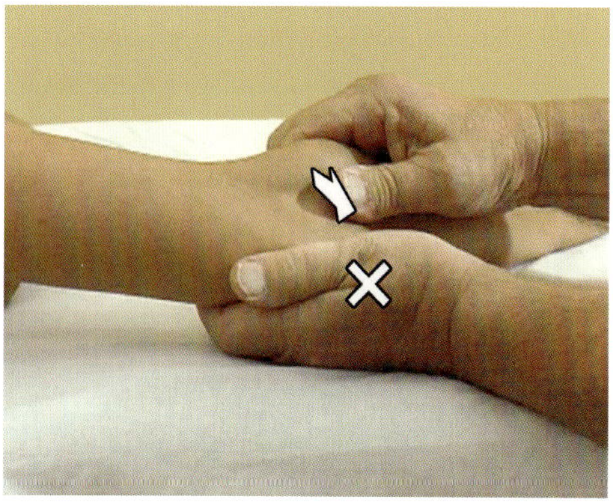

Figure 19d – test and mobilization in resting position

■ Figure 19d: Test and mobilization in resting position

Objective

- To evaluate the quantity and quality of posterior glide joint play in the proximal radio-ulnar joint, including end-feel.
- To increase forearm pronation (Convex Rule).

Starting position

- The ulnar side of the patient's forearm rests on the treatment surface, the elbow flexed, shoulder in abduction.
- Position the joint in its resting position.

Hand placement and fixation

- **Therapist's stable hand (left):** Hold the patient's proximal forearm from the ulnar side; grip around the patient's proximal ulna.
- **Therapist's moving hand (right):** Hold the patient's proximal forearm from the radial side; grip around the patient's proximal radius near the joint space.

Procedure

- Apply a Grade II or III posterior glide movement to the radius.

Proximal radio-ulnar joint posterior glide
for restricted pronation (cont'd)

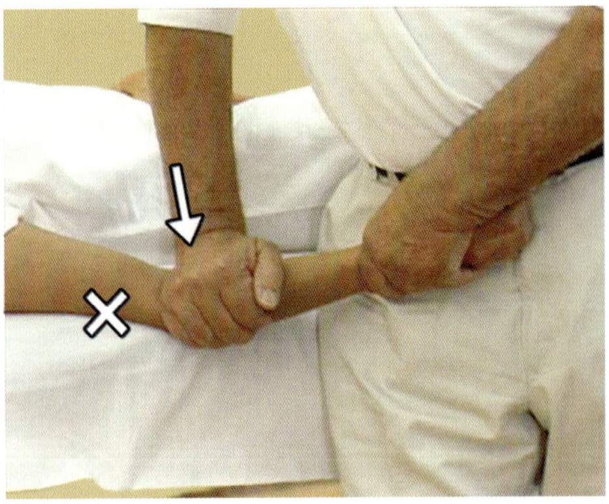

Figure 19e – mobilization in resting position

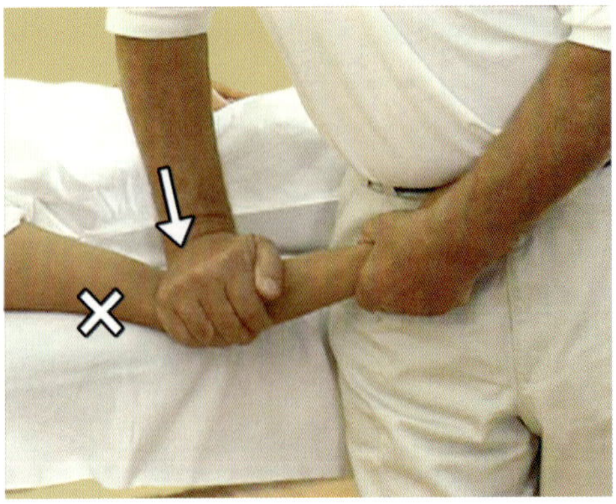

Figure 19f – mobilization in pronation

■ Figure 19e: Mobilization in resting position

Objective

- To increase forearm pronation (Convex Rule).

Starting position

- The posterior side of the patient's arm and proximal ulna rests on the treatment surface, the forearm extends over the edge.
- Position the joint in its resting position.

Hand placement and fixation

- **Fixation:** The ulna is fixated against the treatment surface.
- **Therapist's moving hands:** Hold the patient's radius with both hands; grip with your right hypothenar eminence near the joint space; position your right forearm in line with the treatment plane.

Procedure

- Apply a Grade III posterior glide movement to the proximal radius by bending your knees and leaning your body through your extended arm.

■ Figure 19f: Pronation progression

- Position the forearm near the end range-of-motion into pronation.

Forearm

Humeroradial joint
test

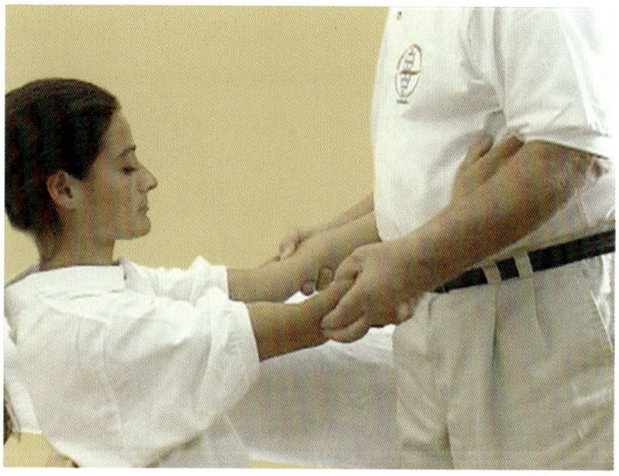

Figure 20 – test bilateral

■ Figure 20: Test bilateral

Objective

- **Position test** for the radial head in relation to the capitulum of the humerus.
- **Mobility test** for the humeroradial joint.

Starting position

- The patient extends both arms forward.

Hand placement and fixation

- **Fixation**: Hold the patient's forearms against your body with your forearms; the patient remains relaxed, so that the soft tissues crossing the joint do not interfere with the test.
- **Therapist's moving hands**: Grip the patient's proximal forearms from the radial side with your palpating index fingers in the humeroradial joint space.

Procedure

- **Position test**: Palpate the distance between the radial head and capitulum of the humerus; palpate from all sides: posterior, lateral, and ventral.
- **Mobility test**: Flex and extend, abduct and adduct the patient's elbows while you palpate the joint space.

Humeroradial joint posterior glide
for restricted extension

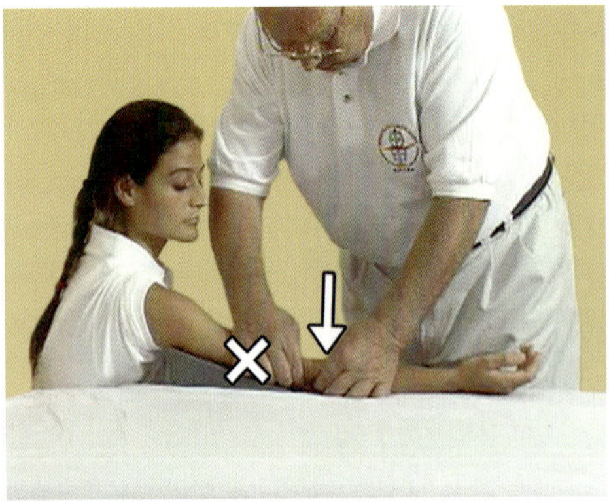

Figure 21a – test
in resting position

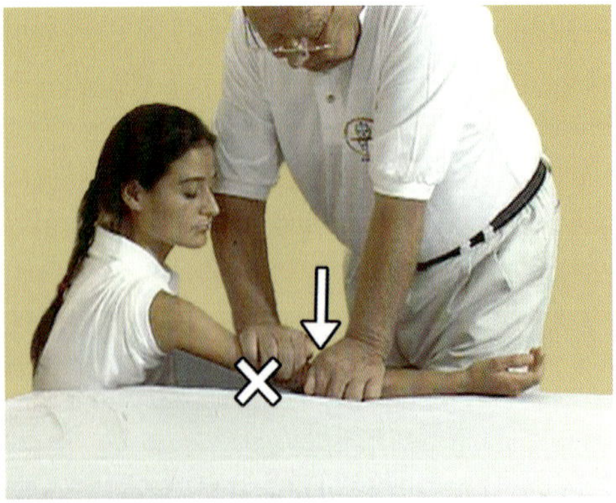

Figure 21b – mobilization
in momentary resting position

■ Figure 21a: Test in resting position

Objective

- To evaluate the quantity and quality of posterior glide movement in the humeroradial joint, including end-feel. Restricted radius-humerus posterior glide affects elbow extension (Concave Rule).

Starting position

- The posterior side of the patient's arm and forearm rests on the treatment surface, the elbow extended as far as possible.

Hand placement and fixation

- **Therapist's stable hand (right):** Hold the distal arm; fixate the distal humerus against the treatment surface.
- **Therapist's moving hand (left):** Hold the patient's proximal radius; grip around the radial head with your thumb and fingers.

Procedure

- Apply a Grade II or III posterior glide movement to the proximal radius.

■ Figure 21b: Mobilization in momentary resting position

- Apply a Grade III posterior glide movement to the radius to increase elbow extension. Position the elbow near the end range-of-motion into elbow extension. Since the resting position of the humeroradial joint is in full extension, with restricted elbow extension the patient will not be able to achieve the resting position.

■ Anterior glide mobilization (not shown)

- Apply a Grade III anterior glide movement to the proximal radius to increase elbow flexion.

Humeroradial joint distal traction
for elbow and forearm hypomobility

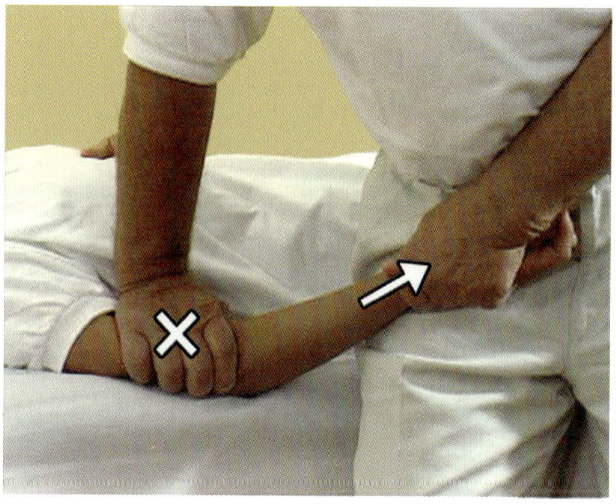

Figure 22 – mobilization in resting position

■ Figure 22: Mobilization in resting position

Objective

- To increase forearm pronation and supination as well as elbow flexion and extension; distal traction movement of the radius in relation to the humerus; stretch the syndesmosis between the ulna and radius.
- To correct a proximal positional fault of the radius in relation to the humerus by moving the radius distally. See figure 20 for position testing technique.

Starting position

- The posterior side of the patient's arm and proximal ulna rests on the treatment surface with the elbow flexed.
- Position the joint in its resting position.

Hand placement and fixation

- **Therapist's stable hand (right):** Grip the patient's distal arm from the anterior side and fixate it against the treatment surface. You may place your palpating finger in the humeroradial joint space.
- **Therapist's moving hand (left):** Hold the patient's distal forearm from the radial side; grip around the patient's distal radius.

Procedure

- Apply a Grade I, II, or III distal traction movement to the radius in relation to the humerus. Facilitate Grade III stretch-mobilization by pulling and turning your body slightly to the left.
- Suitable for early training in manipulative thrust techniques.

■ Mobilization progression (not shown)

- Position the elbow near the end range-of-motion into flexion or extension, pronation or supination.

Humeroradial joint approximation
for elbow and forearm hypomobility

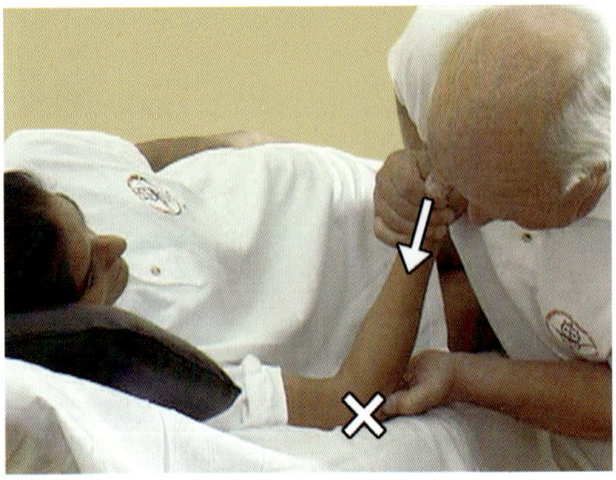

Figure 23 – mobilization in resting position

■ Figure 23: Mobilization in resting position

Objective

- To increase forearm pronation and supination, as well as elbow flexion and extension.
- To correct a distal positional fault of the radius in relation to the humerus by moving the radius proximally. See *Figure 20* for position testing technique.

Starting position

- The posterior side of the patient's arm and proximal ulna rests on the treatment surface with the elbow flexed.
- Position the joint in its resting position.

Hand placement and fixation

- **Therapist's stable hand (left):** Grip the patient's arm and fixate it against the treatment surface; place your palpating finger in the humeroradial joint space.
- **Therapist's moving hand (right):** Hold the patient's distal forearm from the radial side; grip around the patient's distal radius and thumb so that your thenar eminence is in contact with theirs; rest the patient's hand against your shoulder.

Procedure

- Apply a Grade III proximal movement to the radius in relation to the humerus by pushing along the long axis of the radius. Use your shoulder to apply additional force.

■ To correct a radius subluxation in children (not shown)

- Adapt the technique to correct a radius subluxation in children. Grip the child's wrist and forearm with a "handshake" or "thenar to thenar" grip; move the radius proximally while supinating or pronating the forearm.

CHAPTER 12

ELBOW

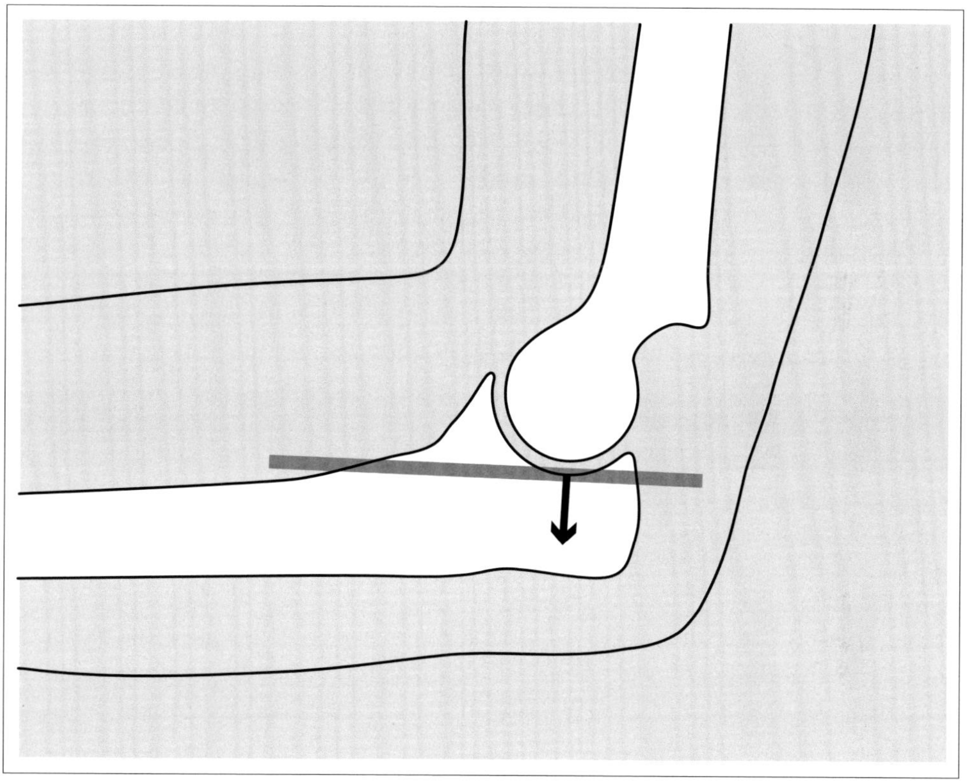

Elbow

12 Elbow

Functional anatomy and movement

The elbow joint (art. cubiti) is an anatomically simple and mechanically compound joint and is divided into three joints:

Humero-ulnar joint
(art. humero-ulnaris)

The humero-ulnar joint is a biaxial saddle joint. The proximal thickened, wrench-shaped, concave trochlear notch of the ulna moves on the trochlea of the humerus.

Humeroradial joint
(art. humeroradialis)

The humeroradial joint belongs anatomically to the elbow, but functionally to the forearm and is described there (See *Chapter 11: Forearm*).

Proximal radio-ulnar joint
(art. radio-ulnaris proximalis)

The proximal radio-ulnar joint belongs anatomically to the elbow, but functionally to the forearm and is described there (See *Chapter 11: Forearm*).

Bony palpation

- Humerus, including the lateral supracondylar crest and lateral epicondyle
- Capitulum of the humerus
- Medial epicondyle
- Olecranon fossa
- Olecranon
- Humero-ulnar joint space
- Ulnar tuberosity
- Ulnar coronoid process

Ligaments

- Ulnar collateral ligament
- Radial collateral ligament

Bone movement and axes

- Flexion - extension: The transverse axis for flexion and extension passes through the trochlea and lies slightly oblique to the longitudinal axis of the upper arm. Therefore, in full extension the lower arm deviates laterally forming the valgus, or carrying angle, at the elbow which varies from 7° to 20°. Hyperextension of 5° to 15° is normal in children and many women because their olecranon process is smaller.
- Abduction - adduction: The humero-ulnar joint is a saddle joint. Therefore, with the elbow in flexion, slight abduction and adduction of the ulna is possible around a dorsal-ventral axis, which passes through the proximal part of the ulna. Abduction and adduction can only be performed passively.

End feel

- Flexion: hard end-feel. Flexion is limited by bone against bone, when the coronoid process of the ulna contacts the coronoid fossa of the humerus. (Active flexion is stopped by approximation of soft tissues on the ventral side of the upper arm and forearm.)
- Extension: hard end-feel. Extension stops when the olecranon contacts the olecranon fossa of the humerus.

Joint movement (gliding)

- Ulna-humerus: Concave Rule
- Radius-humerus: Concave Rule

Treatment plane

- On the concave surface of the ulna
- On the concave surface of the radius

Zero position

- Both the upper arm and forearm lie in the frontal plane with the forearm supinated and the elbow extended

Resting position

- Humero-ulnar joint: elbow joint flexed approximately 70° and the forearm supinated approximately 10°
- Humeroradial joint: the elbow extended and the forearm fully supinated

Close-packed position

- Humero-ulnar joint: the elbow extended and the forearm supinated
- Humeroradial joint: the elbow flexed approximately 90° and the forearm supinated approximately 5°

Capsular pattern

- Flexion - extension. The proportion of these limitations is such that with flexion limited to 90° there is only 10° of limited extension.

■ Elbow examination scheme

(Refer to Chapters 3 and 4 for more information on examination)

Tests of function

1. **Active and passive movements, including stability tests and end-feel**

Flexion	150°
Extension	0° - 15° from zero

2. **Translatoric joint play movements, including end-feel**

Traction - compression	(Figure 24a)
Gliding	
Radial	(Figure 26)
Ulnar	(Figure 27)

3. **Resisted movements**

	OTHER FUNCTIONS
Flexion	
Biceps brachii	Supination
Brachialis	
Brachioradialis	(see Forearm examination scheme)
Extension	
Triceps brachii, long head	Shoulder adduction, extension
Anconeus	

4. **Passive soft tissue movements**
   Physiological
   Accessory

5. **Additional tests**

Trial treatment

Traction	(Figure 24b)

Elbow

■ Elbow techniques

Figure 24a,b	Traction for pain and hypomobility
Figure 25a,b	Traction for restricted flexion and extension
Figure 26	Radial glide for restricted flexion and extension
Figure 27	Ulnar glide for restricted flexion and extension

Elbow

Elbow traction
for pain and hypomobility

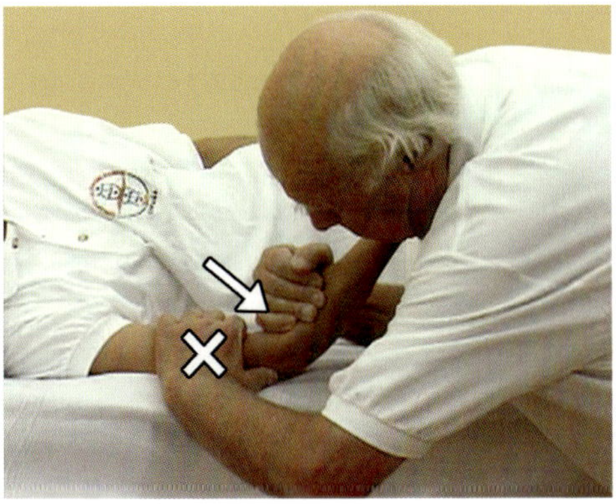
Figure 24a – test and mobilization in resting position

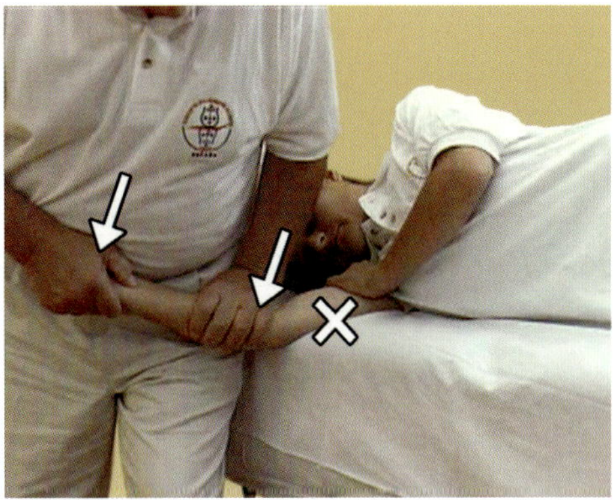
Figure 24b – mobilization in resting position

■ Figure 24a: Test and mobilization in resting position

Objective

- To evaluate the quantity and quality of traction joint play in the humero-ulnar joint, including end-feel.
- To decrease pain or increase range-of-motion in the humero-ulnar joint.

Starting position

- The dorsal side of the patient's humerus rests on the treatment surface.
- Position the joint in its resting position.

Hand placement and fixation

- **Therapist's stable hand (left):** Grip the patient's distal arm from the anterior side and fixate it against the treatment surface; place your palpating finger in the humero-ulna joint space.
- **Therapist's moving hand (right):** Hold the patient's proximal forearm from the ulnar side; grip around the patient's proximal ulna.

Procedure

- Apply a Grade I, II or III traction movement to the ulna. The movement should be approximately at a right angle to the forearm.
- Suitable for early training in manipulative thrust techniques.

■ Figure 24b: Mobilization in resting position

- Enhance the fixation of the humerus by positioning the patient in side-lying on their shoulder and/or by using a strap or wedge.
- Grip the patient's forearm from the anterior side with both of your hands and your hypothenar eminence just distal to the joint space. Hold the patient's forearm against your body. Apply a Grade III traction movement by bending your knees and leaning through your left arm.
- Suitable for early training in manipulative thrust techniques.

Elbow traction
for restricted flexion and extension

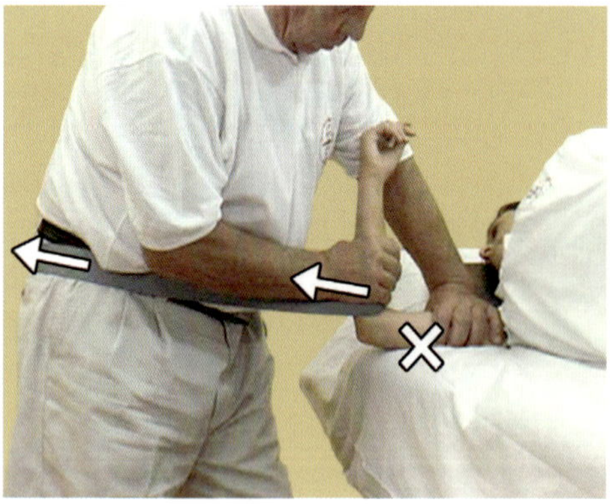

Figure 25a – mobilization in flexion

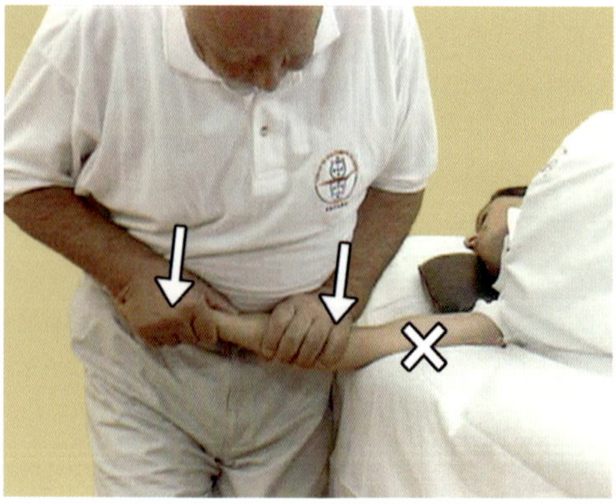

Figure 25b – mobilization in extension

■ Figure 25a: Flexion progression

Objective

- To increase flexion range-of-motion in the humero-ulnar joint.

Starting position

- The posterior side of the patient's humerus rests on the treatment surface; use a strap and position the patient side-lying to improve humerus fixation.
- Position the joint near to its end range-of-motion in flexion.

Hand placement and fixation

- **Therapist's stable hand (left)**: Fixate the patient's humerus against the treatment surface.
- **Therapist's moving hand (right):** Place a strap around the proximal forearm just distal to the joint space and around your body; hold the patient's distal forearm in your hand.

Procedure

- Apply a Grade III posterior/distal traction movement to the ulna at approximately a right angle to the forearm, by shifting your body backwards; move your body and your left hand as one.

■ Figure 25b: Extension progression

- The dorsal side of the patient's humerus rests on the treatment surface.
- Enhance the fixation of the humerus by positioning the patient in side-lying on their shoulder and/or by using a strap or wedge.
- Grip the patient's forearm from the ulnar side with both of your hands and your hypothenar eminence just distal to the joint space; hold the patient's forearm against your body; apply a Grade III posterior traction movement by bending your knees and leaning through your left arm.
- Position the joint near to its end range-of-motion in extension.

Elbow radial glide

for restricted flexion and extension

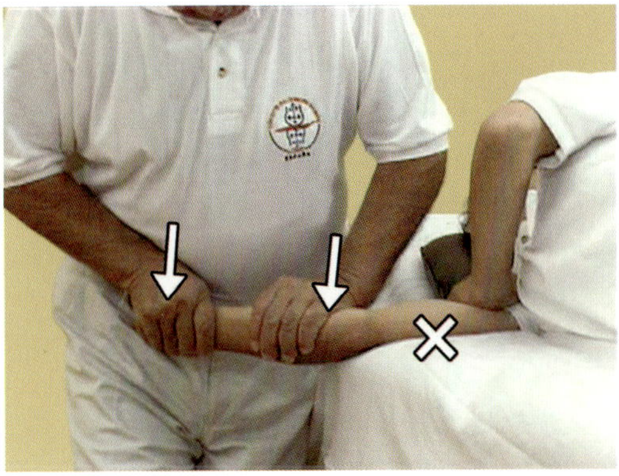

Figure 26 – test and mobilization in resting position

■ Figure 26: Test and mobilization in resting position

Objective

- To evaluate the quantity and quality of radial glide movement in the humero-ulnar joint, including end-feel.
- To increase elbow flexion and extension.

Starting position

- The lateral side of the patient's humerus rests on the treatment surface or wedge.
- Position the joint in its resting position.

Hand placement and fixation

- **Fixation:** The humerus is fixated against the treatment surface.
- **Therapist's moving hands:** Grip the patient's forearm from the ulnar side with both of your hands and your hypothenar eminence just distal to the joint space; hold the patient's forearm against your body.

Procedure

- Apply a Grade II or III radial glide movement to the ulna by bending your knees and leaning through your left arm.

■ Flexion and extension progression (not shown)

- Apply a Grade III radial glide movement to the ulna with the joint positioned near to its end range-of-motion in flexion or extension.

Elbow ulnar glide

for restricted flexion and extension

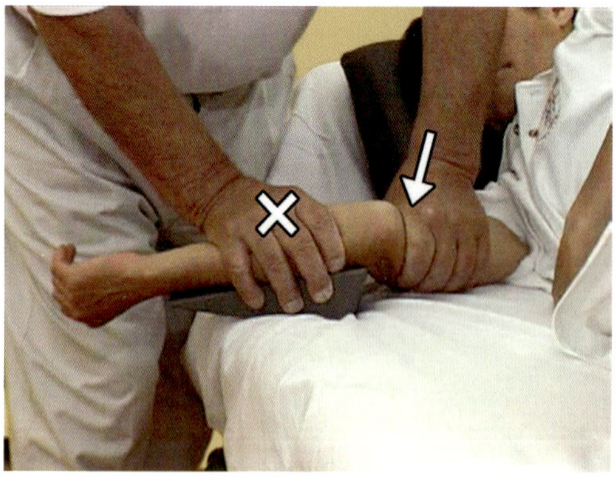

Figure 27 – test and mobilization in resting position

■ Figure 27: Test and mobilization in resting position

Objective

- To evaluate the quantity and quality of ulnar glide joint play in the humero-ulnar joint, including end-feel.
- To increase elbow flexion and extension.

Starting position

- The lateral side of the patient's proximal forearm and humerus contacts the treatment surface; place a wedge under the proximal forearm just distal to the joint space.
- Position the joint in its resting position.

Hand placement and fixation

- **Fixation:** Fixate the proximal forearm against the wedge or sandbag.
- **Therapist's stable hand (right)**: Hold the patient's distal forearm to support the position.
- **Therapist's moving hand (left):** Grip around the patient's distal humerus from the medial side just proximal to the joint space.

Procedure

- Apply a Grade II or III radial movement to the distal humerus, to produce a relative ulnar glide.

■ Flexion and extension progression

- Apply a Grade III radial glide movement to the humerus with the joint positioned close to its end range-of-motion in flexion or extension.

CHAPTER 13

SHOULDER

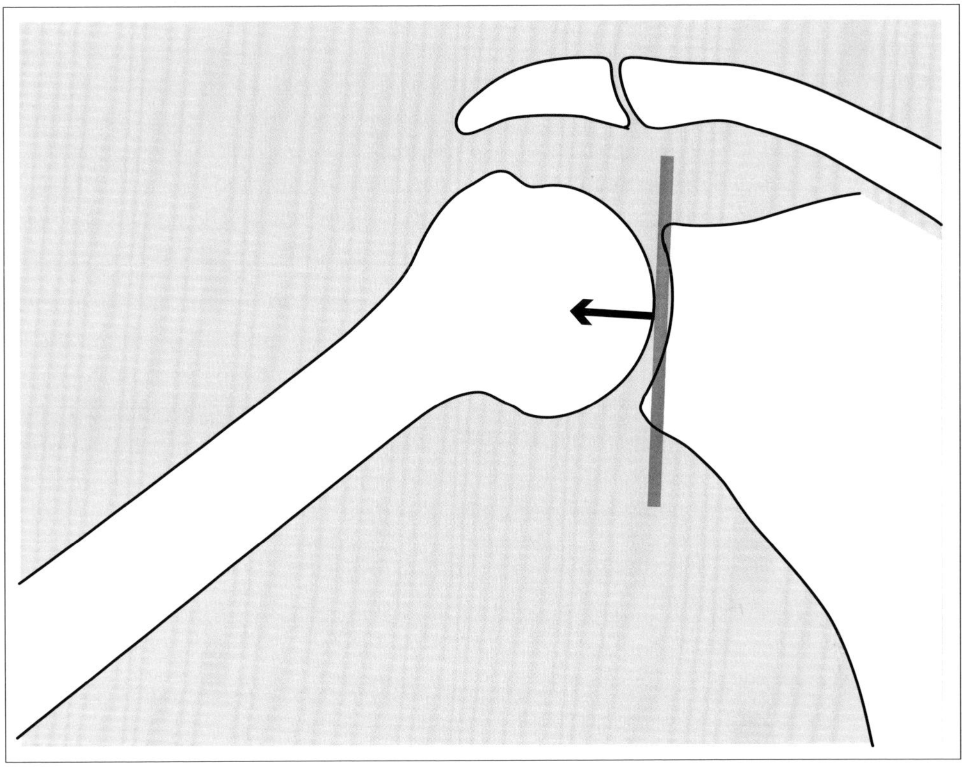

13 Shoulder

Functional anatomy and movement

Glenohumeral joint

(art. humeri)

The glenohumeral joint is an anatomically and mechanically simple triaxial joint (spheroid, unmodified ovoid). The convex surface of the head of the humerus articulates with the concave socket on the scapula.

The joint capsule of the glenohumeral joint is lax. When the arm hangs down in a dependent position, the medial side of the capsule folds loosely (recessus axillaris). This allows the shoulder joint a large range of movement. When the glenohumeral joint is immobilized for a long period of time, adhesions can form in these folds, and must be stretched for the shoulder to regain full mobility.

"Scapulohumeral rhythm" is described in *Chapter 14: Shoulder Girdle*.

Bony palpation

- Humeral head
- Bicipital groove
- Lesser tubercle
- Greater tubercle
- Deltoid tubercle
- Acromion (ventral, dorsal)
- Subacromial space
- Coracoid process
- Spine of scapula
- Infraspinous fossa
- Supraspinous fossa
- 1st rib
- Scapula, inferior angle, medial margin
- Scapula, superior angle, lateral margin

Ligaments

- Glenohumeral (superior, middle and inferior parts)
- Coracohumeral

Bone movement and axes

- Flexion - extension: around a transverse (medial-lateral) axis through the head of the humerus
- Abduction - adduction: around a sagittal (dorsal-ventral) axis through the head of the humerus
- Internal - external rotation: around a longitudinal axis through the length of the humerus

End feel

- Firm

Joint movement (gliding)

- Convex Rule

Treatment plane

- On the concave joint surface of the glenoid fossa of the scapula

Zero position

- The upper arm lies parallel to the trunk with the elbow extended and the thumb pointing ventrally.

Resting position

- Approximately 55° shoulder abduction, 30° horizontal adduction (i.e., the humerus lies in a vertical plane passing through the spine of scapula) and slight external rotation

Close-packed position

- Maximal abduction and external rotation

Capsular pattern

- External rotation - abduction - internal rotation

■ Shoulder examination scheme

(Refer to Chapters 3 and 4 for more information on examination)

Tests of function

1. Active and passive movements, including stability tests and end-feel

With scapula fixated:

Movement in the sagittal plane around a transverse axis

Flexion	65°
Extension	35°

Movement in the frontal plane around a dorsal-ventral axis

Abduction	90°, 120° with lateral rotation
Adduction	8°

Movement in the transverse plane around a longitudinal axis

Horizontal adduction	30°
Medial rotation	90°
Lateral rotation	60°

2. Translatoric joint play movements, including end-feel

Traction - compression	(Figure 28a)
Gliding	
Caudal	(Figure 30a)
Ventral	(Figure 33)
Dorsal	(Figure 35)

3. Resisted movements	OTHER FUNCTIONS
Flexion	
Coracobrachialis	Adduction
Deltoid	Abduction
Pectoralis major	Adduction, horizontal adduction
Biceps brachii	Adduction, elbow flexion
Extension	
Latissimus dorsi	Adduction, internal rotation, shoulder girdle depression (caudal)
Teres major	Adduction, internal rotation
Deltoid	Abduction, horizontal adduction
Triceps brachii	Adduction, elbow extension

Shoulder

Abduction	
Deltoid	Flexion, extension, abduction, horizontal adduction
Supraspinatus	
Adduction	
Teres minor	Extension, lateral rotation
Latissimus dorsi	Extension, medial rotation, shoulder girdle depression (caudal)
Teres major	Extension, medial rotation
Pectoralis major	Internal rotation, horizontal adduction
Lateral rotation	
Teres minor	Adduction
Infraspinatus	
Supraspinatus	Abduction
Medial rotation	
Subscapularis	
Pectoralis major	Horizontal adduction
Latissimus dorsi	Adduction, shoulder girdle depression (caudal)
Teres major Adduction	
Elbow Flexion	
Biceps brachii long head	Can cause pain with humeral rotation
Elbow Extension	
Triceps brachii	May cause pain with shoulder adduction and extension

4. **Passive soft tissue movements**
   Physiological
   Accessory
5. **Additional tests**

Trial treatment

Traction	(Figure 28b)

Shoulder techniques

Figure 28a,b	Traction for pain and hypomobility
Figure 29a,b	Traction for restricted flexion and extension
Figure 30a,b, 31, 32	Caudal glide for restricted abduction
Figure 33	Ventral glide for restricted extension
Figure 34a,b	Ventral glide for restricted extension-external rotation
Figure 35, 36	Dorsal glide for restricted flexion-internal rotation

Shoulder traction
for pain and hypomobility

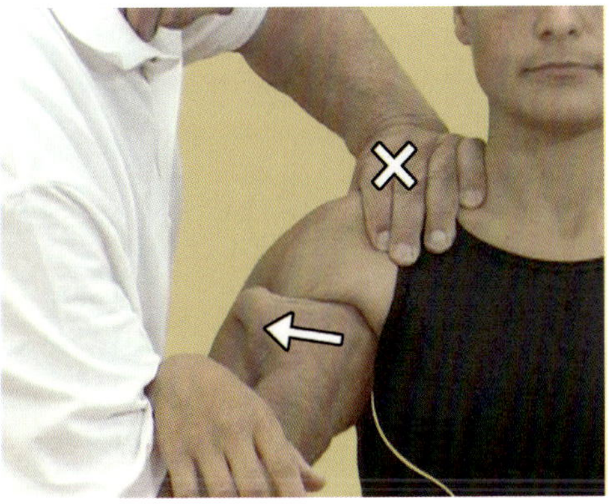

Figure 28a – test and mobilization in resting position

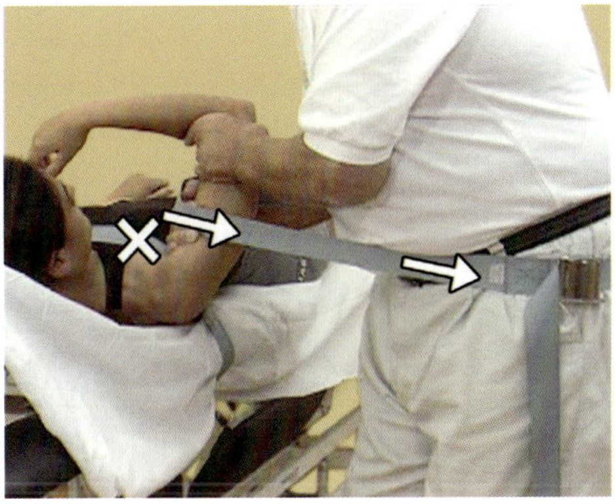

Figure 28b – mobilization in resting position

■ Figure 28a: Test and mobilization in resting position

Objective

- To evaluate the quantity and quality of traction joint play in the glenohumeral joint, including end-feel.
- To decrease pain or increase range-of-motion in the glenohumeral joint.

Starting position

- The patient sits with their forearm resting on your right forearm.

Hand placement and fixation

- **Therapist's stable hand (left):** Grip the patient's shoulder from the posterior-superior side; place your palpating finger (left thumb shown) in the glenohumeral joint space.
- **Therapist's moving hand (right):** Grip the patient's proximal humerus from the medial side.

Procedure

- Apply a Grade I, II, or III traction movement to the glenohumeral joint with a lateral movement of the humerus.
- Suitable for early training in manipulative thrust techniques.

■ Figure 28b: Mobilization in resting position

- The patient lies supine with the shoulder in the resting position and the elbow at approximately 90° of flexion.
- Fixate the patient's thorax and scapula to the treatment surface with a strap.
- Place a strap around the proximal humerus just distal to the joint space and around your body. Grip the humerus with both hands and support it in its resting position.
- Apply a Grade III stretch mobilization by shifting your body weight backward.
- For a manipulative thrust, shift your body weight backward to take up the slack and apply the thrust with your arms.

Shoulder traction
for restricted flexion and extension

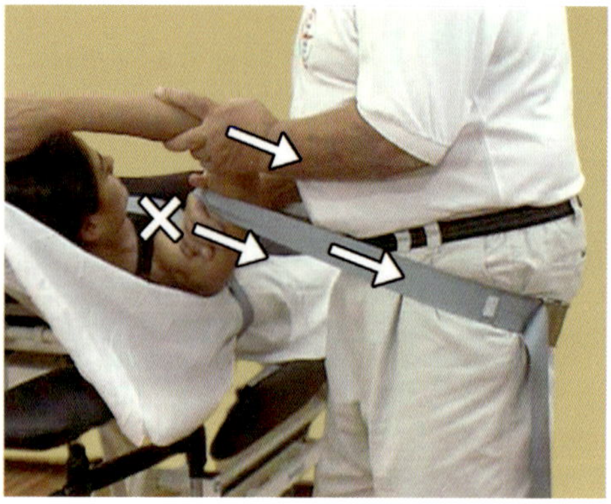

Figure 29a – mobilization in flexion

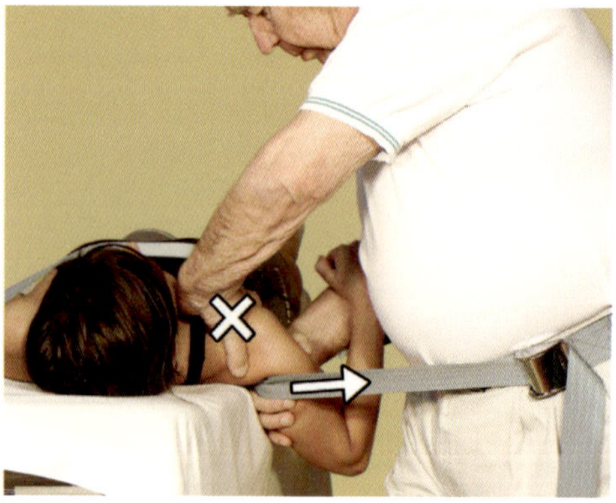

Figure 29b – mobilization in extension

■ Figure 29a: Flexion progression

Objective

- To increase flexion range-of-motion in the glenohumeral joint.

Starting position

- The patient lies supine with the shoulder near its end range-of-motion into flexion and the elbow at approximately 90° flexion.

Hand placement and fixation

- **Fixation**: Fixate the patient's thorax and scapula to the treatment surface with a strap; you may enhance the fixation by pressing your right hand against the lateral border of the scapula.
- **Therapist's moving hands:** Place a strap around the proximal humerus just distal to the joint space and around your body; place your right hand underneath the strap; support the patient's shoulder position by holding the arm with your left hand.

Procedure

- Apply a Grade III traction movement by leaning backward; move your body and your hands together as one.

■ Figure 29b: Extension progression

- Apply a Grade III traction movement with the patient's shoulder positioned near its end range-of-motion in extension.

Shoulder caudal glide
for restricted abduction

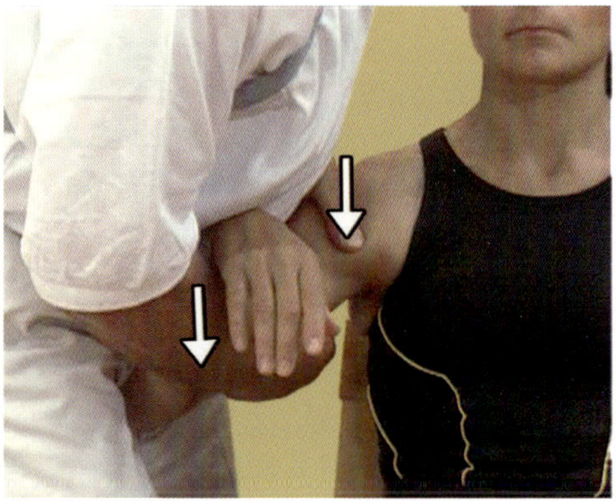

Figure 30a – test and mobilization in resting position

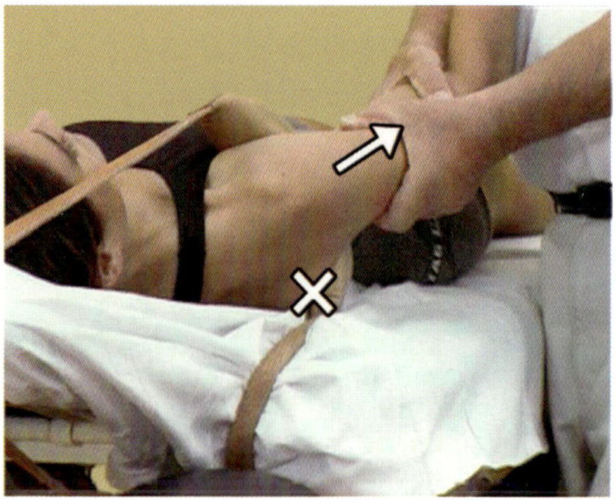

Figure 30b – mobilization in resting position

■ Figure 30a: Test and mobilization in resting position

Objective

- To evaluate the quantity and quality of caudal glide joint play in the glenohumeral joint, including end-feel.
- To increase shoulder abduction range-of-motion with increased humerus caudal glide joint play (Convex Rule).

Starting position

- The patient sits with their forearm resting on your left arm.
- The shoulder is positioned in its resting position.

Hand placement and fixation

- **Fixation:** No external fixation is required.
- **Therapist's moving hands:** Place your left hand on the head of the humerus just distal to the joint space; with your right hand, support the position of the patient's arm.

Procedure

- Apply a Grade II or III caudal glide movement to the glenohumeral joint by pressing down on the head of the humerus with your right hand; your right and left hand move together as one by bending your knees.

■ Figure 30b: Mobilization in resting position

- The patient lies supine with the shoulder in the resting position.
- Fixate the patient's scapula from the axilla with a pommel or stirrup attached to the treatment surface; if necessary, use an additional fixating strap around the patient's chest.
- Grip the humerus with both your hands and support the forearm against your body; apply a Grade III traction movement by shifting your body backward.

■ Alternate technique: See Figure 31

Shoulder caudal glide
for restricted abduction (cont'd)

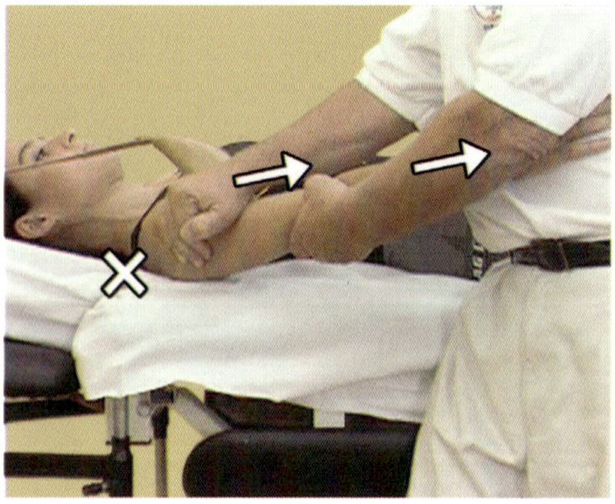

Figure 31 – mobilization in resting position

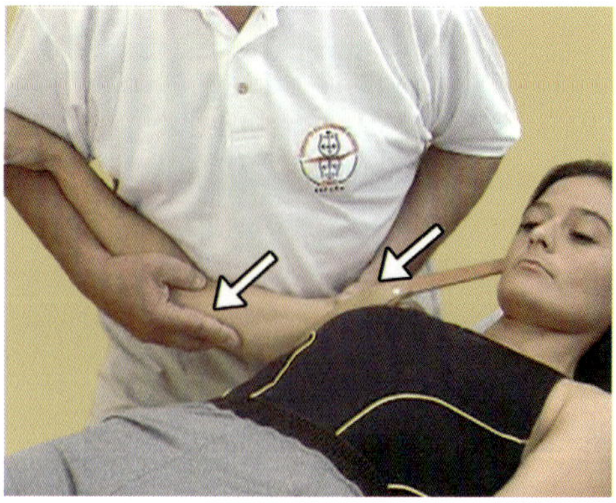

Figure 32 – mobilization in abduction

■ Figure 31: Mobilization in resting position

Objective

- To increase shoulder abduction by increasing humerus caudal glide joint play (Convex Rule).

Starting position

- The patient lies supine.
- Position the joint in its resting position.

Hand placement and fixation

- **Fixation:** Fixate the patient's scapula, from the axilla, with a stirrup or pommel; if necessary, use an additional fixating strap around the patient's chest.
- **Therapist's moving hands:** Place your right hand on the head of the humerus just distal to the joint space; with your left hand and body, support the position of the patient's arm.

Procedure

- Apply a Grade III caudal glide movement to the glenohumeral joint by shifting your body backward while you press the head of the humerus in a caudal direction with your right hand; your hands and body move together as one.

■ Figure 32: Abduction progression

- The shoulder is positioned near the end range-of-motion into abduction.
- Adapt the same technique, but grip from the cranial side of the humerus; apply a Grade III caudal glide movement by shifting your body forward (Convex Rule).

Shoulder ventral glide
for restricted extension

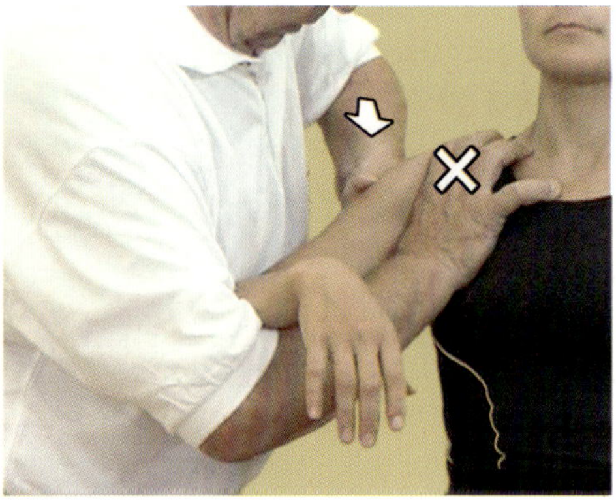

Figure 33 – test and mobilization in resting position

■ Figure 33: Test and mobilization in resting position

Objective

- To evaluate the quantity and quality of ventral glide joint play in the glenohumeral joint, including end-feel.
- To increase shoulder extension range-of-motion with increased humerus ventral glide joint play (Convex Rule).

Starting position

- The patient sits with their forearm resting on your right forearm.
- The shoulder is positioned in its resting position.

Hand placement and fixation

- **Therapist's stable hand (right)**: Fixate the patient's scapula from the ventral side, with firm pressure in the area of the acromion and coracoid process.
- **Therapist's moving hand (left):** Grip around the patient's arm from the dorsal side just distal to the joint space.

Procedure

- Apply a Grade II or III ventral glide movement to the humerus.

Shoulder ventral glide

for restricted extension-external rotation

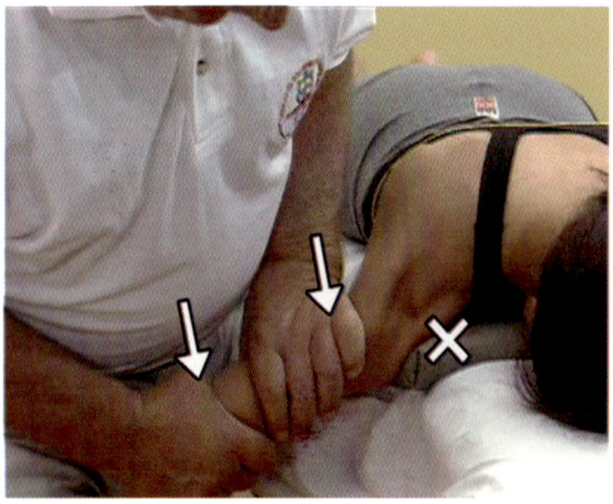

Figure 34a – mobilization in resting position

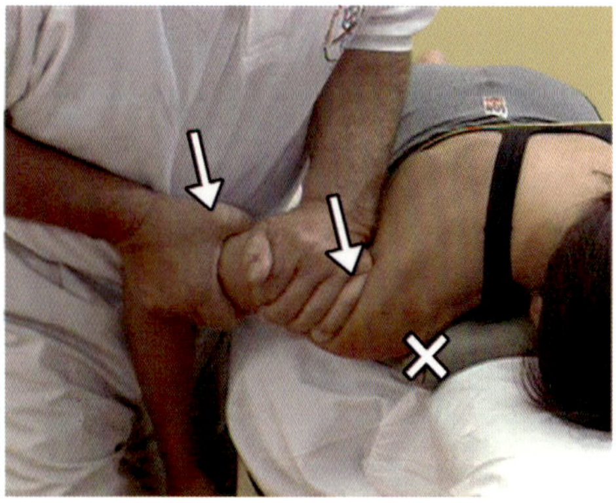

Figure 34b – mobilization in extension

■ Figure 34a: Mobilization in resting position

Objective

- To increase shoulder extension and external rotation with increased humerus ventral glide joint play (Convex Rule).

Starting position

- The patient lies prone with a wedge or sandbag under the coracoid process and the arm beyond the edge of the treatment surface.
- Position the joint in its resting position.

Hand placement and fixation

- **Fixation:** The scapula is fixated by the wedge or sandbag.
- **Therapist's moving hands:** Hold the patient's humerus against your body with both hands; grip with your left hypothenar eminence near the humeral head just distal to the joint space.

Procedure

- Apply a Grade III ventral glide movement to the glenohumeral joint by bending your knees and leaning through your extended left arm; move your hands and body together as one.

■ Figure 34b: Extension progression

- Apply a Grade III ventral glide movement to the glenohumeral joint with the shoulder positioned near its end range-of-motion in extension and external rotation.

Shoulder dorsal glide
for restricted flexion-internal rotation

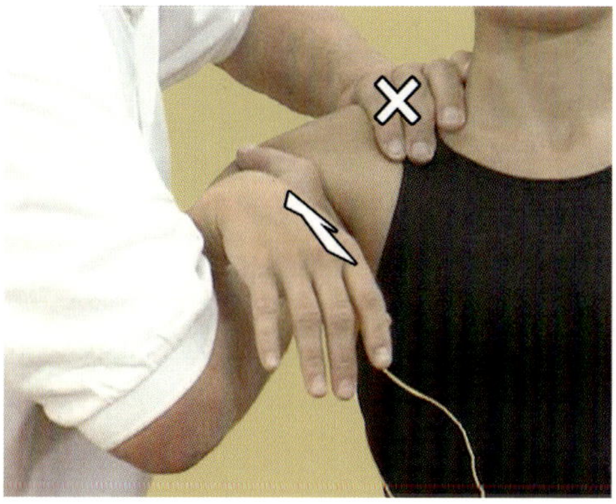
Figure 35 – test and mobilization in resting position

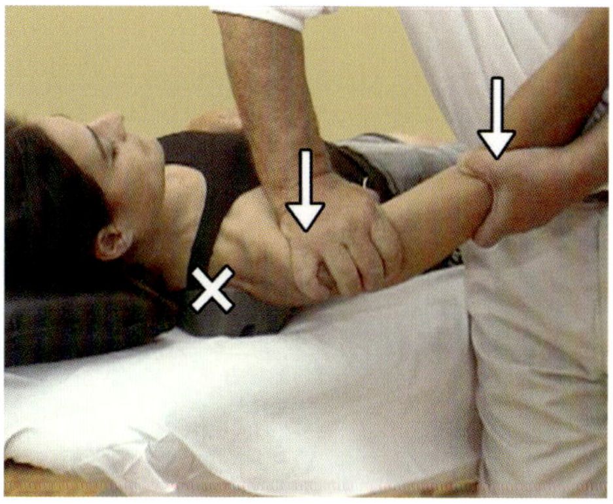
Figure 36 – mobilization in resting position

■ Figure 35: Test and mobilization in resting position

Objective

- To evaluate the quantity and quality of dorsal glide joint play in the glenohumeral joint, including end-feel.
- To increase shoulder flexion and internal rotation with increased humerus dorsal glide joint play (Convex Rule).

Starting position

- The patient sits with their forearm resting on your right forearm.
- The shoulder is positioned in its resting position.

Hand placement and fixation

- **Therapist's stable hand (left)**: Fixate the patient's scapula from the dorsal side with your index finger over the acromion.
- **Therapist's moving hand (right):** Grip around the patient's arm from the medial side just distal to the joint space.

Procedure

- Apply a Grade II or III dorsal glide movement to the humerus.

■ Figure 36: Mobilization in resting position

- The patient lies supine; fixate the patient's scapula with a wedge; hold the patient's humerus against your body with both hands; grip with your right hypothenar eminence near the humeral head just distal to the joint space; apply a Grade III dorsal glide movement to the glenohumeral joint by bending your knees and leaning through your extended right arm; move your hands and body together as one.

Notes

CHAPTER 14

SHOULDER GIRDLE

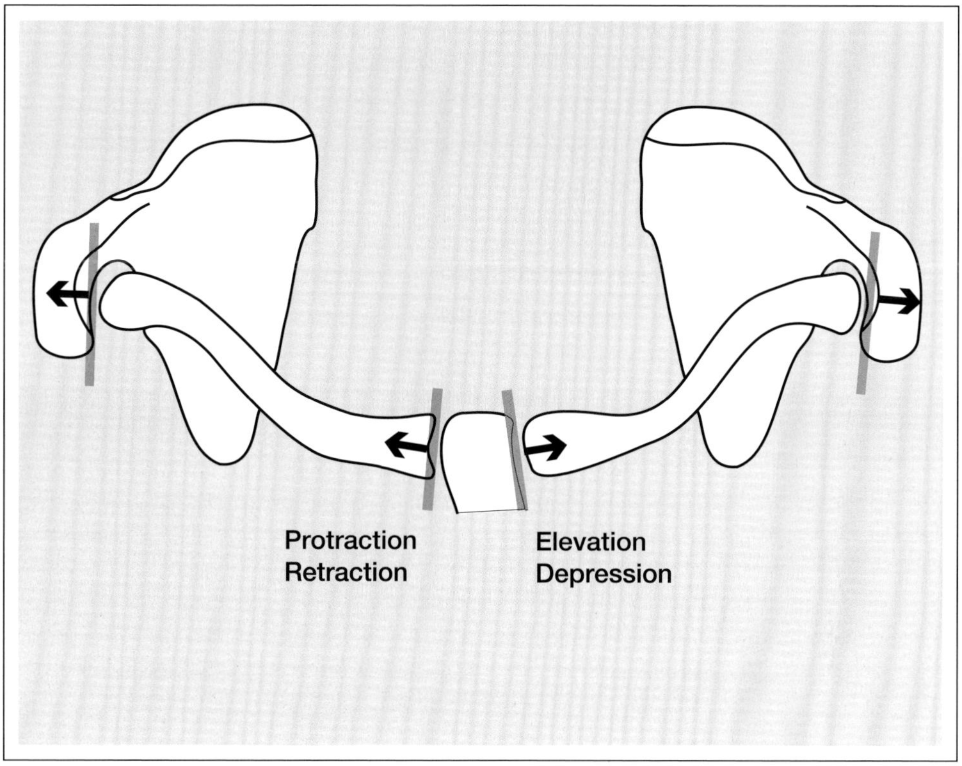

14 Shoulder girdle

(cingulum extremitatis superioris)

Functional anatomy and movement

The shoulder girdle consists of the scapula and clavicle with its connection to the trunk (manubrium sterni) with its joint facets, the clavicular notches (incisura clavicularis sterni).

The scapula is a triangular shaped bone with three borders:

- **The superior border** with the suprascapular notch and its superior transverse scapular ligament
- **The medial border** which is the longest of the three borders
- **The lateral border** which is the thickest border

These borders meet and form three angles: the **superior**, **inferior,** and **lateral angles** with the glenoid fossa located at the lateral angle. The spine of the scapula continues laterally to form the acromion which contains an articular facet for the clavicle cranially and the acromial angle caudally. The coraco-acromial ligament completes the coraco-acromial arch.

The medial or sternal end of the **clavicle** has a facet for articulation with the clavicular notch on the manubrium sterni. The lateral or acromial end has a facet for articulation with the acromion. The clavicle holds the scapula at the required distance from the thorax.

Arm and shoulder girdle movement

The word elevation is used to describe arm movement above the horizontal position. Movement of the entire shoulder girdle (scapula and humerus) enables the arm to elevate, producing flexion or abduction of the upper extremity. The scapula and humerus move together in a coordinated manner to produce what is called the "scapulo-humeral rhythm." Approximately two-thirds of this movement takes place at the glenohumeral joint and the remainder by movement of the scapula. Usually, movement is initiated at the glenohumeral joint and is followed by movement in the other joints. The ratio of humeral to scapular movement is 2:1 and takes place during both abduction and flexion.

At approximately 90° abduction, the greater tubercle of the humerus approaches the coraco-acromial ligament, preventing further movement. The humerus must laterally rotate so the greater tubercle can move dorsally under the coraco-acromial arch - this allows abduction beyond 90°.

Maximal elevation of the arm involves abduction and external rotation of the scapula, elevation and rotation of the clavicle, and flattening of the thoracic kyphosis. Therefore, full elevation of the arm requires that many joints function normally: 1) glenohumeral joint, 2) acromioclavicular joint, 3) sternoclavicular joint, 4) thoracic spine joints, including rib articulations, and 5) the scapulo-thoracic "joint."

The shoulder girdle has two joints: the sternoclavicular joint and the acromioclavicular joint.

■ The sternoclavicular joint

(art. sternoclavicularis, abbreviated SC)

The sternoclavicular joint is an anatomically compound and mechanically simple biaxial joint (sellaris, unmodified sellar). An articular disc divides the joint cavity into two parts. It technically is considered a saddle joint (sellaris), but because there is a lax capsule and the disc is flexible, it is functionally a triaxial joint (spheroid, unmodified ovoid).

Bony palpation

- Sternum
- Medial clavicle
- Sternoclavicular joint space
- Infraclavicular fossa

Ligaments

- Sternoclavicular ligaments (anterior and posterior)
- Interclavicular ligament
- Costoclavicular ligament

Bone movement and axes

For convenience in describing clavicular movements, the clavicle is considered moving on a stationary manubrium sterni around three axes:

- Elevation – depression: around the sagittal (dorso-ventral) axis through the medial end of the clavicle. The clavicle moves with its convex surface around the sagittal axis for cranial and caudal movements.
- Protraction – retraction: around the vertical (cranial-caudal) axis which passes longitudinally through the manubrium sterni. The clavicle's concave surface along with the disc moves around the vertical axis for ventral and dorsal movements.

- Rotation (with shoulder flexion - extension): around the longitudinal axis which passes lengthwise through the clavicle. The anterior border of the clavicle moves cranially (lateral rotation of the clavicle) during shoulder flexion, and caudally (medial rotation of the clavicle) during shoulder extension.

End feel

- Firm

Joint movement (gliding)

- Cranial-caudal movement: Convex Rule
- Dorsal-ventral movement: Concave Rule

Treatment plane

- Elevation - depression: on the concave joint surface of the sternum
- Protraction - retraction: on the concave joint surface of the clavicle

Zero position

- Same as the physiological position in the shoulder girdle.

Resting position

- Same as the physiological position in the shoulder girdle.

Close-packed position

- Arm in full elevation

Capsular pattern

- Unknown

■ The acromioclavicular joint

(art. acromioclavicularis, abbreviated AC)

The acromioclavicular joint is an anatomically simple (or compound when a disc is present) and mechanically compound plane gliding joint. Anatomically the acromion is concave and the clavicle is convex. However, it is functionally a triaxial ball and socket joint (spheroidea) due to its lax capsule and a flexible disc which is usually present.

Bony palpation

- Acromion
- Lateral clavicle
- Acromioclavicular joint space

Ligaments

- Acromioclavicular ligament
- Coracoclavicular ligament (trapezoid and conoid parts)

Bone movement and axes

In describing movements of this joint, one can consider that the scapula moves in relation to a stationary clavicle around three axes. At the same time, the scapula also moves in relation to the thorax. There are three axes of movement for the acromioclavicular joint.

Scapula cranial - caudal: There is very little movement here. A sagittal (dorso-ventral) axis runs through the lateral end of the clavicle. *Figure 37a* (ventral view) shows the clavicular-scapular vertical angle (C-S V) which is approximately 90°. *Figure 37b* illustrates the axis (dark dot) around which the scapula moves. As the inferior angle of the scapula moves laterally, the C-S V angle increases and, as it moves medially, the angle decreases. As a result of these movements, the glenoid cavity will face more cranially (as the C-S V angle increases) or more caudally (as the C-S V angle decreases).

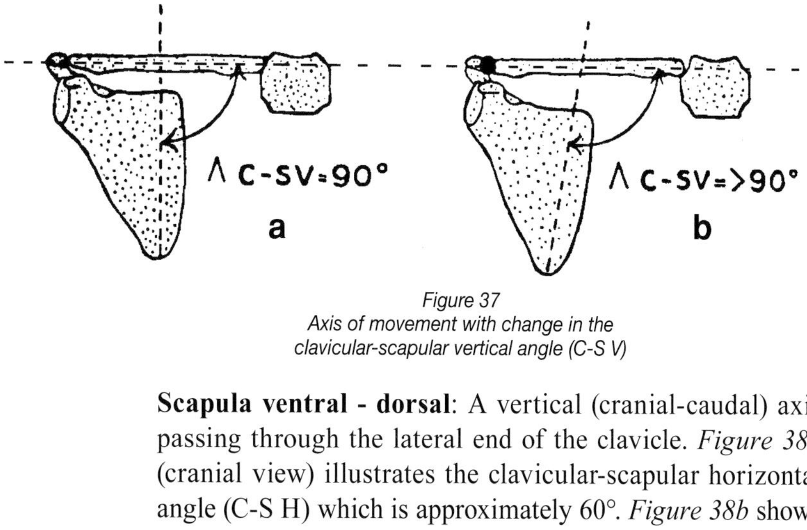

Figure 37
Axis of movement with change in the clavicular-scapular vertical angle (C-S V)

Scapula ventral - dorsal: A vertical (cranial-caudal) axis passing through the lateral end of the clavicle. *Figure 38a* (cranial view) illustrates the clavicular-scapular horizontal angle (C-S H) which is approximately 60°. *Figure 38b* shows the axis (dark dot) around which the scapula moves. When the medial border of the scapula moves away from the thorax ("winging" or abduction of the scapula), the C-S H angle increases (*Figure 38b*). As the medial border of the scapula moves towards the thorax (adduction), the angle decreases. As a result of these movements, the glenoid cavity will face more ventrally (with abduction) or more dorsally (with adduction).

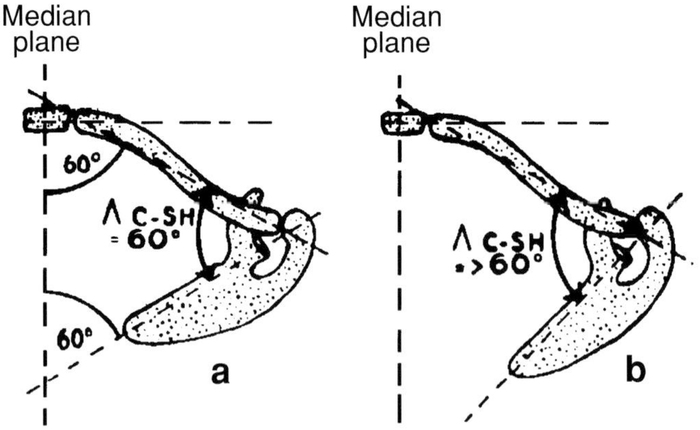

Figure 38
Axis of movement with change in the clavicular-scapular horizontal angle (C-S H)

The **scapula** is positioned more cranially and tightly against the thorax in muscular individuals. In less muscular individuals, the scapula is positioned less tightly against the thorax ("winged") and more caudally. Between these extremes of positions, the scapula lies with the superior angle at the level of the second rib, the inferior angle at the level of the seventh rib, and the medial border approximately five centimeters lateral to the spinous processes. A vertical plane through the scapula forms an angle of approximately 60° with the medial plane (*Figure 38a*).

The superior surface of the **clavicle** lies approximately in the horizontal plane and forms an angle of approximately 60° with the medial plane (*Figure 38a*).

The **clavicular-scapular horizontal angle** (C-S H) is therefore approximately 60° as it forms the third angle of an equilateral triangle (*Figure 38a*).

- **Scapula rotation**: A longitudinal axis which passes lengthwise through the clavicle allows movements of the scapula over the thorax. During lateral rotation the inferior angle moves laterally and forward and the glenoid cavity then faces more cranially and ventrally. With medial rotation, the inferior angle moves medially and backwards, and therefore the glenoid cavity faces more caudally and dorsally.

End feel

- Firm

Joint movement (gliding)

- Retraction - protraction
  Elevation - depression
- Apply the Concave Rule or Convex Rule according to whether the mobilization technique moves the concave or convex surface of the targeted bone.

Treatment plane

- Lies on the concave surface of the acromion

Zero position

- Same as the physiological position in the shoulder girdle.

Resting position

- Same as the physiological position in the shoulder girdle.

Close-packed position

- Arm in 90° abduction

Capsular pattern

- Unknown

Shoulder girdle examination scheme

(Refer to Chapters 3 and 4 for more information on examination)

Tests of function

Sternoclavicular joint

1. Active and passive movements, including stability tests and end-feel

Shoulder girdle

Elevation	45°
Depression	7°
Protraction	30°
Retraction	20°

Clavicle rotation around its longitudinal axis during internal and external rotation of the abducted arm:

Lateral rotation	10°
Medial rotation	10°

2. Translatoric joint play movements, including end-feel

Traction - compression	(Figure 39a)
Gliding	
Cranial	(Figure 39d)
Caudal	(Figure 39e)
Ventral	(Figure 39f)
Dorsal	(Figure 39g)

3. Resisted movements

Shoulder girdle elevation
- *Trapezius*
- *Levator scapula*

Shoulder girdle depression
- *Lower trapezius*
- *Serratus anterior*
- *Latissimus dorsi*
- *Pectoralis minor*
- *Subclavius*

Shoulder girdle protraction
- *Pectoralis major*
- *Pectoralis minor*
- *Serratus anterior*

Shoulder girdle retraction
- *Trapezius*
- *Rhomboids*
- *Latissimus dorsi*

4. Passive soft tissue movements

Physiological

Accessory

5. Additional tests

Acromioclavicular joint

1. **Active and passive movements, including stability tests and end-feel**

   Scapula:

Lateral rotation	25°
Medial rotation	25°

2. **Translatoric joint play movements, including end-feel**

Traction - compression	(adapt from Figure 39a, fixate the clavicle, move the scapula)
Gliding	
Ventral - dorsal	(Figure 40a)
With the scapula	(Figure 41, 42)

3. **Resisted movements**

   Scapula lateral rotation

   Trapezius

   Serratus anterior

   Scapula medial rotation

   Rhomboids

   Levator scapula

4. **Passive soft tissue movements**

   Physiological

   Accessory

5. **Additional tests**

Trial treatment

Sternoclavicular joint	(Figure 39a, 39b)
Acromioclavicular joint	(adapt from Figure 39a, 39b)

Shoulder girdle techniques

Sternoclavicular joint

Figure 39a	Clavicle-sternum traction for pain and hypomobility
Figure 39b,c	Clavicle-sternum traction for hypomobility
Figure 39d,e	Clavicle-sternum cranial and caudal glide for restricted depression and elevation
Figure 39f,g	Clavicle-sternum ventral and dorsal glide for restricted protraction and retraction

Acromioclavicular joint

Figure 40a,b	Clavicle-acromion ventral glide for hypomobility

Scapula

Figure 41, 42	Scapula caudal glide and winging for hypomobility

Clavicle-sternum traction

for pain and hypomobility

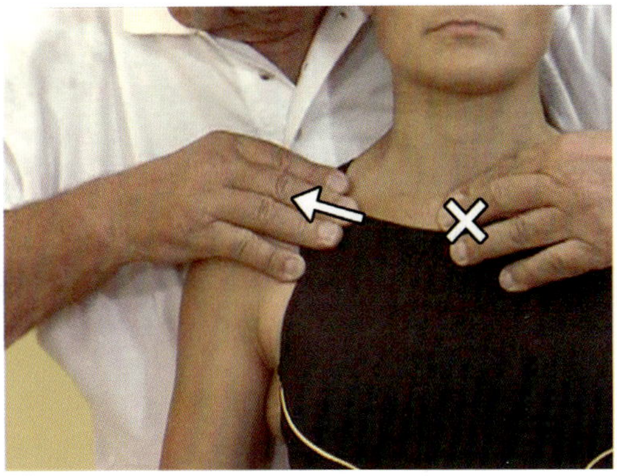

Figure 39a – test and mobilization in resting position

■ Figure 39a: Test and mobilization in resting position

Objective

- To evaluate the quantity and quality of traction joint play in the sternoclavicular joint, including end-feel.
- To decrease pain and increase shoulder girdle mobility with increased sternoclavicular traction joint play.

Starting position

- The patient sits. The sternoclavicular joint is in its resting position.

Hand placement and fixation

- **Therapist's stable hand (left)**: Fixate the patient's sternum and body against your body.
- **Therapist's moving hand (right):** Grip around the patient's clavicle from the ventral side.

Procedure

- Apply a Grade I, II, or III lateral movement to the clavicle to produce a traction movement in the sternoclavicular joint.
- Suitable for early training in manipulative thrust techniques.

Notes

- Adapt hand placement to apply a Grade I, II, or III traction-mobilization or manipulative thrust to the acromio-clavicular joint.

Clavicle-sternum traction

for hypomobility

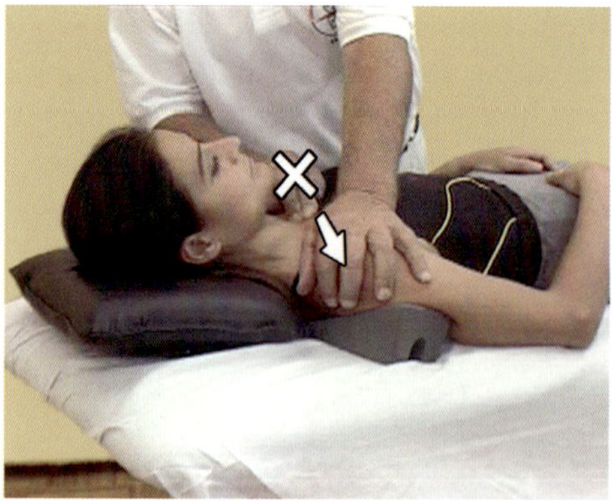

Figure 39b – test and mobilization in resting position

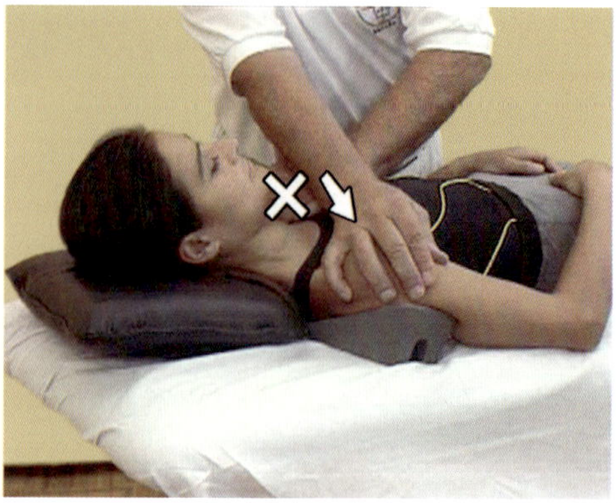

Figure 39c – mobilization in resting position

■ Figure 39b: Test and mobilization in resting position

Objective

- To evaluate the quantity and quality of traction joint play in the sternoclavicular joint, including end-feel.
- To increase shoulder girdle mobility with increased sternoclavicular traction joint play.

Starting position

- The patient lies supine with a sandbag or wedge under the scapula.
- Stand on the side of the patient opposite the targeted sternoclavicular joint.

Hand placement and fixation

- **Therapist's stable hand (right)**: Press the patient's sternum and thorax toward the treatment surface to fixate the sternum.
- **Therapist's moving hand (left):** Grip around the patient's shoulder with your thenar eminence on the lateral clavicle.

Procedure

- Apply a Grade I, II or III traction movement to the clavicle in relation to the sternum.
- Facilitate the movement by leaning through your extended left arm.
- Suitable for early training in manipulative thrust techniques.

■ Figure 39c: Alternate mobilization technique

- Apply a Grade III traction-mobilization or manipulative thrust with the same procedure, switching your left and right hand grips.

Clavicle-sternum cranial and caudal glide

for restricted depression and elevation

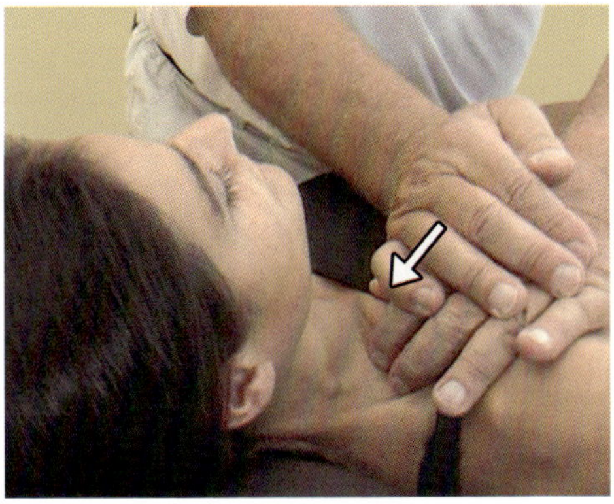

Figure 39d – test and mobilization, cranial

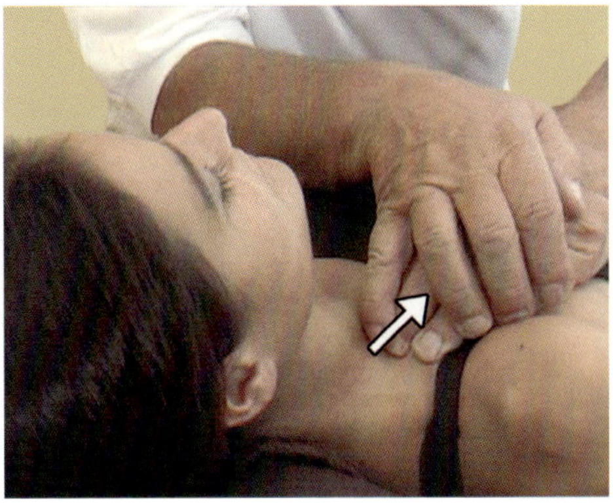

Figure 39e – test and mobilization, caudal

■ Figure 39d: Test and mobilization, cranial

Objective

- To evaluate the quantity and quality of cranial glide joint play in the sternoclavicular joint, including end-feel.
- To increase scapular depression range-of-motion with increased cranial glide joint play in the sternoclavicular joint (Convex Rule).

Starting position

- The patient lies supine.

Hand placement and fixation

- **Fixation**: No external fixation is necessary.
- **Therapist's moving hands:** Place the length of your left thumb and thenar eminence along the caudal surface of the patient's clavicle; place your right hypothenar eminence over your left thumb to reinforce your grip.

Procedure

- Apply a Grade II or III cranial glide movement to the clavicle. When testing, palpate the joint space.

■ Figure 39e: Test and mobilization, caudal

- Apply a Grade III caudal glide movement to increase scapular elevation (Convex Rule). With your left hand, place your finger along the cranial surface of the patient's clavicle; reinforce your grip with the fingers of your right hand. When testing, palpate the joint space.

■ Mobilization progression (not shown)

- Position the shoulder girdle near its end range-of-motion in elevation or depression.

Clavicle-sternum ventral and dorsal glide

for restricted protraction and retraction

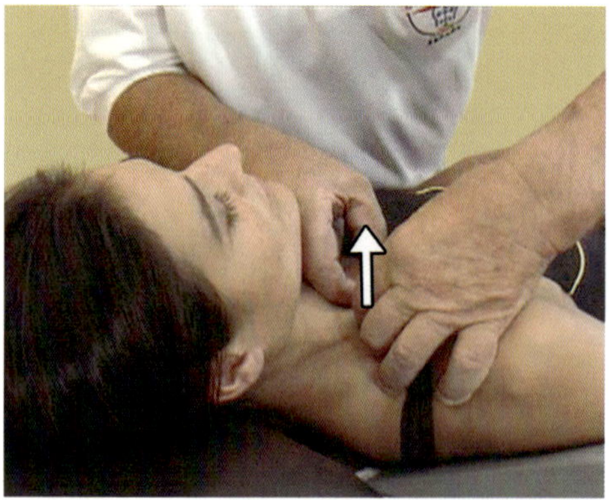

Figure 39f – test and mobilization, ventral

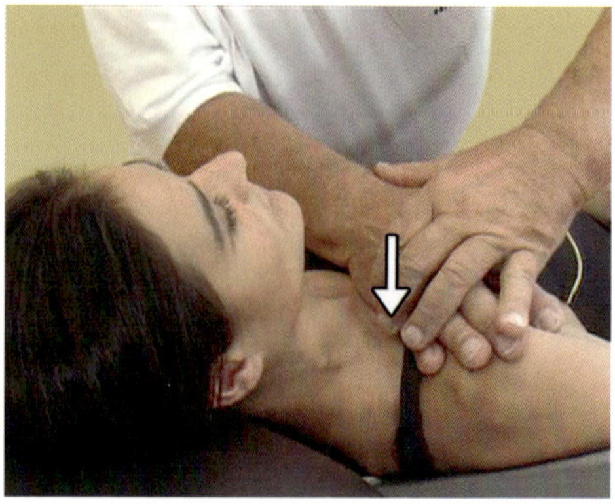

Figure 39g – test and mobilization, dorsal

■ Figure 39f: Test and mobilization, ventral

Objective

- To evaluate the quantity and quality of ventral glide joint play in the sternoclavicular joint, including end-feel.
- To increase scapular protraction range-of-motion by increasing ventral glide joint play in the sternoclavicular joint (Concave Rule).

Starting position

- The patient lies supine.

Hand placement and fixation

- **Fixation**: No external fixation is necessary. You may fixate the sternum with your left hand (not shown).
- **Therapist's moving hands:** Grip around the clavicle with your fingers.

Procedure

- Lift the clavicle in an anterior direction to apply a Grade II or III ventral glide joint play movement (shown). When testing, use your right hand to palpate in the joint space rather than to fixate the sternum (not shown).

■ Figure 39g: Test and mobilization, dorsal

- Apply a Grade III dorsal glide movement to the clavicle to increase scapular retraction (Concave Rule). Place the ulnar part of your right hand along the ventral surface of the patient's clavicle; use your left hand to reinforce your grip; lean through your arms to apply the dorsal glide movement to the clavicle. When testing, palpate the joint space.

■ Mobilization progression (not shown)

- Position the shoulder girdle near its end range-of-motion into protraction or retraction.

Clavicle-acromion ventral glide
for hypomobility

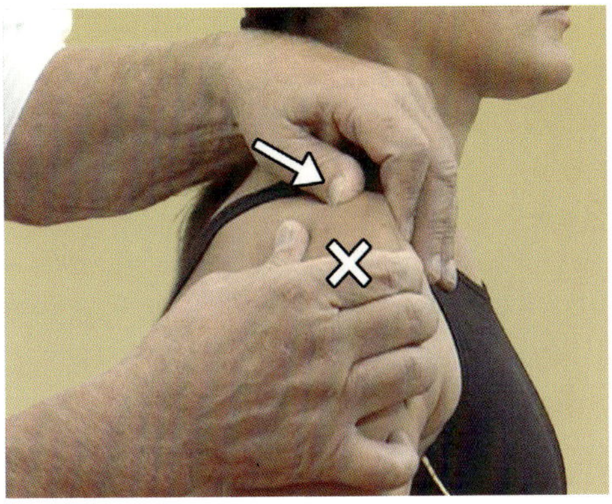

Figure 40a – test and mobilization in resting position

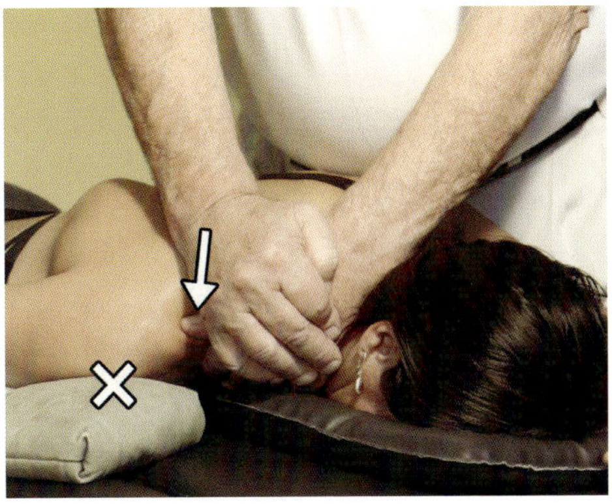

Figure 40b – mobilization in resting position

■ Figure 40a: Test and mobilization in resting position

Objective

- To evaluate the quantity and quality of ventral glide joint play in the acromioclavicular joint, including end-feel.
- To increase shoulder girdle mobility with increased ventral glide joint play in the acromioclavicular joint.

Starting position

- The patient sits. The acromioclavicular joint is in its resting position.

Hand placement and fixation

- **Therapist's stable hand (right)**: Fixate the patient's scapula by gripping the acromion or corocoid process from the ventral side, and the spine of the scapula from the dorsal side.
- **Therapist's moving hand (left):** Grip around the clavicle with your thumb and fingers just proximal to the joint space.

Procedure

- Press the clavicle in a ventral direction to apply a Grade II or III ventral glide movement (shown). When testing, use your right index finger to palpate in the joint space (not shown).

■ Figure 40b: Alternate mobilization technique

- Apply a Grade III ventral glide movement to the clavicle. The patient lies prone; fixate the scapula with a sandbag under the acromion, taking care that the sandbag does not contact the clavicle; place your left thumb and thenar eminence along the clavicle from the dorsal side; place your right hand over your left thumb to reinforce your grip; lean through your extended arms.

Scapula caudal glide and winging
for hypomobility

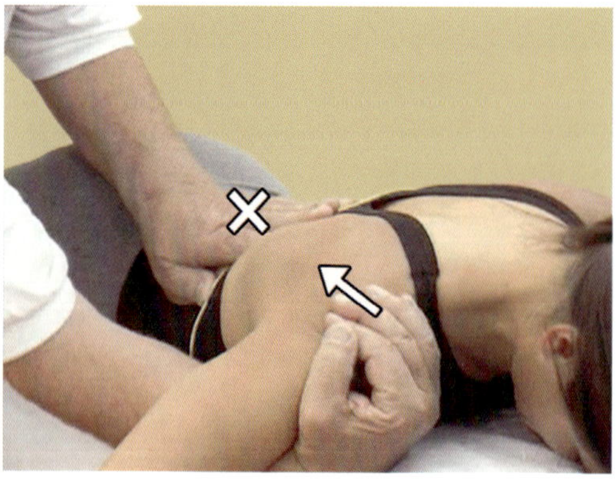

Figure 41 – mobilization caudal
in resting position

■ Figure 41: Mobilization caudal in resting position

Objective

- To increase shoulder girdle mobility by increasing caudal glide in the "scapulo-thoracic" articulation.
- To increase mobility in the sternoclavicular joint.

Starting position

- The patient is prone. The scapula is in its resting position.

Hand placement and fixation

- **Therapist's stable hand (left)**: Place your hand with your index finger against the inferior angle of the scapula.
- **Therapist's moving hand (right):** Grip around the patient's shoulder from the ventral side.

Procedure

- Lift the shoulder with the scapula in a dorsal-caudal direction to apply a Grade III caudal glide movement of the scapula. The inferior angle of the scapula moves upon the fixating right index finger.

Scapula caudal glide and winging
for hypomobility (cont'd)

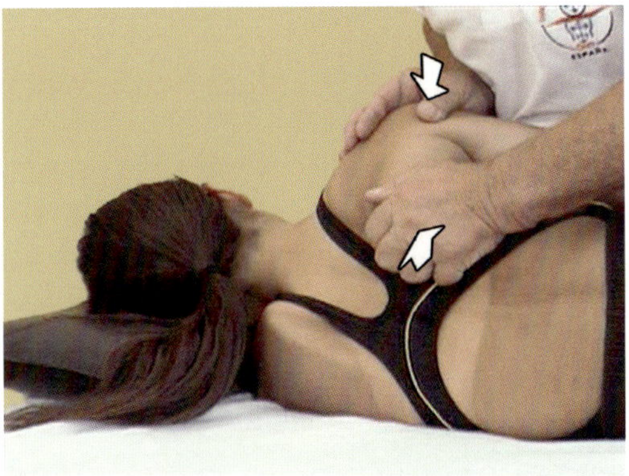

Figure 42 – mobilization winging
in resting position

- **Figure 42: Mobilization winging in resting position**
  - To increase mobility in the acromioclavicular joint.
  - The patient is side-lying; hold the patient's scapula against your body with both hands: your right hand grips the shoulder girdle from the cranial side, your left hand grips the inferior angle of the scapula; apply a Grade III winging mobilization by leaning your body downward on the patient's scapula and lifting the inferior border of the scapula laterally at the same time. This produces a winging movement of the scapula.

- **Alternate mobilization techniques (not shown)**
  - Use the grip described in *Figure 42* to mobilize the scapula in cranial, caudal, medial, and lateral directions. These mobilizations also increase mobility in the sternoclavicular joint.
  - Use the grip described in *Figure 42* to mobilize the scapula into internal and external rotation through the long axis of the clavicle. These mobilizations also increase mobility in the acromioclavicular joint.

■ Notes

CHAPTER 15

TOES

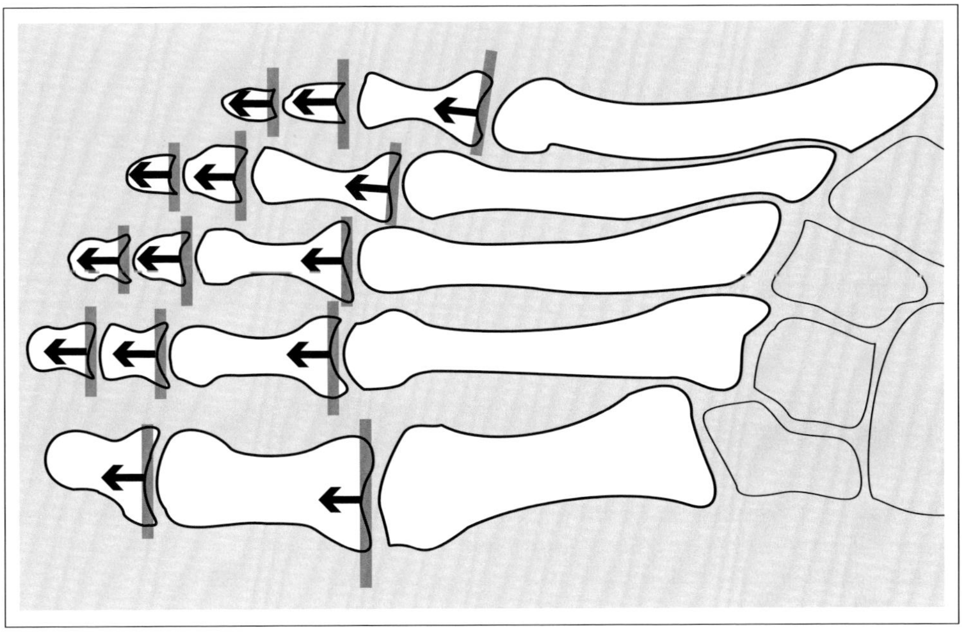

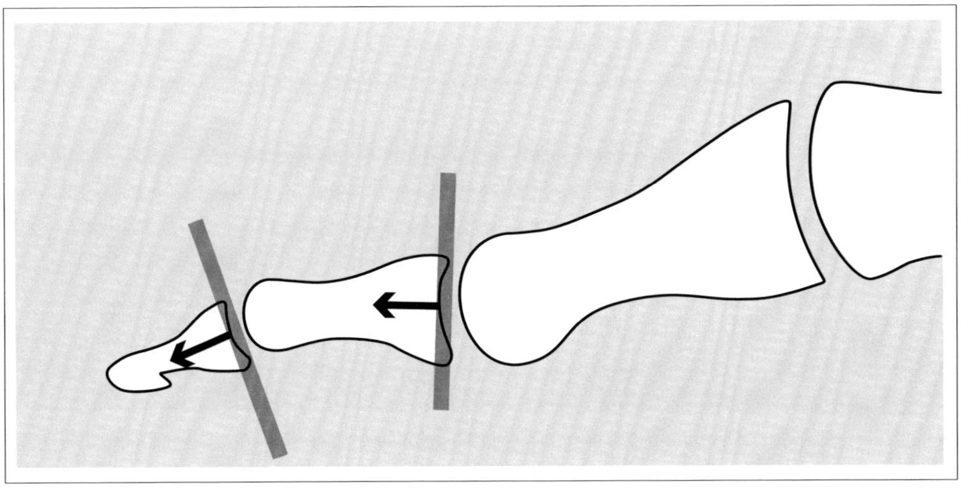

15 Toes

■ Functional anatomy and movement

■ Interphalangeal joints, distal and proximal

(artt. interphalangeals pedis, distalis et proximalis, abbreviated DIP and PIP)

■ Metatarsophalangel joints

(artt. metatarsophalangeae, abbreviated MTP)

The interphalangeal joints of the toe and the metatarsophalangeal joints are anatomically similar to the fingers. Each phalanx has a convex head distally and a concave base proximally. The axes of movement are the same as described for the fingers. Abduction and adduction of the toes around a dorsal-plantar axis results in movement away from and toward the second toe, which is regarded as lying in the middle of the foot.

Bony palpation

- Toe bones
- DIP and PIP joint spaces

Ligaments

- Collateral ligaments

Bone movement and axes

DIP and PIP:

- Flexion - extension: around a tibiofibular axis through the head of the phalanx

MTP:

- Tibial - fibular flexion: around a dorsalplantar axis through the head of the metatarsals. (Also called abduction and adduction movement away from and toward the 2nd toe.)
- Rotation (passive): around a longitudinal axis through the phalanx

End feel

- Firm

Joint movement (gliding)

- Concave Rule

Treatment plane

- Lies on the concave surface at the base of the phalanx.

Zero position

- The longitudinal axes through the metatarsals and corresponding phalangeal bones form a straight line.

Resting position

- *DIP and PIP:* slight flexion
- *MTP:* approximately 10° extension (from zero)

Close-packed position

- *DIP, PIP and MTP I:* maximal extension
- *MTP II-V:* maximal flexion

Capsular pattern

- Restricted in all directions, DIP and PIP extension more limited, MTP slightly more limited in flexion

Toe examination scheme

(Refer to Chapters 3 and 4 for more information on examination)

Tests of function

1. Active and passive movements, including stability tests and end-feel

DIP	Flexion	55°
PIP	Flexion	40°
MTP	Flexion	40°
	Extension from zero	40°
	Abduction	varies greatly with individuals

2. Translatoric joint play movements, including end-feel

Traction - compression	(Figure 43a)
Gliding	
Plantar	(Figure 44a)
Dorsal	(Figure 45a)
Tibial - fibular	(Figure 46a)

3. Resisted Movements

	ACTS ON:
Flexion	
Flexor digitorum brevis	PIP
Flexor digitorum longus	DIP
Flexor hallucis brevis	MTP
Flexor hallucis longus	IP
Flexor digiti minimi brevis	MTP
Lumbricals	MTP flexion; DIP, PIP extension
Extension	
Extensor digitorum	DIP, PIP
Extensor hallucis brevis	MTP
Extensor hallucis longus	IP
Lumbricals	DIP, PIP
Abduction	
Dorsal interossei	MTP
Abductor digiti minimi	MTP
Abductor hallucis	MTP
Adduction	
Adductor hallucis	MTP
Plantar interossei	MTP

4. Passive soft tissue movements

Physiological

Accessory

5. Additional tests

Trial treatment

Traction (Figure 43b)

■ Toe techniques

Figure 43a,b	Traction for pain and hypomobility
Figure 43c,d	Traction for restricted flexion and extension
Figure 44a,b,c	Plantar glide for restricted flexion
Figure 45a,b,c	Dorsal glide for restricted extension
Figure 46a,b,c	Tibial glide for restricted abduction, flexion, and extension

Toe traction

for pain and hypomobility

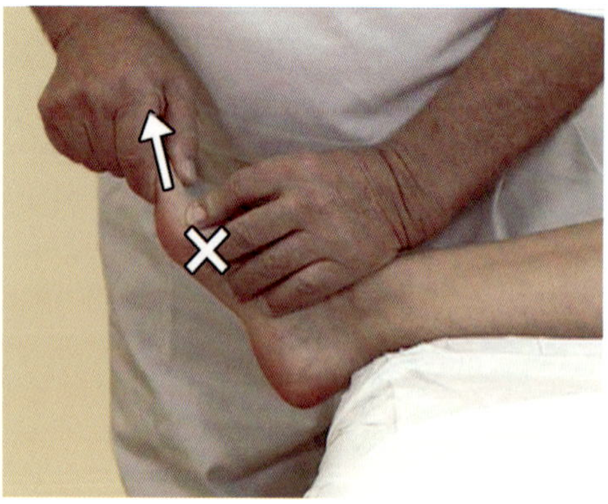

Figure 43a – test and mobilization in resting position

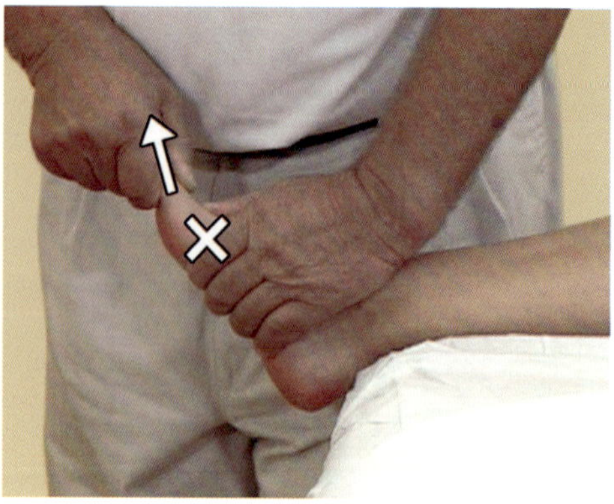

Figure 43b – mobilization in resting position

■ Figure 43a: Test and mobilization in resting position

Objective

- To evaluate the quantity and quality of traction joint play in a DIP, PIP, or MTP joint, including end-feel.
- To decrease pain or increase range of motion in a DIP, PIP, or MTP joint.

Starting position

- The plantar side of the patient's foot faces down.
- Position the targeted DIP, PIP, or MTP joint in its resting position.

Hand placement and fixation

- **Therapist's stable hand (left):** Hold the patient's foot in your hand; grip with your fingers just proximal to the targeted joint space; fixate the patient's foot against your body.
- **Therapist's moving hand (right):** Hold the patient's toe in your hand; grip with your fingers just distal to the targeted joint space.

Procedure

- Apply a Grade I, II or III distal traction movement to the distal phalanx.
- Suitable for early training in manipulative thrust techniques.

■ Figure 43b: Mobilization in resting position

- Improve your "handle" on the toe by gripping with tape, a paper towel, or a tongue depressor taped to the toe.
- Suitable for early training in manipulative thrust techniques.

Toe traction
for restricted flexion and extension

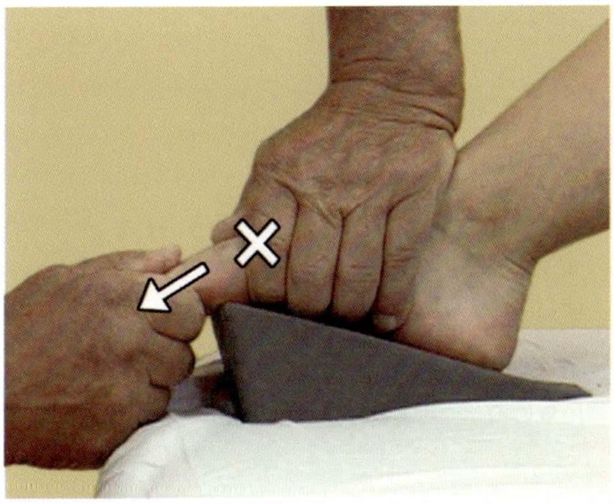

Figure 43c – MTP traction-mobilization in flexion

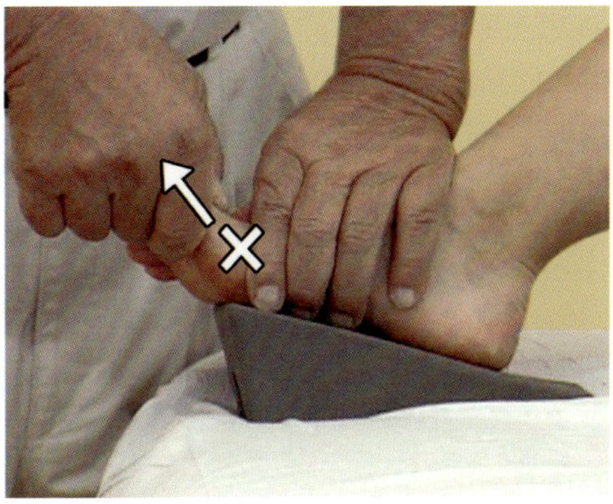

Figure 43d – MTP traction-mobilization in extension

■ Figure 43c: Flexion progression

Objective

- To increase flexion range-of-motion in a DIP, PIP, or MTP joint.

Starting position

- The plantar side of the patient's foot rests on a wedge.
- Position the targeted DIP, PIP, or MTP joint near to its end range-of-motion in flexion.

Hand placement and fixation

- **Therapist's stable hand (left):** Fixate the patient's foot against the wedge with your hand; grip with your fingers or thenar eminence just proximal to the targeted joint space.
- **Therapist's moving hand (right):** Hold the patient's toe in your hand; grip with your fingers just distal to the targeted joint space.

Procedure

- Apply a Grade III distal traction movement to the phalanx.

■ Figure 43d: Extension progression for the MTP joints

- The patient's foot rests on a wedge with the MTP joint positioned near to its end range-of-motion in extension.
- Apply a Grade III distal traction movement to the phalanx.

Toe plantar glide

for restricted flexion

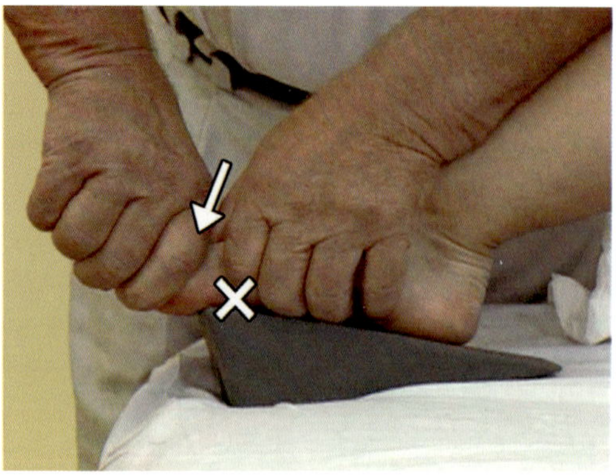

Figure 44a – test and mobilization in resting position

■ Figure 44a: Test and mobilization in resting position

Objective

- To evaluate the quantity and quality of plantar glide joint play in a DIP, PIP, or MTP joint, including end-feel.
- To increase DIP, PIP, or MTP joint flexion (Concave Rule).

Starting position

- The plantar side of the patient's foot rests on a wedge.
- Position the targeted DIP, PIP, or MTP joint in its resting position.

Hand placement and fixation

- **Therapist's stable hand (left):** Fixate the patient's foot against the wedge with your hand; grip the patient's mid-foot with your fingers just proximal to the targeted joint space.
- **Therapist's moving hand (right):** Hold the patient's toe in your hand; grip with your fingers just distal to the targeted joint space.

Procedure

- Apply a Grade II or III plantar glide movement to the phalanx.
- Palpate the joint space with your index finger during the movement.

Toe plantar glide
for restricted flexion (cont'd)

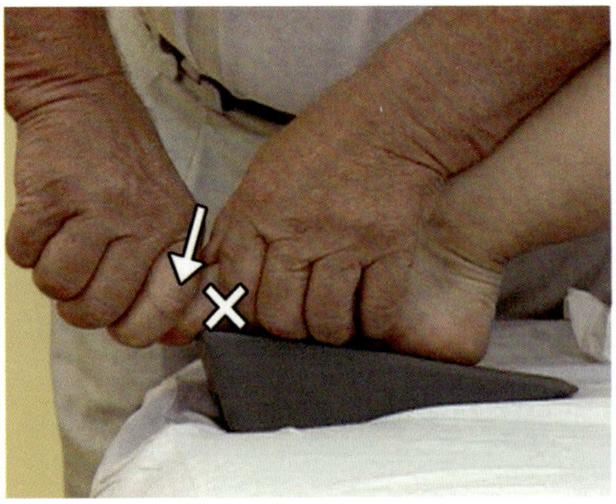

Figure 44b – mobilization in resting position

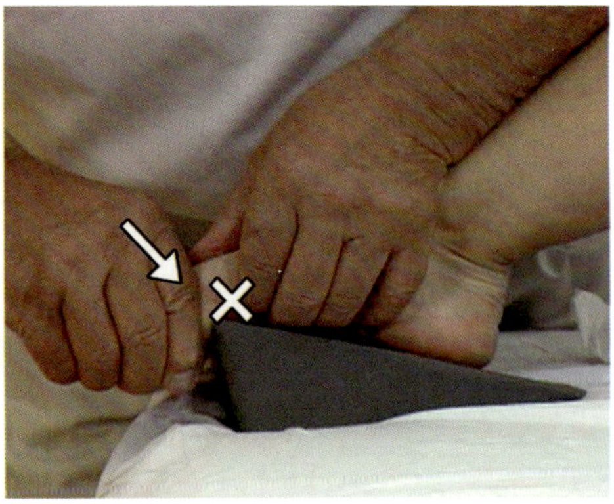

Figure 44c – mobilization in flexion

■ Figure 44b: Mobilization in resting position

Objective

- To increase flexion range-of-motion in a DIP, PIP, or MTP joint (Concave Rule).

Starting position

- The plantar side of the patient's foot rests on a wedge.
- Position the targeted DIP, PIP, or MTP joint in its resting position.

Hand placement and fixation

- **Therapist's stable hand (left):** Fixate the patient's foot against the wedge with your hand; grip with your fingers or thenar eminence just proximal to the targeted joint space.
- **Therapist's moving hand (right):** Hold the patient's toe in your hand; grip with your fingers just distal to the targeted joint space.

Procedure

- Apply a Grade III plantar glide movement to the phalanx.

■ Figure 44c: Flexion progression

- Apply a Grade III plantar glide movement with the targeted toe joint positioned close to its end range-of-motion in flexion.

Toe dorsal glide
for restricted extension

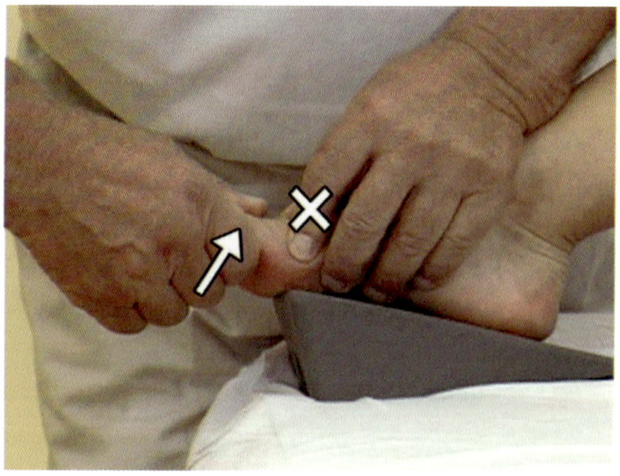

Figure 45a – test and mobilization in resting position

■ Figure 45a: Test and mobilization in resting position

Objective

- To evaluate the quantity and quality of dorsal glide joint play in a DIP, PIP, or MTP joint, including end-feel.
- To increase DIP, PIP, or MTP extension (Concave Rule).

Starting position

- The plantar side of the patient's foot rests on a wedge.
- Position the targeted DIP, PIP, or MTP joint in its resting position.

Hand placement and fixation

- **Therapist's stable hand (left):** Fixate the patient's foot against the wedge with your hand; grip the patient's mid-foot with your fingers just proximal to the targeted joint space.
- **Therapist's moving hand (right):** Hold the patient's toe in your hand; grip with your fingers just distal to the targeted joint space.

Procedure

- Apply a Grade II or III dorsal glide movement to the phalanx.
- Palpate the joint space with your index finger during the movement.

Toe dorsal glide
for restricted extension (cont'd)

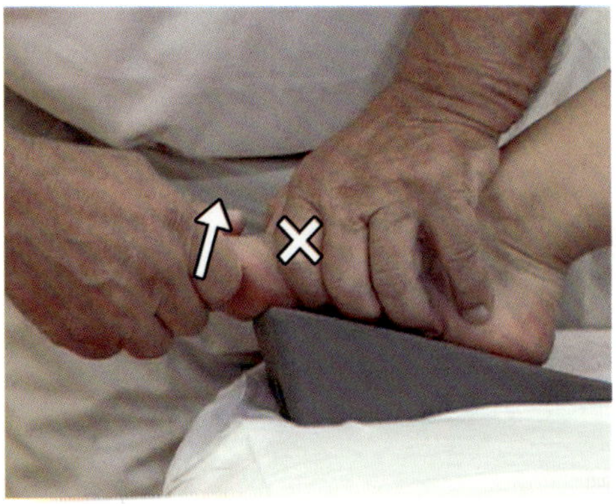

Figure 45b – mobilization in resting position

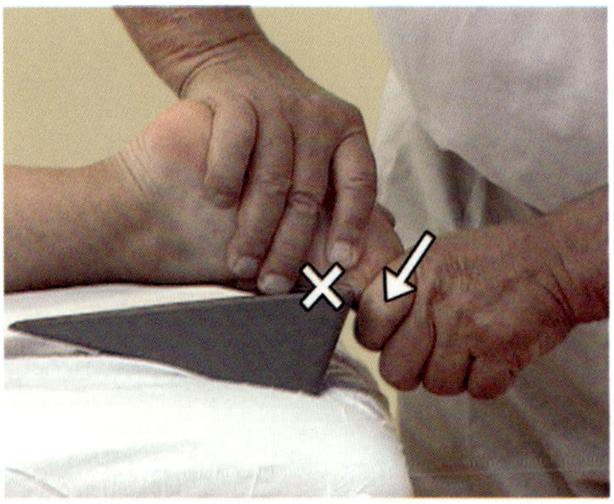

Figure 45c – mobilization in extension

■ Figure 45b: Mobilization in resting position

Objective

- To increase extension range-of-motion in a DIP, PIP, or MTP joint (Concave Rule).

Starting position

- The plantar side of the patient's foot rests on a wedge.
- Position the targeted DIP, PIP, or MTP joint in its resting position.

Hand placement and fixation

- **Therapist's stable hand (left):** Fixate the patient's proximal joint partner against the wedge with your hand; apply pressure with your fingers or thenar eminence just proximal to the targeted joint space.
- **Therapist's moving hand (right):** Hold the patient's toe in your hand; grip with your fingers just distal to the targeted joint space.

Procedure

- Apply a Grade III dorsal glide movement to the phalanx.

■ Figure 45c: Extension progression

- Apply a Grade III dorsal glide movement to the phalanx with the targeted toe joint positioned close to its end range-of-motion in extension. The dorsal side of the patient's foot rests on the wedge.

Toe tibial glide

for restricted abduction, flexion & extension

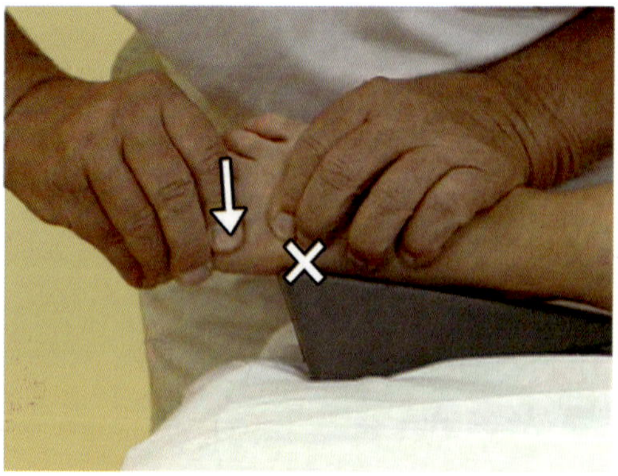

Figure 46a – test and mobilization in resting position

■ Figure 46a: Test and mobilization in resting position

Objective

- To evaluate the quantity and quality of tibial glide joint play in a DIP, PIP, or MTP joint, including end-feel.
- To increase toe flexion, extension, or tibial flexion (abduction) in a MTP joint.

Starting position

- The tibial side of the patient's foot rests on a wedge.
- Position the targeted DIP, PIP, or MTP joint in its resting position.

Hand placement and fixation

- **Therapist's stable hand (left):** Fixate the patient's forefoot against the wedge with your hand; grip with your fingers just proximal to the targeted joint space.
- **Therapist's moving hand (right):** Hold the patient's toe in your hand; grip with your fingers just distal to the targeted joint space; improve your "handle" on the toe by gripping with tape, a paper towel, or a tongue depressor taped to the toe.

Procedure

- Apply a Grade II or III tibial glide movement to the phalanx.
- Palpate the joint space with your index finger during the movement.

■ Toe fibular glide: test for restricted flexion and extension (not shown)

- Follow the same procedure for testing fibular glide joint play. Apply a Grade II or III fibular glide movement.

Toe tibial glide
for restricted abduction, flexion & extension (cont'd)

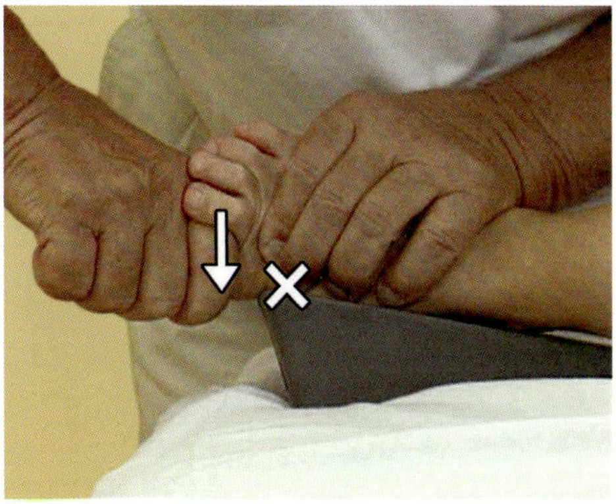
Figure 46b – mobilization in resting position

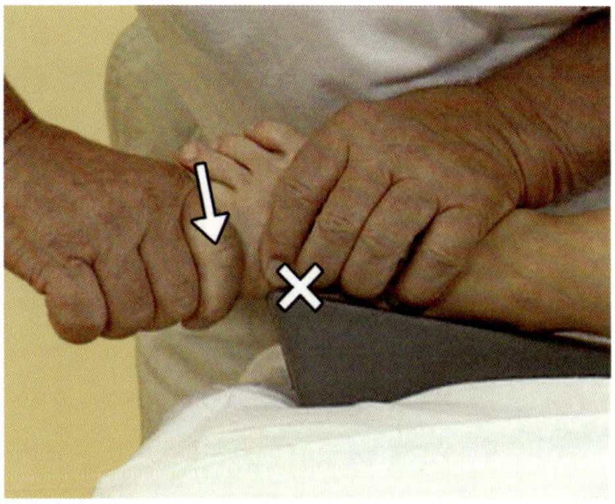
Figure 46c – mobilization in abduction

■ Figure 46b: Mobilization in resting position

Objective

- To increase tibial flexion (abduction) range-of-motion in a MTP joint (Concave Rule).
- To increase flexion or extension range-of-motion in a DIP, PIP, or MTP joint

Starting position

- The tibial side of the patient's foot rests on a wedge.
- Position the targeted DIP, PIP, or MTP joint in its resting position.

Hand placement and fixation

- **Therapist's stable hand (left):** Fixate the patient's forefoot against the wedge with your hand; grip with your fingers just proximal to the targeted joint space.
- **Therapist's moving hand (right):** Hold the patient's toe in your hand; grip with your fingers just distal to the targeted joint space; improve your "handle" on the toe by gripping with tape, a paper towel, or a tongue depressor taped to the toe.

Procedure

- Apply a Grade III tibial glide movement to the phalanx.

■ Figure 46c: Abduction progression

- Apply a Grade III tibial glide movement with the MTP joint positioned near its end range-of-motion toward abduction. In cases of extreme hypomobility, the MTP joint may remain in adduction.

■ Toe fibular glide: mobilization and progression (not shown)

- Follow the same procedure for fibular glide. Apply a Grade III fibular glide movement; may be performed in the resting position and progressed to end range-of-motion positioning into flexion or extension.

■ Notes

CHAPTER 16

METATARSALS

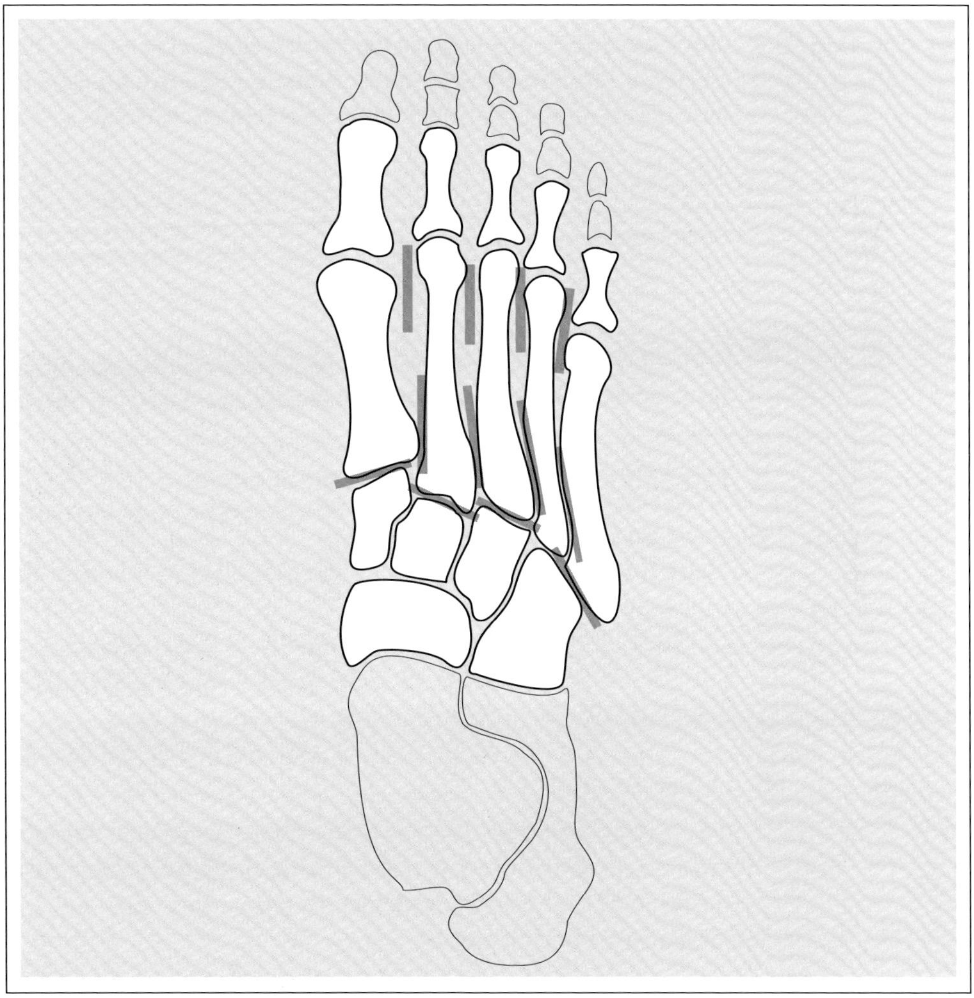

16 Metatarsals

(metatarsus)

Functional anatomy and movement

The metatarsus consists of five metatarsal bones (metatarsalia, abbreviated MT), one for each toe. Each metatarsal bone has a head (caput) or distal end with a convex surface, a body (corpus) and a base (basis) or proximal end with a concave surface.

The metatarsal joints are anatomically simple and mechanically compound plane gliding joints (amphiarthroses, modified sellar). Small gliding movements, synchronized with movements of the foot, take place in the metatarsus.

Proximal metatarsals (intermetatarsal joints)

Plane joints lie between the bases of the MT bones I-V.

Tarsometatarsals (tarsometatarsal joints)

Joints which are almost plane lie between the base of the metatarsal bones (functionally concave) and the adjacent row of tarsal bones (functionally convex). *Figure 49* illustrates how the MT bones I, II, and III articulate with the three cuneiform bones: (medial "C1", intermediate "C2", and lateral "C3") and that the MT bones IV and V together articulate with the cuboid.

Distal metatarsals

There are no joints between the heads of the metatarsals. The metatarsal heads are joined together by the deep transverse metatarsal ligaments. Their movements follow the movements of the proximal metatarsals, but with greater range.

Bony palpation

- Metatarsal bones I-V
- Distal row of tarsals (cuneiform I-III, cuboid)
- Joint spaces of tarsometatarsal joints I-V

Ligaments

- Metatarsal ligaments (dorsal, interosseous and plantar)
- Tarsometatarsal ligaments (plantar and dorsal)
- Interosseous cuneometatarsal ligaments

Bone movement and axes

Intermetatarsal joints:

- There are no defined axes for the small movements that occur in these joints. Intermetatarsal joint movements increase and decrease the curve of the transverse metatarsal arch.

  As the curve of the transverse metatarsal arch increases, the metatarsals glide in a plantar direction with relation to metatarsal II.

  As the curve of the transverse metatarsal arch decreases, the metatarsals glide in a dorsal direction with relation to metatarsal II.

Tarsometatarsal joints:

- Plantar - dorsal flexion: around a tibiofibular axis through the distal part of the cuneiform I-III and the cuboid.

End feel

- Firm

Joint movement (gliding)

- Concave rule

Treatment plane

- *Distal and proximal intermetatarsal I-V:* parallel between the metatarsals
- *Tarsometatarsal:* on the concave joint surface at the base of the metatarsal

Zero position:

- Unknown

Resting position

- Unknown

Close-packed position

- Unknown

Capsular pattern

- Unknown

Metatarsal examination scheme

(Refer to Chapters 3 and 4 for more information on examination)

Tests of function

1. **Active and passive movements, including stability tests and end-feel**
   Tarsometatarsal joints I-V
   Flexion - extension — very slight movement
2. **Translatoric joint play movements, including end-feel**
   Tarsometatarsal joint I-V
   Traction - compression — (Figures 6a, 7a – adapt from Metacarpals)
   Distal intermetatarsal
   Gliding plantar - dorsal — (Figure 47a)
   Proximal intermetatarsal
   Gliding plantar - dorsal — (Figure 48a)

Trial treatment

Tarsometatarsal traction — (Figures 6b, 7b – adapt from Metacarpals)

Metatarsal techniques

Figure 47a,b	Distal intermetatarsal plantar glide for hypomobility
Figure 48a,b	Proximal intermetatarsal plantar glide for hypomobility

Recommended mobilization sequence for the metatarsals

1. Proximal intermetatarsal plantar glide (Figure 48)
2. Distal intermetatarsal glide (Figure 47)

Distal intermetatarsal plantar glide
for hypomobility

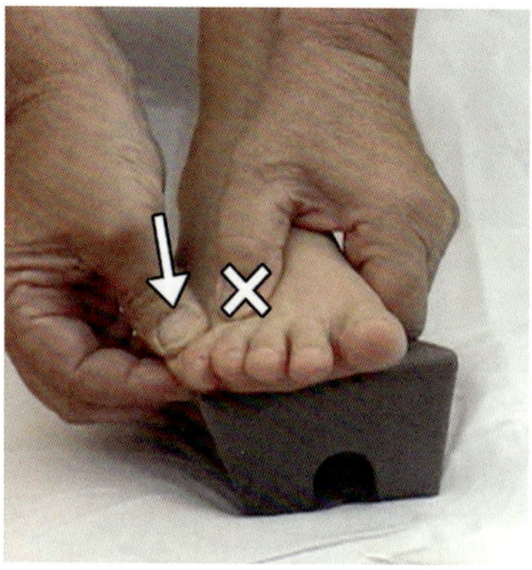

Figure 47a – test

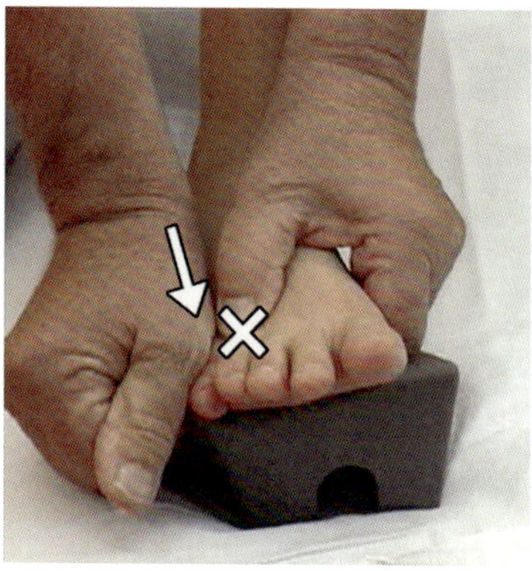

Figure 47b – mobilization

■ Figure 47a: Test

Objective

- To evaluate the quantity and quality of metatarsal plantar glide joint play, including end-feel.

Starting position

- The plantar side of the patient's foot rests on the treatment surface or a wedge, with the targeted metatarsal extending over the lateral edge.

Hand placement and fixation:

- **Fixation:** The medial metatarsal is supported on a wedge (MT IV shown) or with the therapist's hand.
- **Therapist's stable hand (left):** Hold the patient's foot from the medial side; place your palpating finger in the targeted syndesmosis (MT IV-V shown).
- **Therapist's moving hand (right):** Grip around the patient's targeted metatarsal (MT V shown).

Procedure

- Apply a Grade II or III plantar glide movement to the targeted metatarsal (MT V shown).

■ Figure 47b: Mobilization

- Fixate metatarsal IV with your thumb or thenar eminence on the dorsal surface of the foot; apply a Grade III plantar glide movement with your right thenar eminence pressing down on the targeted metatarsal (MT V shown) to increase metatarsal mobility and stretch the syndesmosis.

■ Alternate mobilization technique (not shown)

- Use the same grip; apply a Grade III dorsal glide movement.

Proximal intermetatarsal plantar glide

for hypomobility

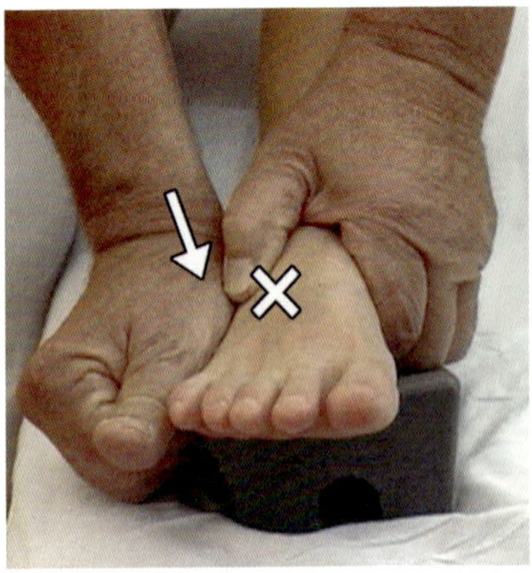

Figure 48a – test

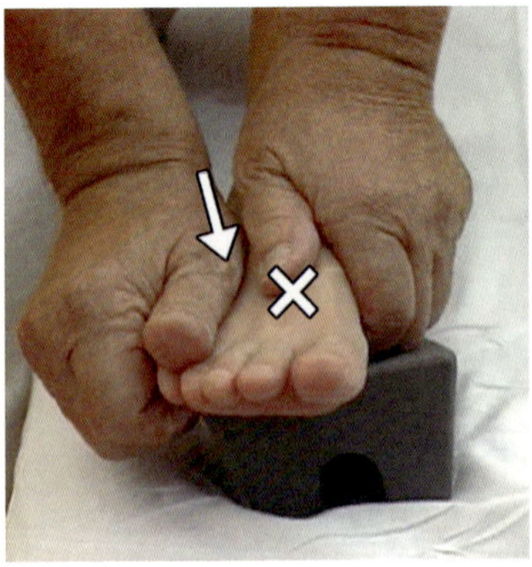

Figure 48b – mobilization

■ Figure 48a: Test

Objective

- To evaluate the quantity and quality of metatarsal plantar glide joint play, including end-feel.

Starting position

- The plantar side of the patient's foot rests on the treatment surface or a wedge, with the targeted metatarsal extending over the lateral edge.

Hand placement and fixation:

- **Fixation:** The medial metatarsal is supported on a wedge (metatarsal IV shown) or with the therapist's hand.
- **Therapist's stable hand (left):** Hold the patient's foot from the medial side; place your palpating finger in the targeted joint space (metatarsal IV-V shown).
- **Therapist's moving hand (right):** Grip around the patient's proximal metatarsal (metatarsal V shown).

Procedure

- Apply a Grade II or III plantar glide movement to the targeted metatarsal (metatarsal V shown).

■ Figure 48b: Mobilization

- Fixate metatarsal III with your thumb or thenar eminence on the dorsal surface of the foot; apply a Grade III plantar glide movement with your right thenar eminence pressing down on the base of the targeted metatarsal (metatarsal IV shown) to increase forefoot mobility by increasing intermetatarsal plantar glide.

■ Mobilization (not shown)

- With modified hand placement the lateral tarsometatarsal joints can be treated with traction (adapt from Metacarpals).
- Suitable for early training in manipulative thrust techniques.

CHAPTER 17

FOOT & ANKLE

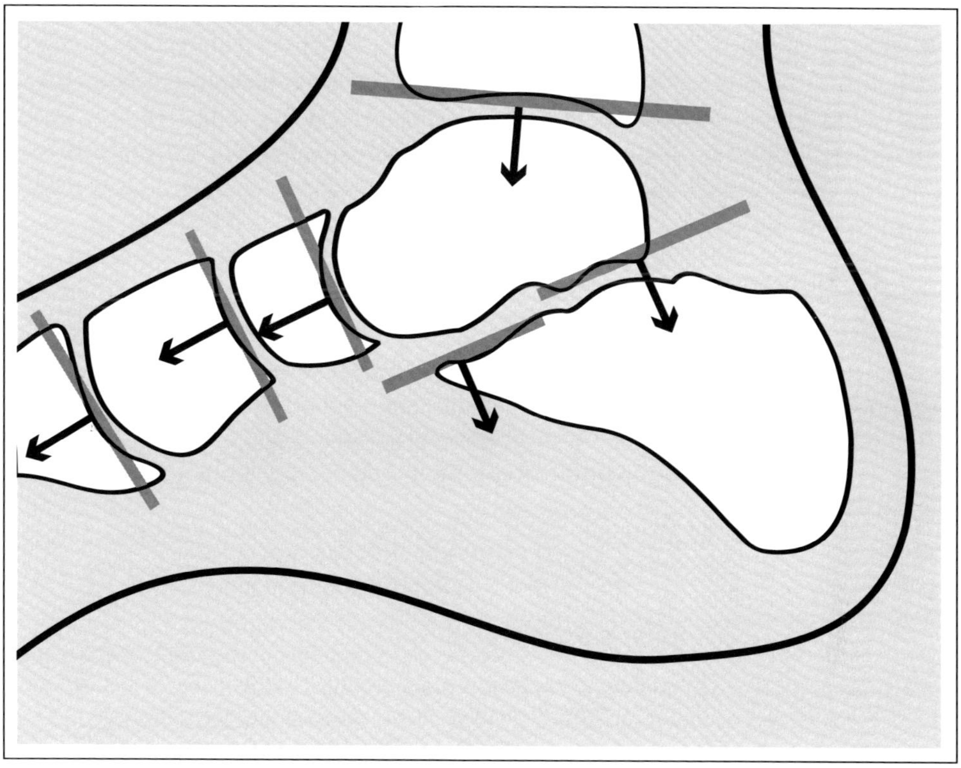

17 Foot and ankle

Functional anatomy and movement

The foot (*tarsus*) consists of seven tarsal bones (see *Figure 49*). The bones of the foot are:

- three cuneiform bones (*ossa cuneiformia I, II* and *III*)
- cuboid (*os cuboideum*)
- navicular (scaphoid = *os naviculare*)
- talus (*astragalus*)
- calcaneus.

The ankle joint (*art. talocruralis*) includes the talus articulating with the distal aspect of the tibia and fibula.

Tarsal joints

For testing and treatment purposes, we divide the tarsal joints into the following functional units:

Cuneonavicular joint

The cuneonavicular joint consists of three convex facets on the navicular and three concave facets on the cuneiform bones.

Cuboid-3rd cuneiform/navicular

Medially, the slightly convex cuboid articulates with the concave 3rd cuneiform and navicular.

Calcaneocuboid joint

The calcaneocuboid joint has a saddle-shaped joint surface. The concave surface on the cuboid guides movement for flexion and extension. The convex surface on the cuboid guides movement for abduction and adduction.

Talonavicular joint

The convex anterior surface of the talus articulates with the corresponding concave surface of the navicular.

Talocalcaneal joint, anterior and middle

The convex inferior/anterior surfaces of the talus articulate with the corresponding concave surfaces on the calcaneus.

Subtalar joint (talocalcaneal joint, posterior)

The subtalar joint is an anatomically simple and mechanically compound joint. The concave surface on the inferior/posterior surface of the talus articulates with a corresponding convex surface on the superior calcaneus.

■ Talocrural joint

The talocrural joint, between the talus and the distal surfaces of the tibia and fibula, is an anatomically and mechanically simple uniaxial joint (ginglymus, modified sellar). The trochlear surface of the talus is broader anteriorly so that during foot dorsal flexion the talus pushes the ankle mortise apart. In this position the talus fits tightly in the recess created by the tibia, fibula and the tibiofibular syndesmosis, which restricts movement of the talus and makes the joint more stable.

Foot

Bony palpation

- Cuneiform I, II and III
- Navicular
- Cuboid
- Calcaneus
- Talus
- Joint spaces between the tarsal bones
- Navicular tuberosity
- Sustentaculum tali
- Medial malleolus
- Lateral malleolus

Ligaments

- Plantar and dorsal cuneonavicular ligaments
- Plantar and dorsal intercuneiform ligaments
- Interosseous tarsal ligaments
- Cuboideonavicular (plantar and dorsal) ligaments
- Cuneocuboid (plantar and dorsal) ligaments
- Calcaneocuboid ligament (lateral half of the bifurcate ligament)
- Long plantar ligament
- Calcaneonavicular ligament (medial half of the bifurcate ligament)
- Talocalcaneal ligaments (lateral, medial, and interosseous ligaments)
- Deltoid ligament (medially)
- Calcaneofibular ligament (laterally)
- Talofibular ligament (anterior and posterior)

Bone movements and axes (see Figure 49)

- Plantar-dorsal flexion occurs primarily at the talocrural joint around a tibiofibular axis through the convex joint partner (talus).
- Pronation-supination occurs primarily in the forefoot around a longitudinal axis through metatarsal II. This movement is much greater when performed passively.
- Inversion-eversion occurs primarily between the talus and calcaneus and the talus and navicular around an oblique axis through the calcaneus and talus. Inversion is the combined movement of supination-adduction-plantar flexion; eversion is the combined movement of pronation-abduction-dorsal flexion.

Joint movement (gliding)

- Apply the Concave Rule or Convex Rule according to whether the mobilization technique moves the concave or convex surface of the targeted bone.

Treatment plane

- Lies on the concave surface of the targeted joint.

Zero position:

- The fibular side of the foot forms a right angle with the longitudinal axis through the leg.
- A line from the anterior superior iliac spine through the patella passes through the second toe.

Resting position:

- Approximately 10° plantar flexion and midway between maximal inversion and eversion.

Close-packed position:

- Metatarsus and tarsus: maximal inversion
- Talocrural joint: maximal dorsal flexion

Capsular pattern:

- Plantar flexion - dorsal flexion

Foot

Foot examination scheme

(Refer to Chapters 3 and 4 for more information on examination)

Tests of function

1. **Active and passive movements, including stability tests and end-feel**

Tarsal joints

Flexion	
Extension	
Pronation	10°
Supination	20°

Subtalar joints

Inversion	40°
Eversion	20°

2. **Translatoric joint play movements, including end-feel**

Tarsal joints

Traction - compression		(Figure 50a, 50b)
Gliding	Plantar	(Figure 50a, 51a, 52a, 53a)
	Dorsal	(Figure 50c, 50d)

Subtalar joints

Traction - compression		(Figure 54a)
Gliding	Distal	(Figure 54c)
	Tibial	(Figure 55a)
	Fibular	(Figure 55c)

3. **Resisted movements**

Eversion
Peronei

Inversion
Tibialis posterior
Triceps surae

4. **Passive soft tissue movements**

Physiological
Accessory

5. **Additional tests**

Trial treatment

Tarsal joints: traction	(Figure 50a Note, 51b Note)
Subtalar joint: traction	(Figure 54b)

■ Ankle examination scheme

Tests of function

Talocrural joint

1. **Active and passive movements, including stability and end-feel**

Plantar flexion	40°
Dorsal flexion	20°

2. **Translatoric joint play movements, including end-feel**

Traction - compression	(Figure 56a)
Gliding	
Anterior	(Figure 57a)
Posterior	(Figure 59a)

3. **Resisted movements**

Plantar flexion

Triceps surae

Flexor hallucis longus

Flexor digitorum longus

Dorsal flexion

Tibialis anterior

Extensor hallucis longus

Extensor digitorum longus

4. **Passive soft tissue movements**

Physiological

Accessory

5. **Additional tests**

Trial treatment

Talocrural joint traction	(Figure 56b)

Foot and ankle glide tests
Recommended sequence

■ **Figure 49: Recommended glide test sequence for the foot and ankle**

Foot

Movements in the middle of the foot (distally)

Fixate the third and second cuneiforms and move:

1. Metatarsal III
2. Metatarsal II

Movements on the medial side of the foot .... (Figure 50a)

Fixate the first cuneiform and move:

3. Metatarsal I

Fixate navicular and move:

4. The first, second, and third cuneiforms

Fixate talus and move:

5. Navicular

Movements on the lateral side of the foot around the cuboid

Fixate cuboid and move:

6. Metatarsals IV and V ....(Figure 51a)

Fixate the navicular and the third cuneiform from the medial side and move:

7. Cuboid ....(Figure 52a)

Fixate calcaneus and move:

8. Cuboid ....(Figure 53a)

Movements between the talus and calcaneus

Fixate talus and move:

9. Calcaneus...(Figure 55a)

Movements in the ankle joint

Fixate the leg and move:

10. Talus, or ....(Figure 56a)
11. Fixate the talus and move the leg ....(Figure 57a)

Foot

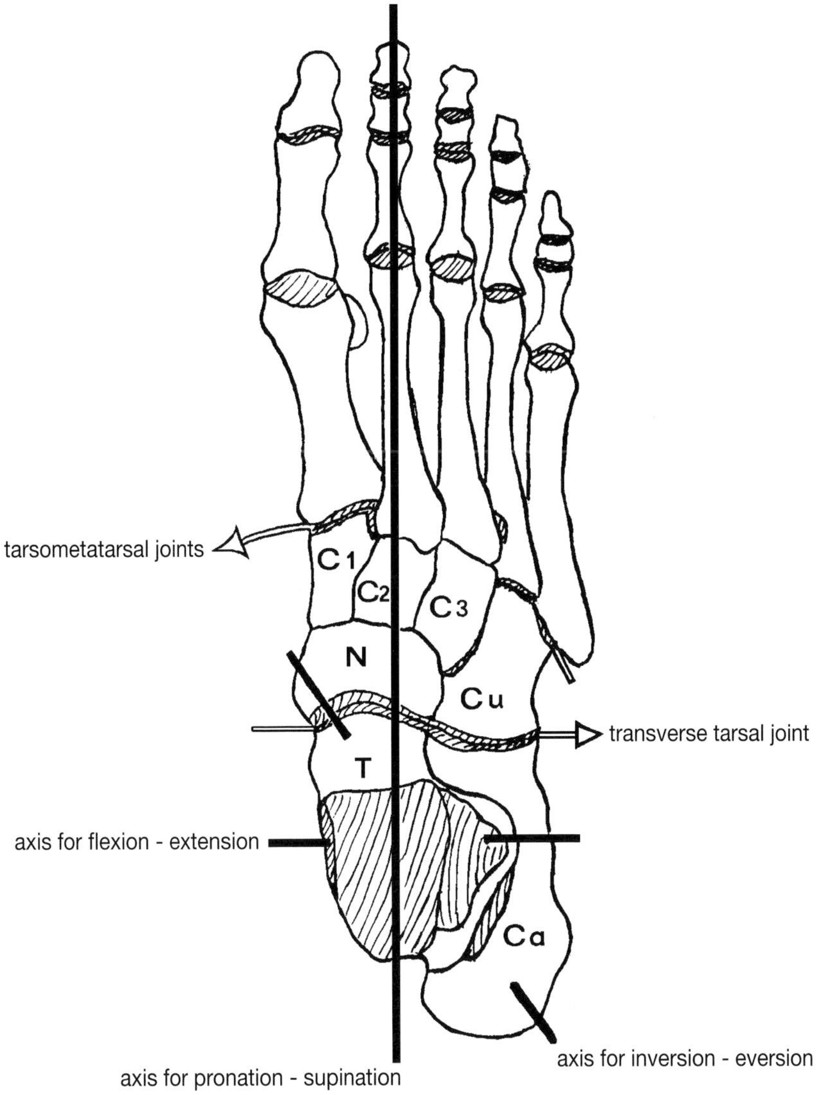

Figure 49
Tarsal bones and axes
(dorsal aspect of the right foot)

C1	=	*cuneiform I*
C2	=	*cuneiform II*
C3	=	*cuneiform III*
Cu	=	*cuboid*
N	=	*navicular*
T	=	*talus*
Ca	=	*calcaneus*

■ Foot and ankle techniques

Figure 49	Foot and ankle glide tests recommended sequence
Figure 49	Tarsal bones and axes

Cuneonavicular

Figure 50a,b	Plantar glide for restricted plantar flexion

Talonavicular

Figure 50c,d	Dorsal glide for restricted dorsal flexion

Metatarsals IV/V-cuboid

Figure 51a,b	Plantar glide for restricted plantar flexion

Cuboid-cuneiform III

Figure 52a,b	Plantar glide for hypomobility

Calcaneocuboid

Figure 53a,b	Plantar glide for hypomobility

Talocalcaneal

Figure 54a,b	Distal traction for pain and hypomobility
Figure 54c	Distal glide for hypomobility
(not shown)	Proximal glide for hypomobility
Figure 55a,b	Tibial glide for hypomobility
Figure 55c,d	Fibular glide for hypomobility

Talocrural

Figure 56a,b,c	Traction for pain and hypomobility
Figure 57a,b; 58a,b	Anterior glide for restricted plantar flexion
Figure 59a,b,c	Posterior glide for restricted dorsal flexion

Cuneonavicular plantar glide

for restricted plantar flexion

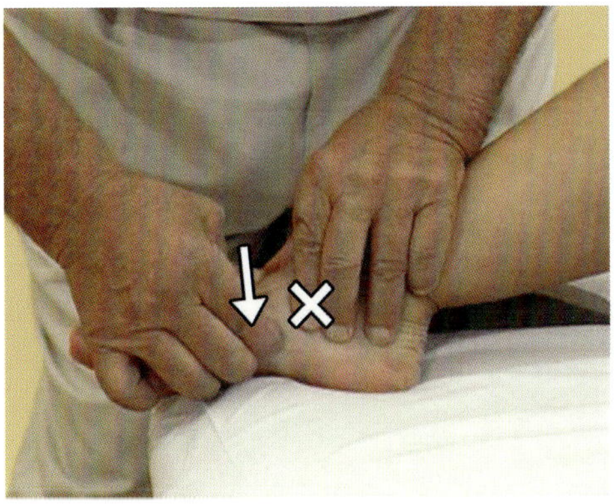

Figure 50a – test and mobilization in resting position

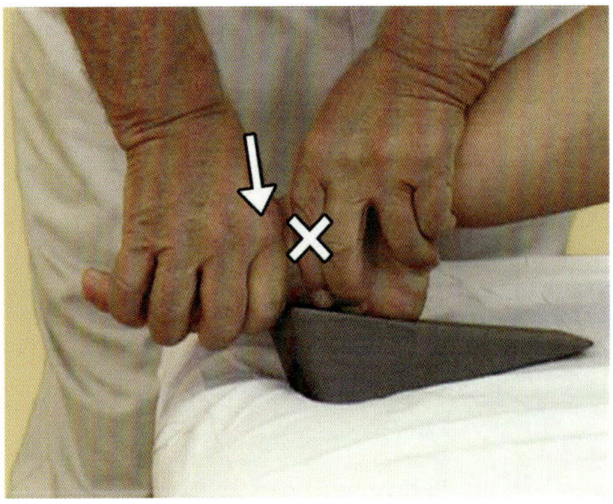

Figure 50b – mobilization in resting position

■ Figure 50a: Test and mobilization in resting position

Objective

- To evaluate the quantity and quality of plantar glide joint play of the cuneiform in relation to the navicular, including end-feel.
- To increase foot plantar flexion range-of-motion (Concave Rule).

Starting position

- The patient's foot rests on the treatment surface.
- Position the joint in its resting position.

Hand placement and fixation

- **Therapist's stable hand (left):** Hold the patient's foot; grip the patient's navicular bone with your fingers; fixate the patient's foot against treatment surface.
- **Therapist's moving hand (right):** Hold the patient's forefoot; grip the 1st cuneiform with your fingers just distal to the joint space.

Procedure

- Apply a Grade II or III plantar glide movement to the cuneiform bone.
- During testing and mobilization, palpate the joint with your left index finger.
- Use the same procedure to mobilize the 1st MT - 1st cuneiform and the talonavicular joint.
- With modified hand placement, all joints on the medial side of the foot can be tested and treated with traction mobilization and manipulative thrust.

■ Figure 50b: Mobilization in resting position

- Rest the plantar side of the patient's foot, including the navicular, on the wedge.
- Hold the patient's foot with your right hand; grip with your index finger and second metacarpal over the first cuneiform.
- Apply a Grade III plantar glide movement by leaning with your body over your extended arm.

Navicular-talus dorsal glide
for restricted dorsal flexion

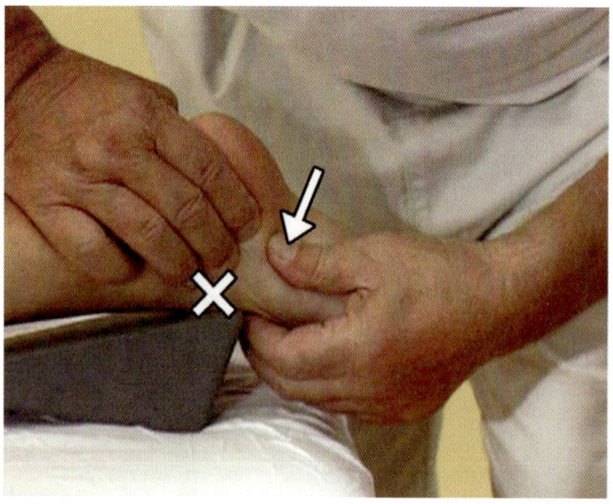

Figure 50c – test and mobilization in resting position

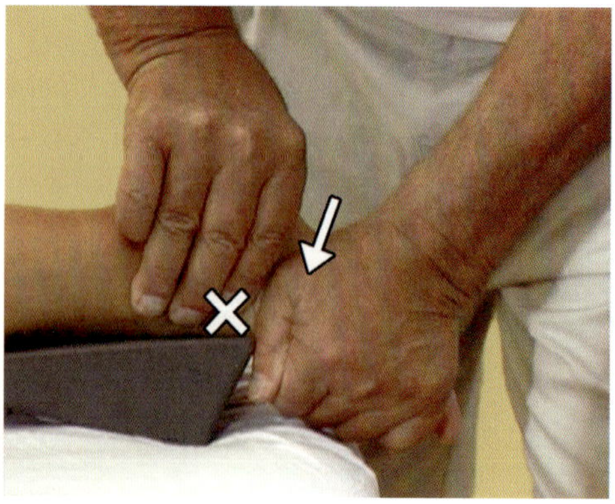

Figure 50d – mobilization in resting position

■ Figure 50c: Test and mobilization in resting position

Objective

- To evaluate the quantity and quality of dorsal glide joint play of the navicular in relation to the talus, including end-feel.
- To increase foot dorsal flexion range-of-motion (Concave Rule).

Starting position

- The anterior side of the patient's leg rests on the treatment wedge.
- Position the joint in its resting position.

Hand placement and fixation

- **Therapist's stable hand (right):** Hold the patient's distal leg against the wedge; place your palpating finger in the joint space.
- **Therapist's moving hand (left):** Hold the patient's mid-foot in your hand; grip with your fingers surrounding the navicular bone.

Procedure

- Apply a Grade II or III dorsal glide movement to the navicular bone.

Note

- Use the same procedure to mobilize the cuneiform - MT I and cuneionavicular joint, with modified hand placement.

■ Figure 50d: Mobilization in resting position

- Hold the patient's foot with your left hand; grip with your index finger and second metacarpal or thenar eminence over the navicular bone.
- Apply a Grade III dorsal glide movement by leaning with your body through your arm.

Metatarsals IV/V-cuboid plantar glide

for restricted plantar flexion

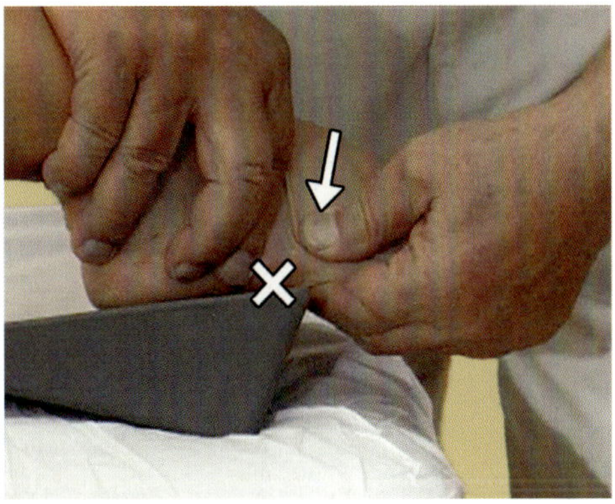

Figure 51a – test in resting position

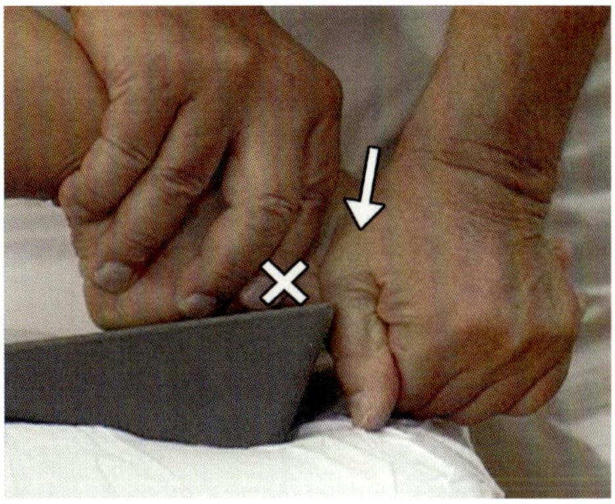

Figure 51b – mobilization in resting position

Foot

■ Figure 51a: Test in resting position

Objective

- To evaluate the quantity and quality of plantar glide joint play of metatarsals IV and V in relation to the cuboid, including end-feel.
- To increase foot plantar flexion range-of-motion (Concave Rule).

Starting position

- The plantar side of the patient's foot rests on a treatment wedge or sandbag.
- Position the joint in its resting position.

Hand placement and fixation.

- **Therapist's stable hand (right):** Fixate the patient's cuboid against the treatment surface.
- **Therapist's moving hand (left):** Hold the patient's forefoot; grip the bases of metatarsals IV and V with your fingers.

Procedure

- Apply a Grade I, II or III plantar glide movement to metatarsals IV/V.
- With modified hand placement, all joints on the lateral side of the foot can be tested and treated with traction and manipulative thrust techniques.

■ Figure 51b: Mobilization in resting position

- Use your right hand to fixate the cuboid bone on a wedge with metatarsals IV and V extending just past the edge.
- Grip the metatarsals with your left hand, with your thenar eminence over the bases of the metatarsals.
- Apply a Grade III plantar glide movement by leaning your body over your extended arm.
- With modified hand placement, suitable for early training in manipulative traction-thrust techniques.

Foot

Cuboid-cuneiform III plantar glide
for hypomobility

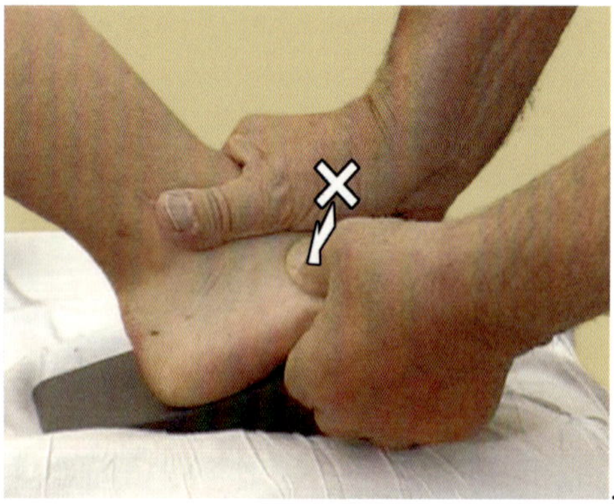

Figure 52a – test and mobilization in resting position

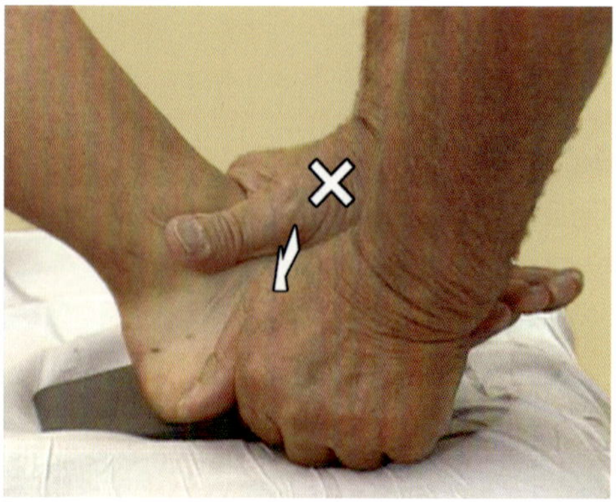

Figure 52b – mobilization in resting position

■ Figure 52a: Test and mobilization in resting position

Objective

- To evaluate the quantity and quality of plantar glide joint play of the cuboid in relation to the cuneiform III and navicular bones, including end-feel.
- To increase mid-foot mobility.

Starting position

- The tibial-plantar side of the patient's foot rests on the treatment wedge.
- Position the joint in its resting position.

Hand placement and fixation

- **Therapist's stable hand (right):** Fixate the patient's cuneiform III and navicular against the treatment surface with your thenar eminence and fingers.
- **Therapist's moving hand (left):** Hold the patient's forefoot; grip the patient's cuboid with your fingers.

Procedure

- Apply a Grade II or III plantar glide movement to the cuboid.

■ Figure 52b: Mobilization in resting position

- Use your right hand to fixate the patient's foot on a wedge or sandbag with cuboid extending just past the edge.
- Grip the cuboid with your thenar eminence and fingers from the fibular side.
- Apply a Grade III plantar glide movement by leaning your body over your extended arm.

Cuboid-calcaneus plantar glide
for hypomobility

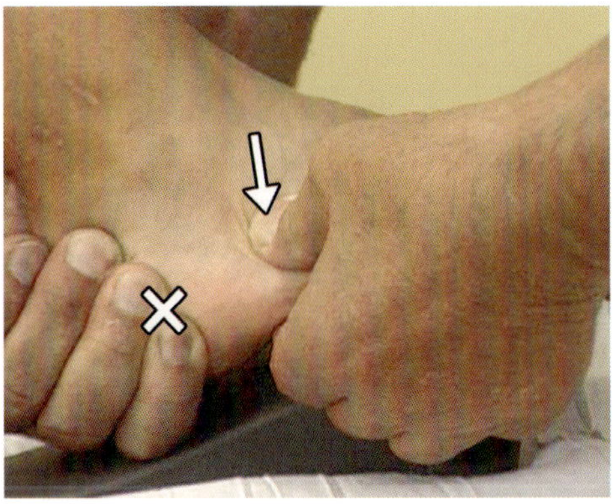

Figure 53a – test and mobilization in resting position

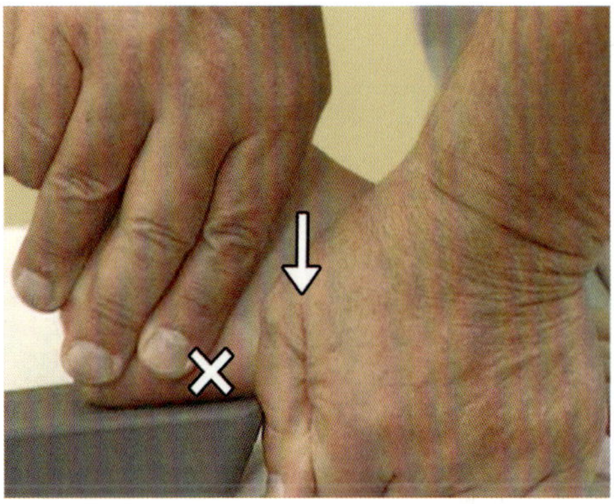

Figure 53b – mobilization in resting position

Foot

■ Figure 53a: Test and mobilization in resting position

Objective

- To evaluate the quantity and quality of plantar glide joint play of the cuboid in relation to the calcaneus, including end-feel.
- To increase mid-foot mobility.

Starting position

- The tibial-plantar side of the patient's foot rests on the treatment wedge.
- Position the joint in its resting position.

Hand placement and fixation

- **Therapist's stable hand (right):** Fixate the patient's calcaneus against the treatment wedge.
- **Therapist's moving hand (left):** Hold the patient's forefoot; grip the cuboid with your fingers.

Procedure

- Apply a Grade II or III plantar glide movement to the cuboid.

■ Figure 53b: Mobilization in resting position

- Use your right hand to fixate the patient's calcaneus on a wedge with the cuboid extending just past the edge.
- Grip the cuboid with your left hand, with your thenar eminence and fingers.
- Apply a Grade III plantar glide movement by leaning your body over your extended arm.

Calcaneus-talus distal traction

for pain and hypomobility

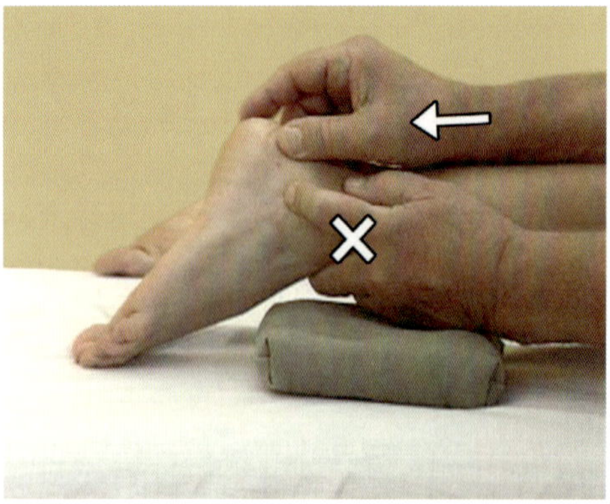

Figure 54a – test and mobilization in resting position

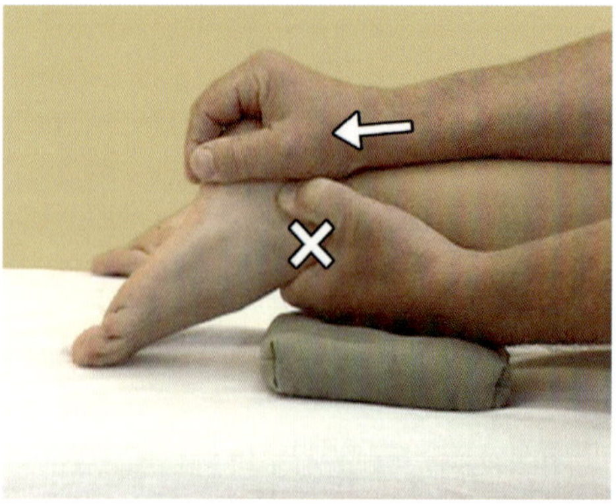

Figure 54b – mobilization in resting position

■ Figure 54a: Test and mobilization in resting position

Objective

- To evaluate the quantity and quality of distal traction joint play of the calcaneus in relation to the talus, including end-feel.
- To decrease pain or increase foot inversion or eversion range-of-motion.

Starting position

- The anterior side of the patient's leg and the dorsal side of the foot rests on the treatment surface.
- Position the subtalar joint in its resting position.

Hand placement and fixation

- **Therapist's stable hand (left):** Hold the patient's distal leg against the treatment surface; place your palpating finger in the joint space.
- **Therapist's moving hand (right):** Grip the patient's calcaneus with your fingers, rest your forearm on the patient's leg.

Procedure

- Apply a Grade I, II, or III distal traction movement to the calcaneus parallel to the long axis of the leg.

■ Figure 54b: Mobilization in resting position

- Hold the patient's distal leg with your left hand; grip around the talus from the ventral side.
- Apply a Grade III distal traction movement to the calcaneus in relation to the talus.
- Suitable for early training in manipulative thrust techniques.

Calcaneus-talus distal glide

for hypomobility

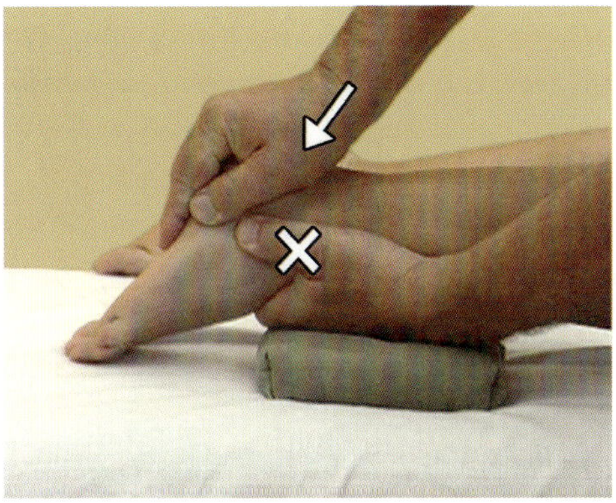

Figure 54c – test and mobilization in resting position

■ Figure 54c: Test and mobilization in resting position

Objective

- To evaluate the quantity and quality of distal glide joint play of the calcaneus in relation to the talus, including end-feel.
- To increase foot inversion and eversion.

Starting position

- The anterior side of the patient's leg and the dorsal side of the foot rests on the treatment surface.
- Position the subtalar joint in its resting position.

Hand placement and fixation

- **Therapist's stable hand (left):** Hold the patient's distal leg with your left hand; grip around the talus from the ventral side; place your palpating finger in the joint space.
- **Therapist's moving hand (right):** Grip the patient's calcaneus with your thenar eminence and fingers; position your forearm parallel to the sole of the foot.

Procedure

- Apply a Grade II or III distal glide movement to the calcaneus, parallel to the sole of the foot towards the toes.

■ Calcaneus-talus proximal glide (not shown)

- Reverse your grip to apply a Grade II or III proximal glide movement to the calcaneus away from the toes.

Calcaneus-talus tibial glide

for hypomobility

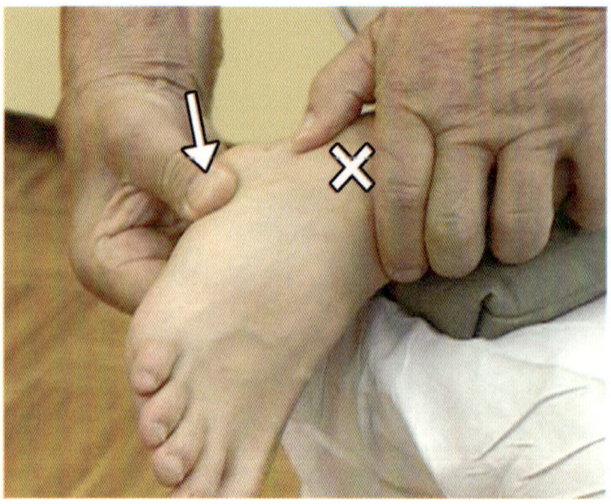

Figure 55a – test and mobilization in resting position

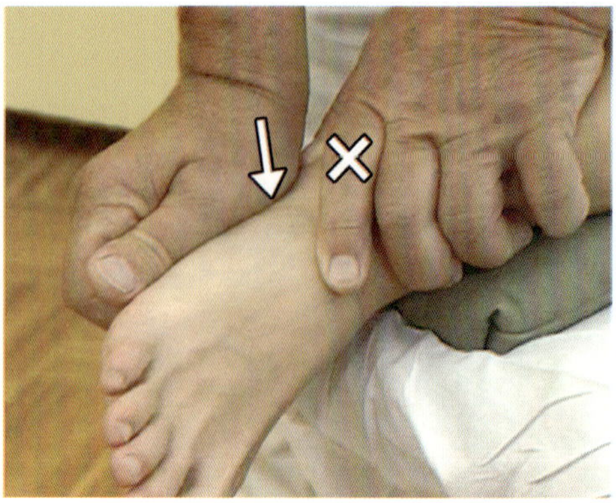

Figure 55b – mobilization in resting position

Foot

■ Figure 55a: Test and mobilization in resting position

Objective

- To evaluate the quantity and quality of tibial glide joint play in the anterior part of the talocalcaneal joint, including end-feel.
- To increase foot inversion range-of-motion (Concave Rule).

Starting position

- The tibial side of the patient's leg rests on the treatment surface.
- Position the subtalar joint in its resting position.

Hand placement and fixation

- **Therapist's stable hand (left):** Hold the patient's distal leg with your left hand; grip around the talus; place your palpating finger in the joint space.
- **Therapist's moving hand (right):** Grip the distal aspect of the patient's calcaneus with your fingers.

Procedure

- Apply a Grade II or III tibial glide movement to the calcaneus.

Note

- Use the same procedure to test tibial glide movement in the posterior part of the talocalcaneal joint. Restricted tibial glide joint play in the posterior part of the talocalcaneal joint is associated with restricted eversion (Convex Rule).

■ Figure 55b: Mobilization in resting position

- Hold the patient's distal leg with your left hand; grip around the calcaneus with your thenar eminence and fingers on the fibular side of the calcaneus.
- Apply a Grade III tibial glide movement to the calcaneus by leaning your body through your extended arm.

Calcaneus-talus fibular glide

for hypomobility

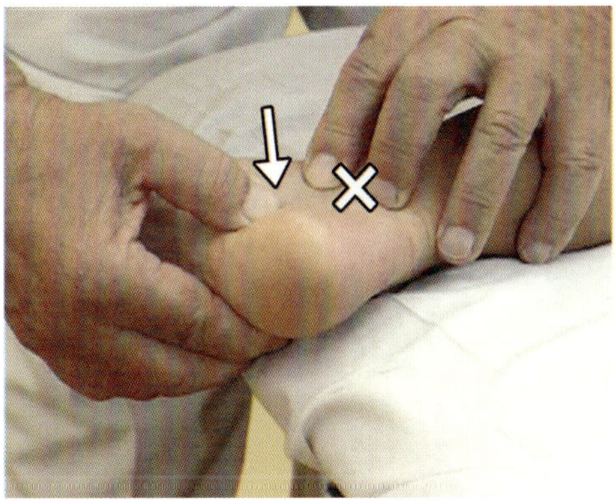
Figure 55c – test and mobilization in resting position

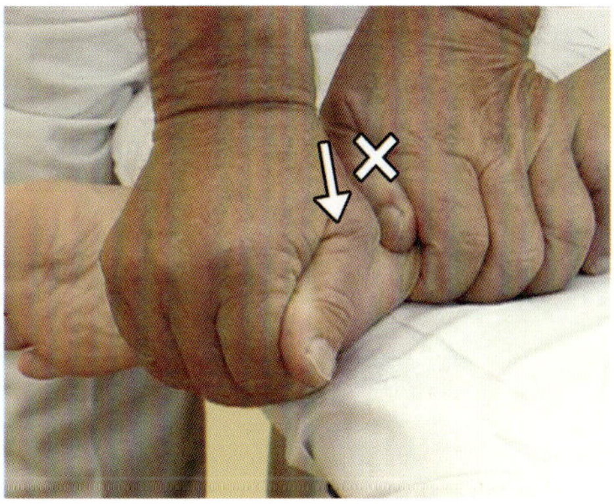
Figure 55d – mobilization in resting position

■ Figure 55c: Test and mobilization in resting position

Objective

- To evaluate the quantity and quality of fibular glide joint play in the posterior part of the talocalcaneal joint, including end-feel.
- To increase foot inversion range-of-motion (Convex Rule).

Starting position

- The fibular side of the patient's leg rests on the treatment surface.
- Position the subtalar joint in its resting position.

Hand placement and fixation

- **Therapist's stable hand (left):** Hold the patient's distal leg with your left hand; grip around the talus; place your palpating finger in the joint space.
- **Therapist's moving hand (right):** Grip the distal aspect of the patient's calcaneus with your fingers.

Procedure

- Apply a Grade II or III fibular glide movement to the calcaneus.

Note

- Use the same procedure to test fibular glide movement in the anterior part of the talocalcaneal joint. Restricted fibular glide movement in the anterior part of the talocalcaneal joint is associated with restricted eversion (Concave Rule).

■ Figure 55d: Mobilization in resting position

- Grip around the talus with your fingers.
- Apply a Grade III fibular glide movement to the calcaneus by leaning your body through your extended arm.

Talocrural traction
for pain and hypomobility

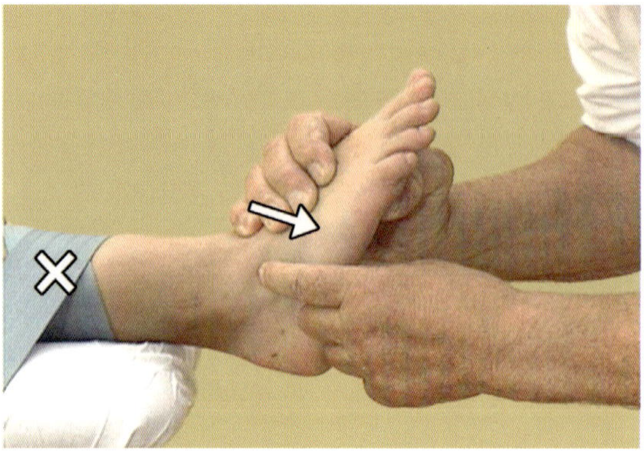

Figure 56a – test and mobilization in resting position

■ Figure 56a: Test and mobilization in resting position

Objective

- To evaluate the quantity and quality of distal traction joint play between the talus and tibia/fibula, including end-feel.
- To decrease pain or increase foot dorsal and plantar flexion range-of-motion.

Starting position

- The posterior side of the patient's leg rests on the treatment surface with the foot extended beyond the edge.
- Position the talocrural joint in its resting position.

Hand placement and fixation

- **Fixation**: Fixate the distal leg against the treatment surface with a strap.
- **Therapist's stable hand (left):** Place your palpating finger in the joint space.
- **Therapist's moving hand (right):** Grip the patient's midfoot from the tibial side with your little finger over the dorsal talus; position your forearm in line with the patient's leg.

Procedure

- Apply a Grade I, II, or III distal traction movement to the talus, parallel to the line of the leg.

Talocrural traction
for hypomobility (cont'd)

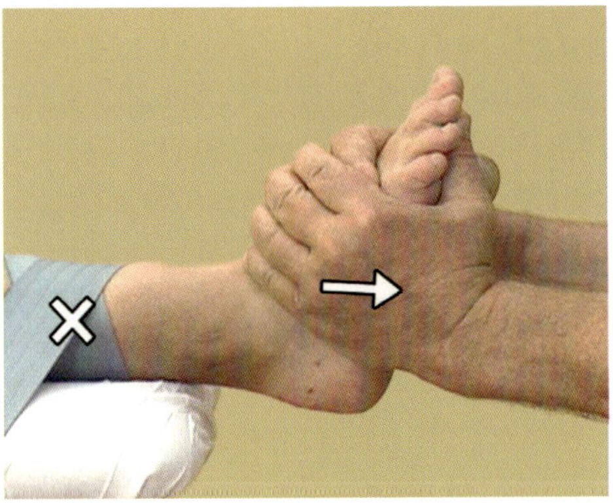

Figure 56b – mobilization in resting position

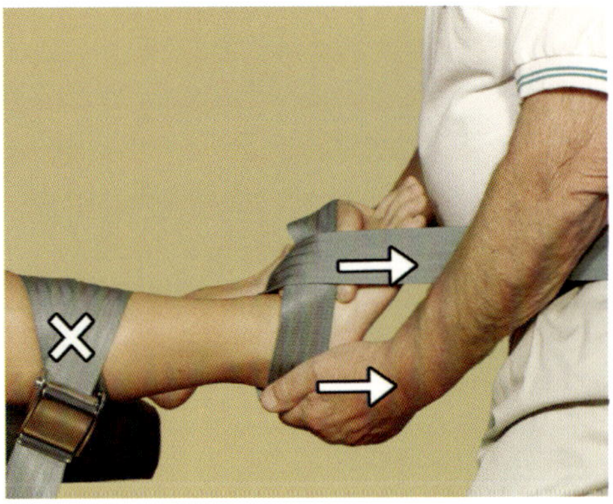

Figure 56c – mobilization in resting position

Figure 56b: Mobilization in resting position

Objective

- To decrease pain or increase range-of-motion between the talus and tibia/fibula.

Starting position

- The posterior side of the patient's leg rests on the treatment surface with the foot extended beyond the edge.
- Position the talocrural joint in its resting position.

Hand placement and fixation

- **Fixation**: Fixate the distal leg against the treatment surface with a strap.
- **Therapist's moving hand (right):** Grip the patient's midfoot from the tibial side with your little finger over the dorsal talus; position your forearm in line with the patient's leg; supplement your grip with your left hand.

Procedure

- Apply a Grade III distal traction movement to the talus parallel to the line of the leg. Take up the slack by shifting your body weight backward. Apply the mobilization by leaning back further and/or pulling with your arms.
- Suitable for early training in manipulative thrust techniques. Take up the slack with your body and apply the thrust with your arms.

Figure 56c: Alternate mobilization technique in resting position

- For Grade III traction treatment of longer durations, use a mobilization strap. By attaching the mobilization strap with the "figure-8" positioned on the anterior, posterior, medial, or lateral aspect of the ankle, you can alter the effect of the mobilization.
- Suitable for early training in manipulative thrust techniques. Take up the slack with your body and apply the thrust with your arms.

Talocrural anterior glide
for restricted plantar flexion

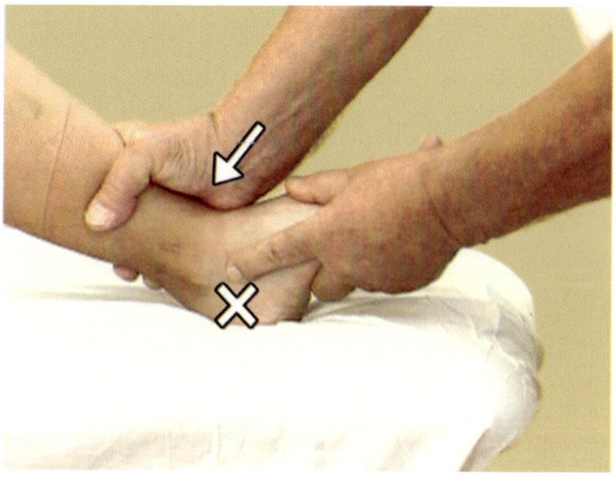

Figure 57a – test and mobilization in resting position

■ Figure 57a: Test and mobilization in resting position

Objective

- To evaluate the quantity and quality of anterior glide joint play of the talus in relation to the tibia/fibula.
- To increase foot plantar flexion range-of-motion (Convex Rule).

Starting position

- The patient's heel rests on the treatment surface with a bent knee.
- Position the talocrural joint in its resting position.

Hand placement and fixation

- **Fixation**: The calcaneus and, indirectly, the talus are fixated against the table.
- **Therapist's stable hand (left):** Hold the patient's foot with your hand; place your palpating finger in the joint space.
- **Therapist's moving hand (right):** Grip the distal aspect of the patient's lower leg with the heel of your hand just proximal to the joint space.

Procedure

- Apply a Grade II or III dorsal glide movement to the tibia/fibula to produce a relative anterior glide movement of the talus.

Talocrural anterior glide
for restricted plantar flexion (cont'd)

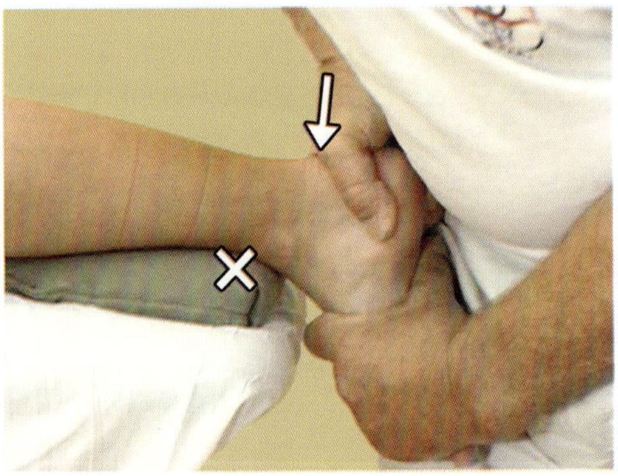

Figure 57b – mobilization in resting position

Foot

- **Figure 57b Mobilization in resting position**
  - The patient's anterior leg rests on the treatment surface or sandbag with the foot extended beyond the edge. Position the talocrural joint in its resting position.
  - Grip the mid-foot from the tibial side with your left index finger around the dorsal talus; maintain a Grade I distal traction.
  - Grip around the dorsal calcaneus with your right hand; position your forearm in line with the treatment plane. Your left hand holds around the patient's midfoot.
  - Apply a Grade III anterior glide movement to the talus by leaning your body over your extended arms and by bending your knees.
- **Plantar progression (not shown)**
  - Position the foot near its end range-of-motion into plantar flexion.
  - Apply a Grade III anterior glide movement to the talus (Convex Rule)

Foot

Talocrural anterior glide

for restricted plantar flexion (cont'd)

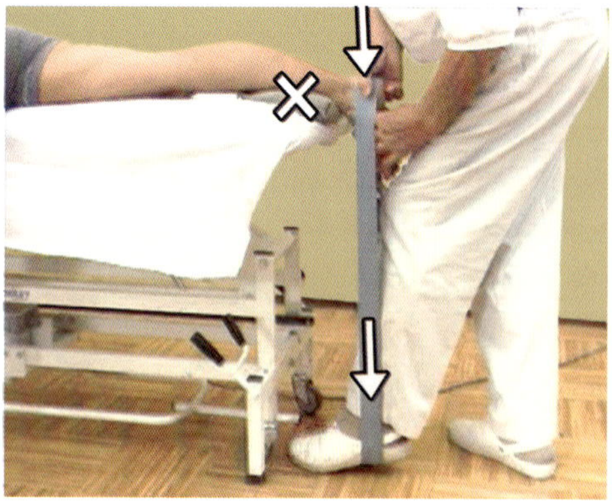

Figure 58a – mobilization in resting position

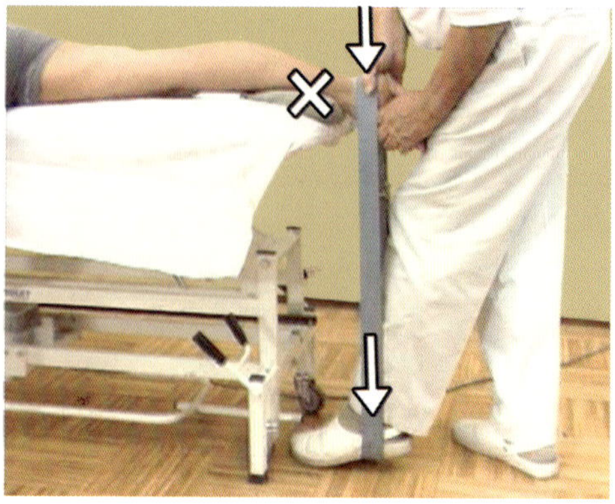

Figure 58b – mobilization in plantar flexion

■ Figure 58a: Mobilization in resting position

Objective

- To increase plantar flexion by increasing anterior glide of the talus on the tibia/ fibula (Convex Rule).

Starting position

- The anterior side of the patient's leg rests on the treatment surface or sandbag with the foot extended over the edge.
- Position the talocrural joint in its resting position.

Hand placement and fixation

- **Fixation**: The distal tibia and fibula are fixated against the treatment surface.
- **Therapist's moving hands:** With your left hand, grip the patient's midfoot from the tibial side with your index finger over the dorsal talus; with your right hand, grip around the posterior talus; position your right forearm in line with the treatment plane; maintain a Grade I distal traction.

Procedure

- Apply a Grade III anterior glide movement to the talus. For treatment of longer duration, use a traction strap: your heel applies the gliding force while your hands guide the movement.

■ Figure 58b: Plantar flexion progression

- Position the ankle near the end range-of-motion into plantar flexion.
- Apply a Grade III anterior glide movement to the talus (Convex Rule).

Talocrural posterior glide
for restricted dorsal flexion

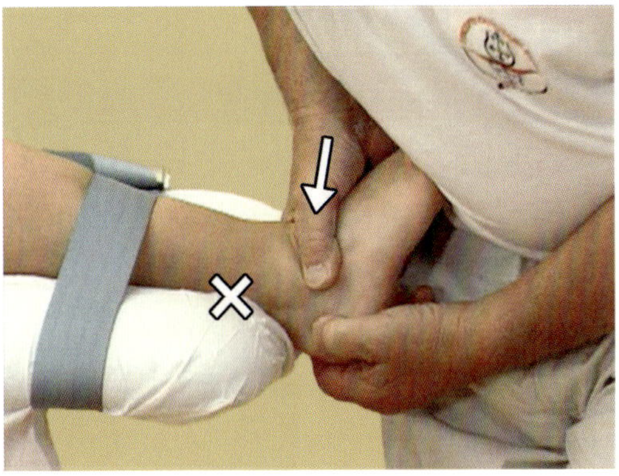

Figure 59a – Mobilization in resting position

Foot

■ Figure 59a: Mobilization in resting position

Objective

- To increase dorsal flexion by increasing dorsal glide of the talus on the tibia/fibula (Convex Rule).

Starting position

- The posterior side of the patient's leg rests on the treatment surface or wedge with the foot extended beyond the edge.
- Position the talocrural joint in its resting position.

Hand placement and fixation

- **Fixation**: Fixate the distal leg against the treatment surface with a strap.
- **Therapist's moving hands:** With your left hand, grip around the talus and calcaneus from the fibular side; with your right hand, grip around the anterior talus and forefoot; position your right forearm in line with the treatment plane; maintain a Grade I distal traction.

Procedure

- Apply a Grade III posterior glide movement to the talus.

■ Dorsal flexion progression (not shown)

- Position the ankle near the end range-of-motion into dorsal flexion.

Talocrural posterior glide

for restricted dorsal flexion (cont'd)

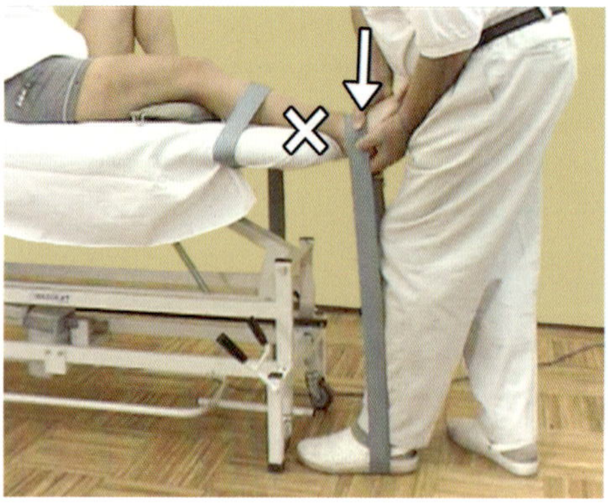

Figure 59b – mobilization in resting position

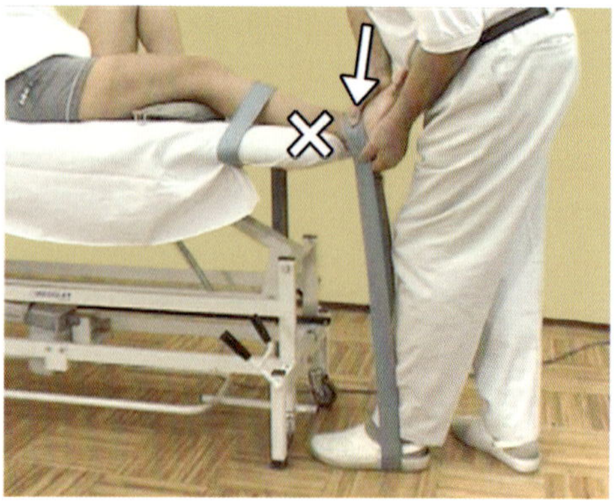

Figure 59c – mobilization in dorsal flexion

■ Figure 59b: Mobilization in resting position, alternate technique

Objective

- To increase foot dorsal flexion (Convex Rule).

Starting position

- The posterior side of the patient's leg rests on the treatment surface or sandbag with the foot extended over the edge.
- Position the talocrural joint in its resting position.

Hand placement and fixation

- **Fixation**: The distal tibia and fibula are fixated against the treatment surface.
- **Therapist's moving hands:** With your right hand, grip the patient's midfoot from the tibial side with your web space over the dorsal talus; with your left hand, grip around the posterior talus; position your right forearm in line with the treatment plane; maintain a Grade I distal traction.

Procedure

- Apply a Grade III dorsal glide movement to the talus. For treatment of longer duration, use a traction strap: your heel applies the gliding force while your hands guide the movement.

■ Figure 59c: Dorsal flexion progression, alternate technique

- Position the ankle near the end range-of-motion into dorsal flexion.
- Apply a Grade III posterior glide movement to the talus.

CHAPTER 18

LEG

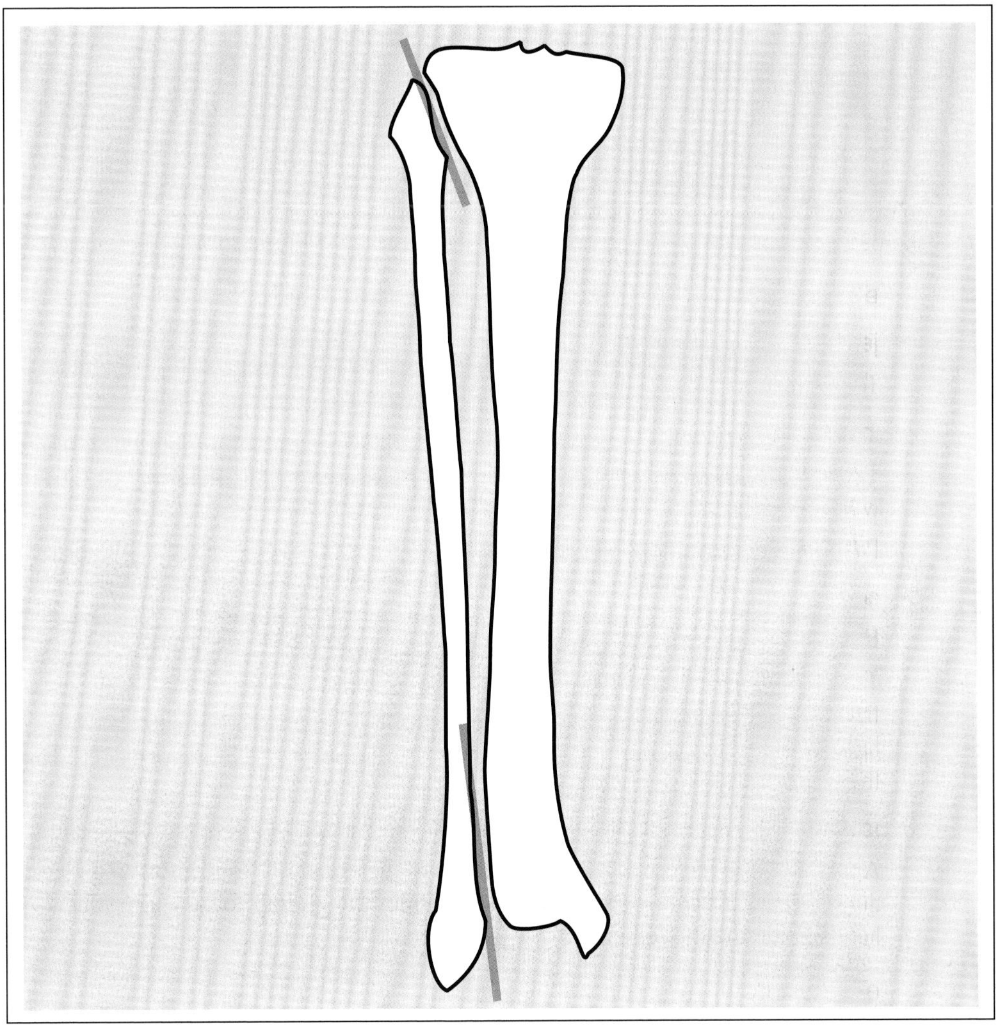

Leg

18 Leg

(crus)

Functional anatomy and movement

The leg consists of the tibia and fibula with the crural interosseous membrane.

Distal tibiofibular syndesmosis
(syndesmosis tibiofibularis distalis)

The distal tibiofibular syndesmosis has little movement.

"Long" syndesmosis
(syndesmosis tibiofibularis)

The "long" syndesmosis extends along the interosseous borders of the tibia and fibula with the interosseous membrane, and allows slight movement of the fibula in relation to the tibia.

Proximal tibiofibular joint
(art. tibiofibularis)

The proximal tibiofibular joint is an anatomically simple and mechanically compound joint and may communicate with the knee joint via the subpopliteal recess. According to MacConaill, the proximal tibiofibular joint is a sellar joint when it is considered as a functional unit with the distal syndesmosis.

Bony palpation

- Proximal end of the fibula (head of fibula)
- Proximal tibiofibular joint space
- Distal end of the fibula (lateral malleolus)
- Medial malleolus

Ligaments

Distal tibiofibular:

- Tibiofibular (anterior and posterior) ligaments
- Talofibular (anterior and posterior) ligaments

Proximal tibiofibular:

- Anterior and posterior ligaments

Bone movement and axes

Isolated active movements of the fibula do not take place. However, movement of the fibula does take place with foot and ankle movements.

- **Inversion of the foot:** The head of the fibula glides distally and slightly dorsally. This movement is considered to be lateral rotation by some authors.
- **Eversion of the foot:** The head of the fibula glides proximally and slightly ventrally (medial rotation).
- **Dorsal flexion of the ankle:** The fibula glides slightly proximally.
- **Plantar flexion of the ankle:** The fibula glides slightly distally.

End feel

- Firm

Joint movement (gliding)

- *Proximal tibiofibular joint:* Concave Rule — The articular surface of the head of the fibula is concave, while the articular surface of the tibial condyle is convex.

Treatment plane

- *Proximal tibiofibular joint:* on the concave joint surface of the head of the fibula

Zero position

- Same as for knee, foot and ankle

Resting position

- Approximately 10° ankle plantar flexion

Close-packed position

- Maximal dorsal flexion in the ankle joint

Leg examination scheme

(Refer to Chapters 3 and 4 for more information on examination)

Tests of function

1. **Active and passive movements, including stability tests and end-feel**
2. **Translatoric joint play movements, including end-feel**

   Gliding

   Distal tibiofibular syndesmosis (Figure 60a)

   Posterior-anterior glide of the lateral malleolus

   Proximal tibiofibular joint

   Anterior glide of the fibular head (Figure 61a)

   Posterior glide of the fibular head (Figure 61c)
3. **Resisted movements**

   (see Ankle examination scheme and Knee examination scheme)
4. **Passive soft tissue movements**

   Physiological

   Accessory
5. **Additional tests**

Trial treatment

Distal tibiofibular syndesmosis (Figure 60b)

Proximal tibiofibular joint (Figure 61b)

Leg

Leg techniques

Distal tibiofibular joint

Figure 60a,b Fibula posterior glide for hypomobility

Proximal tibiofibular joint

Figure 61a,b Fibula anterior glide for hypomobility

Figure 61c,d Fibula posterior glide test and mobilization

Leg

Distal fibula posterior glide
for hypomobility

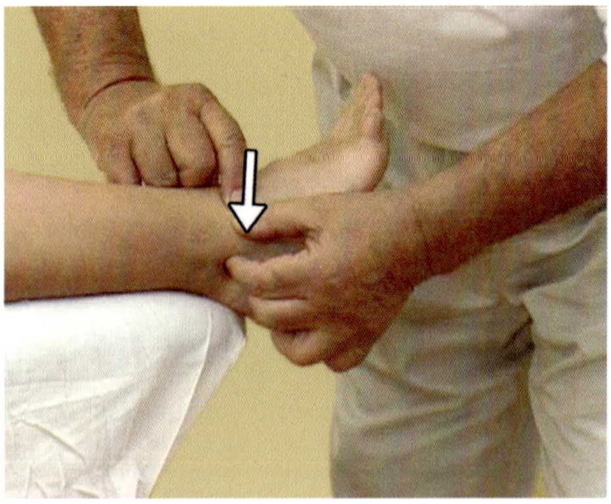

Figure 60a – test and mobilization in resting position

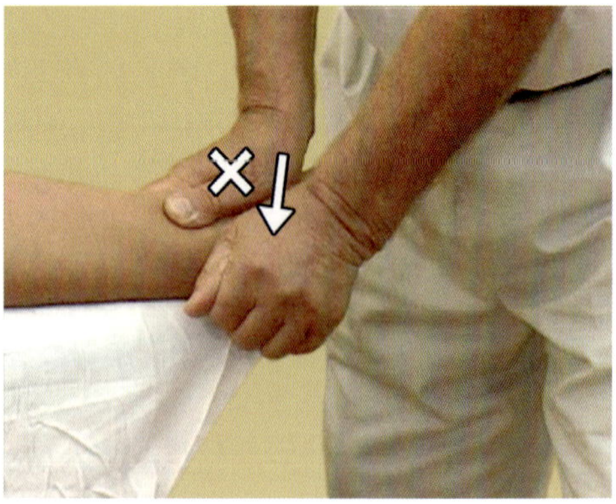

Figure 60b – mobilization in resting position

■ Figure 60a: Test and mobilization in resting position

Objective

- To evaluate the quantity and quality of posterior glide joint play in the tibiofibular syndesmosis, including end-feel.
- To increase tibiofibular mobility.

Starting position

- The posterior side of the patient's leg rests on the treatment surface, with the ankle off the edge in the resting position.

Hand placement and fixation

- **Fixation and therapist's stable hand (right):** The patient's tibia is fixated by the treatment surface; place your palpating finger in the joint space.
- **Therapist's moving hand (left):** Grip around the patient's lateral malleolus with your fingers and thumb.

Procedure

- Press the patient's lateral malleolus in a dorsal direction to apply a Grade II or III posterior glide movement to the fibula.

■ Figure 60b: Mobilization in resting position

- Apply a Grade III posterior glide movement to the fibula.
- Adapt the same procedure with the patient in prone for restricted fibular anterior glide.

Proximal fibula anterior glide

for hypomobility

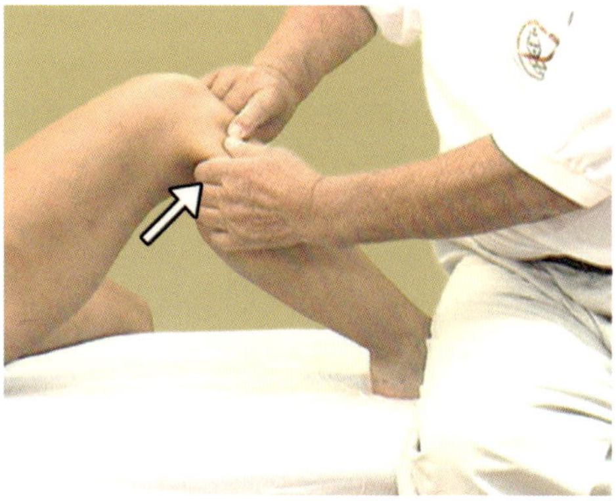

Figure 61a – test and mobilization in resting position

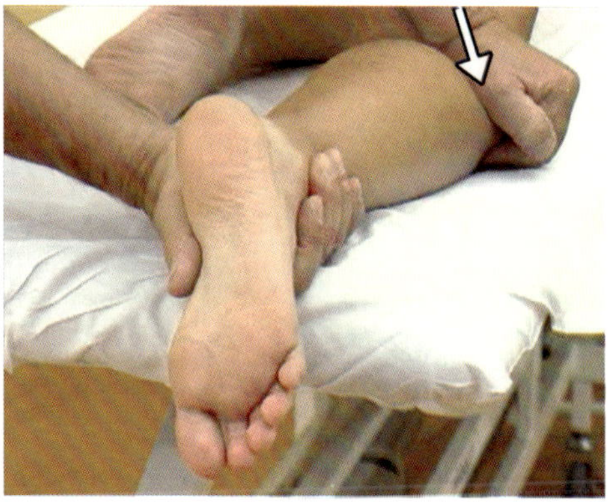

Figure 61b – mobilization in resting position

■ Figure 61a: Test and mobilization in resting position

Objective

- To evaluate the quantity and quality of anterior glide joint play in the proximal tibiofibular joint, including end-feel.
- To increase knee and ankle mobility.

Starting position

- The patient lies supine with the knee flexed.

Hand placement and fixation

- **Fixation and therapist's stable hand (right):** Hold around the patient's proximal tibia; enhance fixation of the tibia by sitting on the patient's foot.
- **Therapist's moving hand (left):** Grip around the patient's fibular head with your fingers and thumb.

Procedure

- Pull the fibular head in an anterior-lateral direction to apply a Grade II or III anterior glide movement in line with the treatment plane.

■ Figure 61b: Mobilization in resting position

- The patient is on their hands and knees with their foot over the end of the treatment surface; with your right hand, grip around the distal tibia; with your left hand and fingers; grip around the fibular head and apply a Grade III anterior-lateral glide movement.
- Be careful to avoid pressure on the fibular nerve.

Proximal fibula posterior glide

test and mobilization

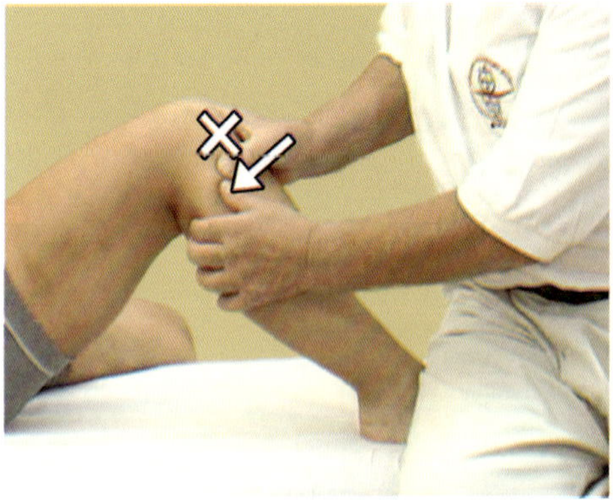

Figure 61c – test and mobilization in resting position

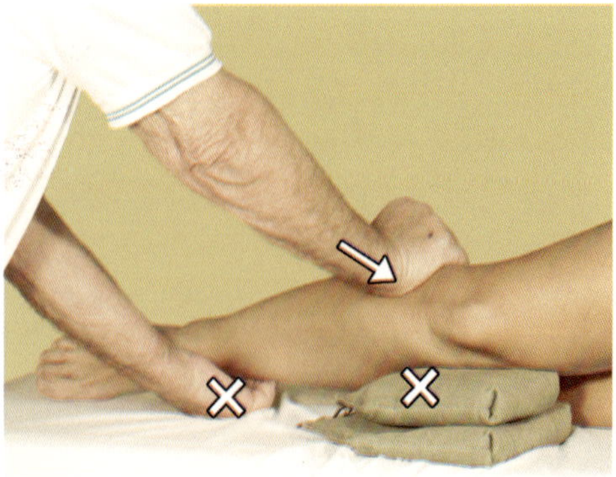

Figure 61d – mobilization in resting position

■ Figure 61c: Test and mobilization in resting position

Objective

- To evaluate the quantity and quality of posterior glide joint play in the proximal tibiofibular joint, including end-feel.
- To increase knee and ankle mobility.

Starting position

- The patient lies supine with the knee flexed.

Hand placement and fixation

- **Fixation and therapist's stable hand (right):** Hold around the patient's proximal tibia; enhance fixation of the tibia by sitting on the patient's foot.
- **Therapist's moving hand (left):** Grip around the patient's fibular head with your fingers and thumb.

Procedure

- Push the fibular head in an posterior-medial direction to apply a Grade II or III posterior glide movement in line with the treatment plane.

■ Figure 61d: Mobilization in resting position

- The tibial side of the patient's leg rests on the treatment surface; with your left hand, fixate the distal tibia against the treatment surface; with your right hand, grip around the fibular head.
- Apply a Grade III posterior-medial glide movement in line with the treatment plane; be careful to avoid pressure on the fibular nerve.

CHAPTER 19

KNEE

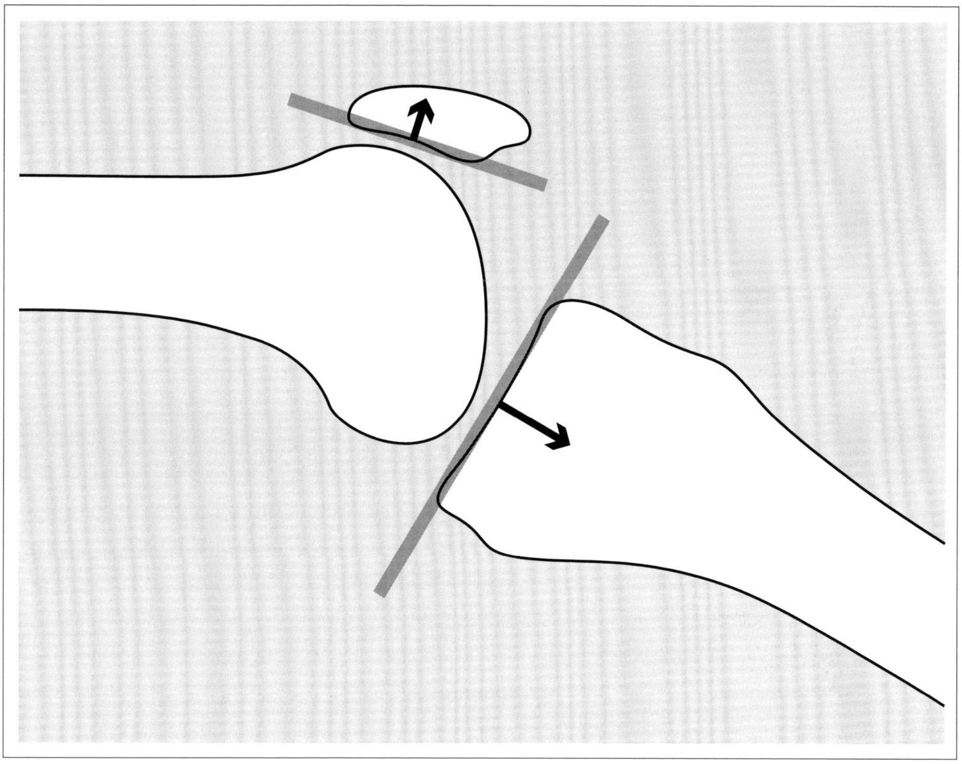

Knee

19 Knee

Functional anatomy and movement

Tibiofemoral joint
(art. genu)

The knee joint is an anatomically compound and mechanically simple biaxial joint (modified ovoid). It is mechanically compound when the tibiofibular joint is included. The distal end of the femur (convex surface) has two facets (medial and lateral condyles) for the menisci (semilunar cartilages). The proximal end of the tibia has two concave joint surfaces, separated by the intercondylar eminence for articulation with the menisci.

Patellofemoral joint

The distal end of the femur also has a convex facet for articulation with the concave patella.

Bony palpation

Anterior
- Femur
- Patella
- Knee joint space and menisci
- Tibial tuberosity
- Iliotibial tubercle

Medial
- Tibial plateau
- Medial femoral condyle
- Knee joint space
- Adductor tubercle

Lateral
- Lateral tibial plateau
- Lateral femoral condyle
- Knee joint space
- Fibular head

Posterior
- Medial femoral condyle
- Lateral femoral condyle
- Fibular head

Ligaments

- Anterior and posterior cruciate ligaments (intra-articular)
- Tibial collateral ligament (also, attaches to the medial meniscus and joint capsule)
- Fibular collateral ligament (attaches to the lateral part of the fibular head; not attached to the lateral meniscus or joint capsule)
- Patellar ligament (patellar tendon)
- Transverse ligament
- Meniscotibial (coronary) ligaments (medial and lateral). The medial meniscotibial ligament extends from the medial meniscus to the proximal medial aspect of the tibia and also to the tibial collateral ligament. The lateral meniscotibial ligament extends from the lateral meniscus to the proximal lateral aspect of the tibia; it has a greater laxity than the medial meniscotibial ligament.

Bone movement and axes

Tibiofemoral joint:

- Flexion - extension: around a tibiofibular axis through the femoral condyles
- Internal - external rotation between the menisci and tibia: around a longitudinal axis through the medial intercondylar eminence. Rotation is greatest at 90° flexion.
- Abduction - adduction (passive lateral movement): around an anterior-posterior axis through the femur. Abduction and adduction are greatest at 30° flexion.

When the knee is in full extension, the collateral ligaments become taut. This provides stability to the knee in standing and limits rotation and lateral movements in the knee.

Patellofemoral joint:

- Proximal and distal gliding during knee flexion and extension

End feel

Tibiofemoral joint:

- Extension: firm
- Flexion: soft

Patellar-femoral joint

- Firm in all directions

Joint movement (gliding)

- Concave Rule

  During flexion and extension, a combined movement of rolling and gliding takes place between the femur and menisci. Simultaneously, the menisci are pushed slightly dorsally on the tibia during flexion and ventrally with extension.

  Isolated rotation can only occur in a normal knee when the knee is in some degree of flexion. During knee extension, the tibia rotates into external rotation.

  The patella glides proximally on the femur during knee extension due to the quadriceps femoris contraction.

Treatment plane

- *Tibiofemoral joint:* on the concave joint surface of the tibia
- *Patellofemoral joint:* on the concave posterior joint surface of the patella

Zero position

- The longitudinal axes passing through the femur and tibia meet in the frontal plane and form a laterally facing angle of approximately 170° (valgus).

Resting position

- 25° to 40° flexion

Close-packed position

- Maximal knee extension

Capsular pattern

- Flexion - extension: The proportion of these limitations is such that, with 90° of limited flexion, there is only 5° of limited extension.
- Rotation is limited only when there is marked limitation of both flexion and extension.

■ Knee examination scheme

(Refer to Chapters 3 and 4 for more information on examination)

Tests of function

1. Active and passive movements, including stability tests and end-feel

Flexion	160°
Extension from zero	5°
Lateral rotation at 90° knee flexion	45°
Medial rotation at 90° knee flexion	15°
Abduction (passive)	
Adduction (passive)	
Stability tests (passive)	(Figure 62a, b, c, d)
Meniscus tests (passive)	(Figure 63a, b, c, d)

2. Translatoric joint play movement, including end-feel

Traction - compression	(Figure 64a)
Gliding	
Posterior - anterior	(Figure 66a, b)
Lateral	(Figure 69)
Medial	(Figure 70)
Patella distal	(Figure 71a)

3. Resisted movements

	OTHER FUNCTIONS
Flexion	
Biceps femoris	Lateral rotation
Semitendinosus	Medial rotation
Semimembranosus	Medial rotation
Gastrocnemius	Ankle plantar flexion
Popliteus	Medial rotation
Extension	
Rectus femoris	Hip flexion
Vastus lateralis, medialis, intermedius	
Lateral Rotation	
Tensor fasciae latae	Extension
Biceps femoris	Flexion
Medial Rotation	
Sartorius	Flexion; hip lateral rotation
Gracilis	Flexion; hip medial rotation
Semitendinosus	Hip adduction, extension
Semimembranosus	Hip adduction, extension
Popliteus	Flexion

4. Passive soft tissue movements

Physiological

Accessory

5. Additional tests

Trial treatment

Traction (Figure 64b)

Knee

Knee techniques

Knee

Figure 62a,b	Lateral stability test
Figure 62c,d	Medial stability test
Figure 63a,b	Meniscus test in adduction
Figure 63c,d	Meniscus test in abduction
Figure 64a,b,c	Traction for pain and hypomobility
Figure 65a,b	Traction for hypomobility (alternate technique)
Figure 66a,b	Posterior and anterior glide test
Figure 66c,d	Posterior glide for restricted flexion
Figure 66e,f	Posterior glide for restricted flexion (supine)
Figure 67a,b	Posterior glide for restricted flexion (prone)
Figure 68a,b	Anterior glide for restricted extension
Figure 69	Lateral glide for restricted flexion and extension
Figure 70	Medial glide for restricted flexion and extension

Patella

Figure 71a,b	Distal glide
Figure 71c,d	Medial and lateral glide

Knee lateral stability
test

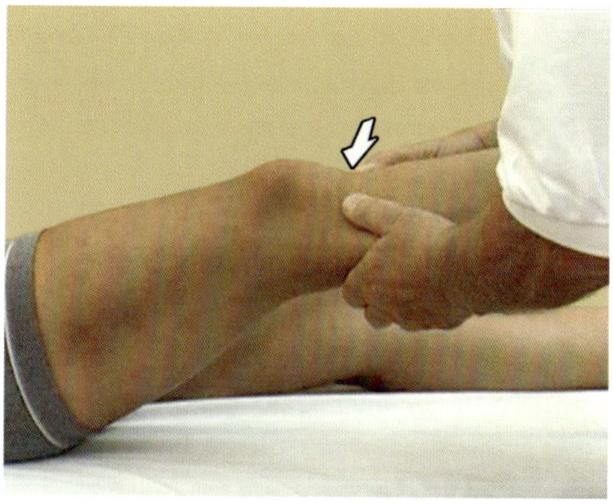

Figure 62a – stability test in slight flexion

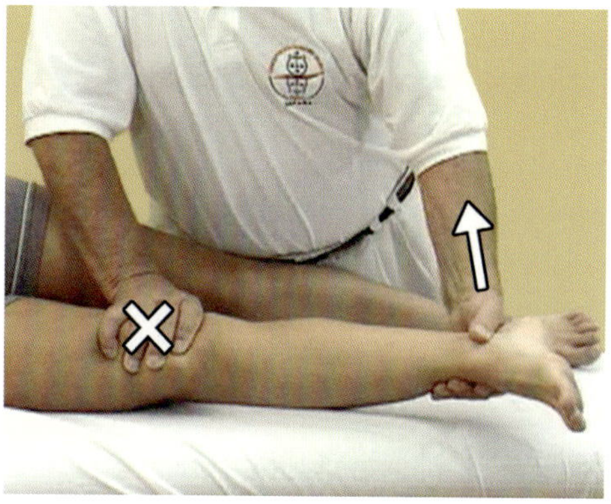

Figure 62b – stability test in zero position

■ Figure 62a: Stability test in slight flexion

Objective

- To test for ligamentous and capsular integrity in the lateral compartment of the knee.
- To evaluate the quantity and quality of lateral joint play in the knee, including hypermobility.

Starting position

- The patient is supine with the knee slightly flexed and the lower leg beyond the edge of the treatment surface.

Hand placement and fixation

- **Fixation:** Grip the patient's lower leg between your body and upper arm.
- **Therapist's moving hands:** Grip the patient's knee from both sides.

Procedure

- Apply a Grade II or III lateral movement to the knee; test for end-feel gently and with caution; the patient's thigh should move slightly during the test.

■ Figure 62b: Stability test in the zero position

- The lateral side of the patient's leg rests on the treatment surface; with your right hand, fixate the patient's extended knee against the treatment surface; with your left hand, grip the patient's distal leg and move it in a medial direction to produce lateral gapping. Tests ligamentous and capsular integrity in the lateral compartment of the knee.
- The stability test is normal if the end-feel is very firm (i.e., firm "+"), there is very little movement, and there is no pain.

Knee medial stability
test

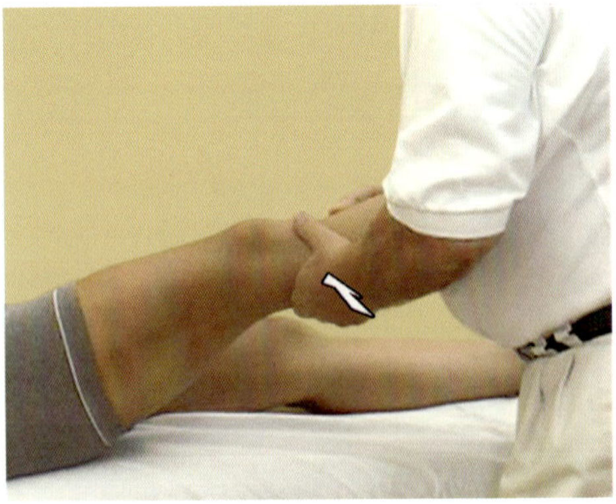

Figure 62c – stability test in slight flexion

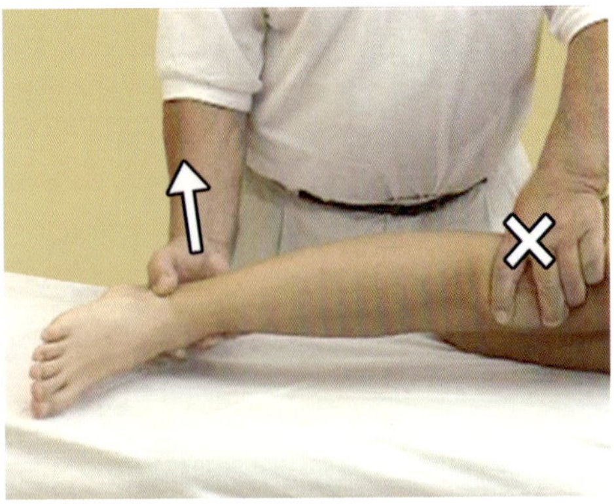

Figure 62d – stability test in zero position

■ Figure 62c: Stability test in slight flexion

Objective

- To test for ligamentous and capsular integrity in the medial compartment of the knee.
- To evaluate the quantity and quality of medial joint play in the knee, including hypermobility.

Starting position

- The patient is supine with the knee slightly flexed and the lower leg beyond the edge of the treatment surface.

Hand placement and fixation

- **Fixation:** Grip the patient's lower leg between your body and upper arm.
- **Therapist's moving hands:** Grip the patient's knee from both sides.

Procedure

- Apply a Grade II or III medial movement to the knee; test for end-feel gently and with caution; the patient's thigh should move slightly during the test.

■ Figure 62d: Stability test in the zero position

- The medial side of the patient's leg faces the treatment surface; with your left hand, fixate the patient's extended knee against the treatment surface; with your right hand, grip the patient's distal leg and move it in a lateral direction to produce medial gapping. Tests ligamentous and capsular integrity in the medial compartment of the knee.
- The stability test is normal if the end-feel is very firm (i.e., firm "+"), there is very little movement, and there is no pain.

Knee

Knee meniscus
test in adduction

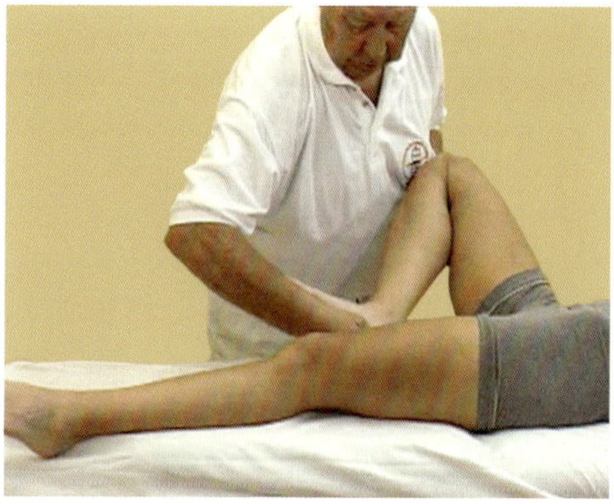

Figure 63a – meniscus test
in adduction/external rotation

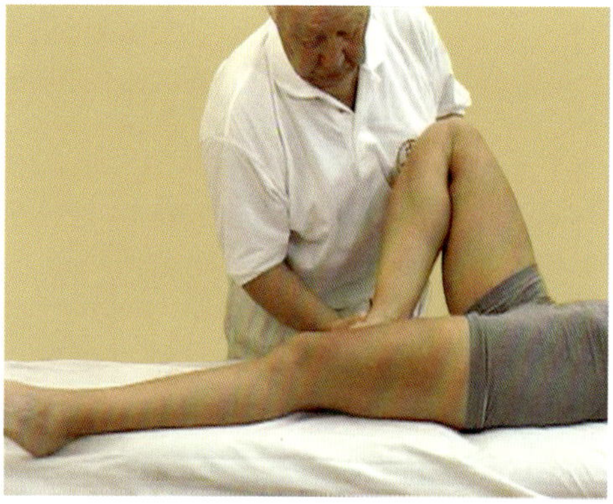

Figure 63b – meniscus test
in adduction/internal rotation

■ Figure 63a: Meniscus test in adduction/external rotation

Objective

- To test for integrity of the knee meniscus. The test is positive if there are joint noises (e.g., snapping, popping), restricted movement, or pain.

Starting position

- The patient is supine with the knee and hip in the resting position (not shown).

Hand placement and fixation

- **Therapist's hand placement:** With your left hand, grip the patient's knee from the anterior side to guide and control hip position; palpate in the medial joint space; with your right hand, grip the patient's foot.

Procedure

- Adduct and externally rotate the lower leg; gently maintain the adduction/ external rotation force while you move the knee into full flexion (pictured) and back again into full extension; the hip should not adduct nor abduct during the test.

Note

- With positive findings, refer the patient to an orthopedist for further examination.

■ Figure 63b: Meniscus test in adduction/internal rotation

- Adduct and internally rotate the lower leg; gently maintain the adduction/ internal rotation force while you move the knee into full flexion and back again into full extension.

Knee meniscus
test in abduction

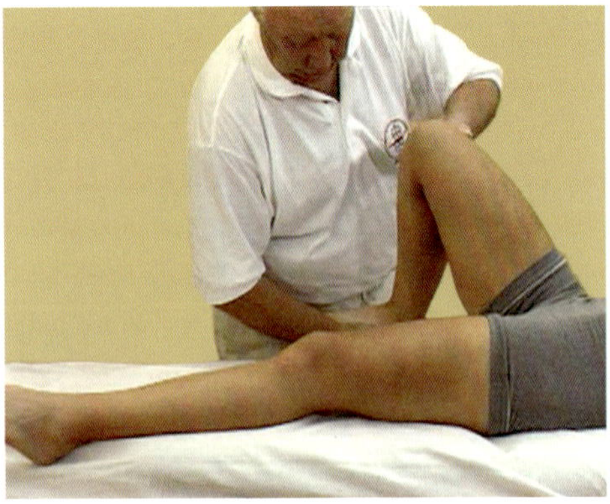

Figure 63c – meniscus test
in abduction/external rotation

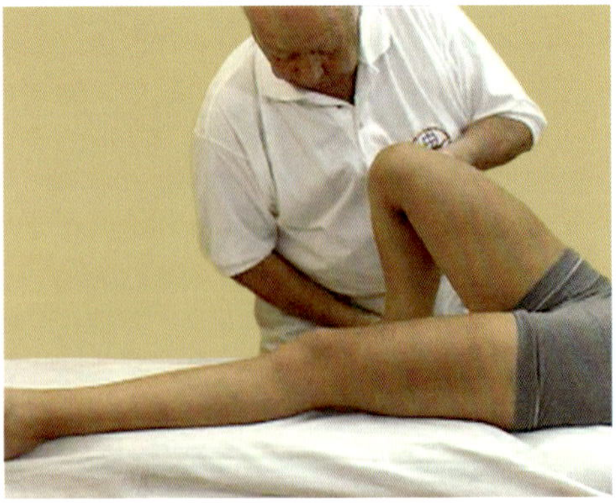

Figure 63d – meniscus test
in abduction/internal rotation

Knee

■ Figure 63c: Meniscus test in abduction/external rotation

Objective

- To test for integrity of the knee meniscus. The test is positive if there are joint noises (e.g., snapping, popping), restricted movement or pain.

Starting position

- The patient is supine with the knee and hip in the resting position (not shown).

Hand placement and fixation

- **Therapist's hand placement:** With your left hand, grip the patient's knee from the anterior side to guide and control hip position; palpate in the medial joint space, with your right hand, grip the patient's foot.

Procedure

- Abduct and externally rotate the lower leg; gently maintain the abduction/ external rotation force while you move the knee into full flexion (pictured) and back again into full extension; the hip should not adduct nor abduct during the test.

Note

- With positive findings, refer the patient to an orthopedist for further examination.

■ Figure 63d: Meniscus test in abduction/internal rotation

- Abduct and internally rotate the lower leg; gently maintain the abduction/ internal rotation force while you move the knee into full flexion and back again into full extension.

Knee traction
for pain and hypomobility

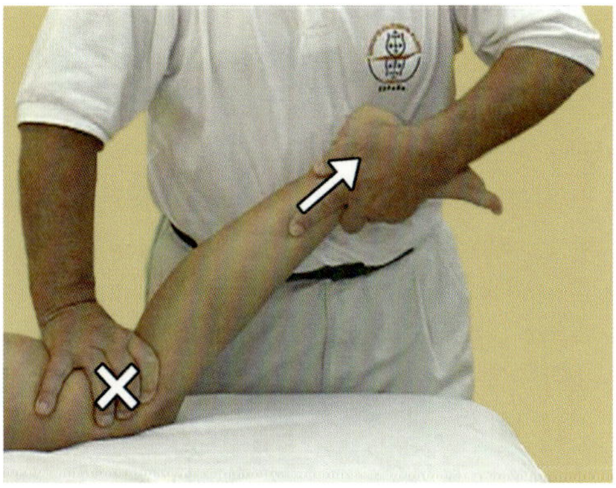

Figure 64a – test and mobilization in resting position

■ Figure 64a: Test and mobilization in resting position

Objective

- To evaluate the quantity and quality of traction joint play in the knee, including end-feel.
- To decrease pain or increase knee mobility.

Starting position

- The patient lies prone with the anterior side of the thigh on the treatment surface.
- Position the knee in its resting position.

Hand placement and fixation

- **Therapist's stable hand (right):** Fixate the patient's distal thigh against the treatment surface; place your palpating finger in the joint space.
- **Therapist's moving hand (left):** Grip the patient's leg above the ankle joint; position your forearm in line with the patient's lower leg.

Procedure

- Apply a Grade I, II, or III traction movement in line with the lower leg.
- Suitable for early training in manipulative thrust techniques.

Knee traction
for hypomobility

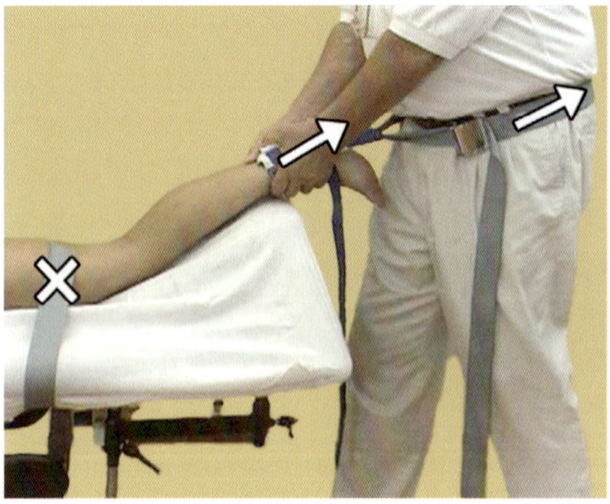

Figure 64b – mobilization in resting position

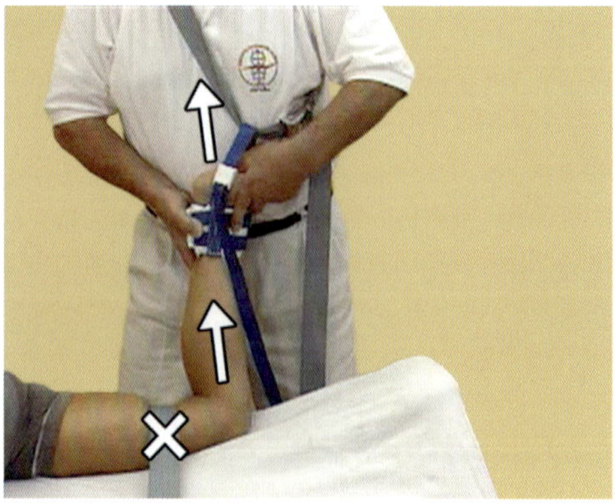

Figure 64c – mobilization in flexion

■ Figure 64b: Mobilization in resting position

Objective

- To increase knee mobility.

Starting position

- The patient lies prone with the anterior side of the thigh on the treatment surface.
- Position the knee in its resting position.

Hand placement and fixation

- **Fixation:** Fixate the patient's distal thigh against the treatment surface with a strap.
- **Therapist's moving hands:** Grip above the patient's ankle joint with both hands; for longer treatments, enhance your grip by using a traction cuff and/or a strap around your body and hands.

Procedure

- Apply a Grade III traction movement in line with the lower leg by shifting your body weight backward. Apply the mobilization by leaning back further and/or pulling with your arms.
- Suitable for early training in manipulative thrust techniques. Take up the slack with your body and apply the thrust with your arms.

■ Figure 64c: Flexion progression

- Position the joint near to its end range-of-motion in flexion; adapt the technique by positioning the traction strap over your shoulder.
- Apply a Grade III traction movement by extending your bent knees; palpate in the joint space.

Knee traction

for hypomobility (alternate technique)

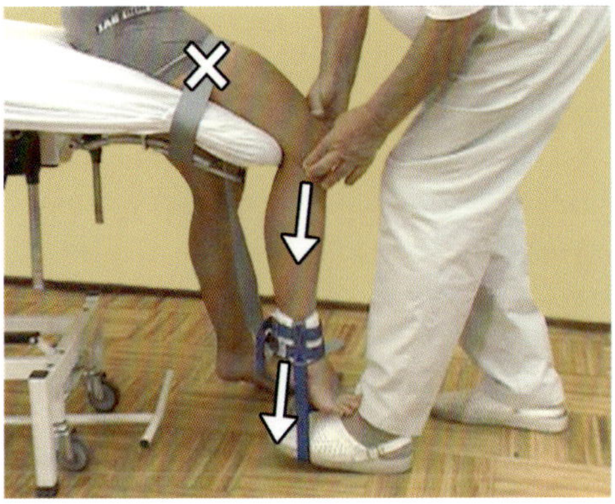

Figure 65a – mobilization in resting position

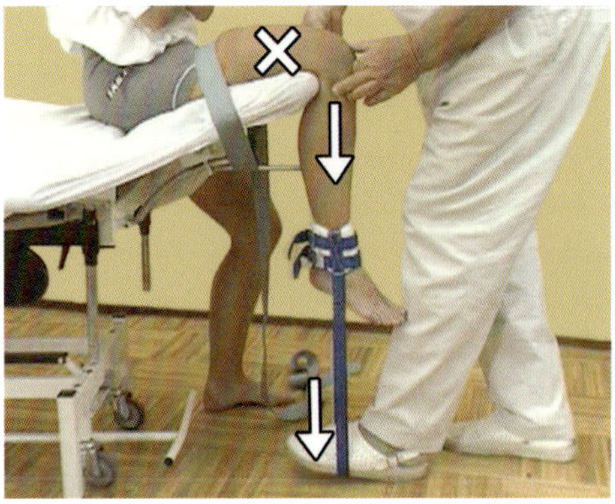

Figure 65b – mobilization in flexion

■ Figure 65a: Mobilization in resting position

Objective

- To increase knee mobility.

Starting position

- The patient sits on the treatment table with the knee over the edge.
- Position the knee in its resting position.

Hand placement and fixation

- **Fixation:** Fixate the patient's proximal thigh against the treatment surface with a strap; the patient's distal thigh is fixated by the edge of the treatment surface.
- **Therapist's moving hands:** Attach a traction strap above the patient's ankle with its stirrup adjusted just above the floor; put your foot in the stirrup.

Procedure

- Apply a Grade III traction movement in line with the lower leg by pressing the traction stirrup down with your foot; keep your heel on the floor; palpate in the joint space.

■ Figure 65b: Flexion progression

- Position the joint near to its end range-of-motion in flexion. Control the position of the knee by raising or lowering the end of the treatment table. Apply a Grade III traction movement to the lower leg.

Knee posterior and anterior glide
test

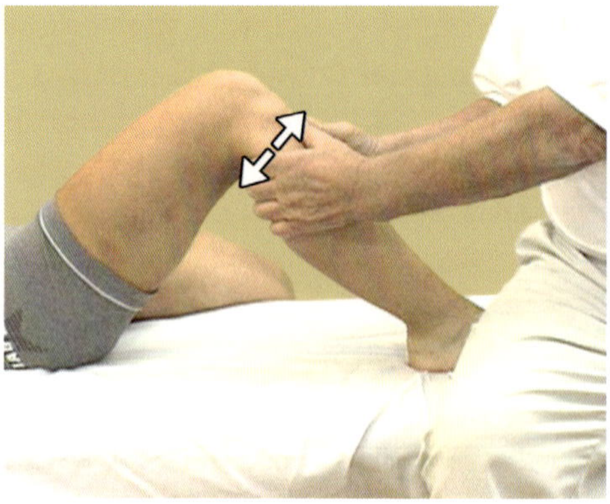

Figure 66a – test in mid-range-of-motion

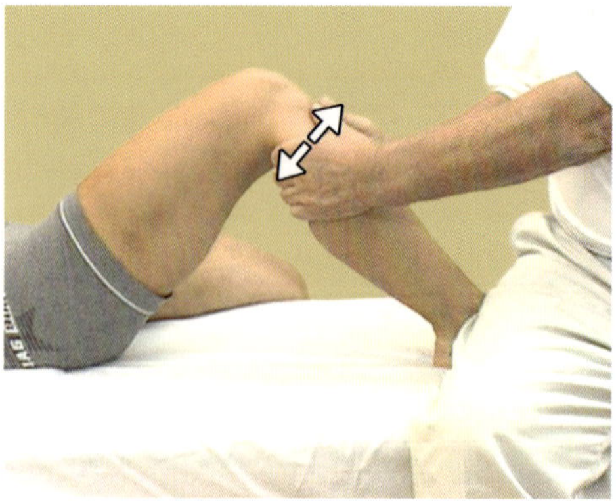

Figure 66b – test in internal rotation

■ Figure 66a: Test in mid-range-of-motion

Objective

- To evaluate the quantity and quality of posterior and anterior glide joint play in the knee, including end-feel. Restricted posterior glide is associated with restricted knee flexion; restricted anterior glide is associated with restricted knee extension.

Starting position

- The patient lies supine.
- Position the knee at about 90° flexion. This technique is difficult to perform with the patient's knee in the resting position.

Hand placement and fixation

- **Fixation:** No external fixation of the femur is necessary; the foot is fixated on the treatment surface by the weight of the patient's thigh; enhance fixation of the patient's foot by sitting on it.
- **Therapist's moving hands:** Grip below the patient's knee with both hands; you may palpate the joint space with your thumbs.

Procedure

- Apply a Grade II or III posterior or anterior glide movement to the tibia by leaning through your arms and shifting your body forward and backward.

■ Figure 66b: Test in internal rotation

- Position the joint close to its end range-of-motion in internal rotation.
- **Ligamentous stability test:** Posterior glide tests the posterior cruciate; anterior glide tests the anterior cruciate. With intact cruciate ligaments, range-of-motion into posterior and anterior glide is less with the lower leg internally rotated than when the leg is in a neutral position or externally rotated.

Knee posterior glide
for restricted flexion

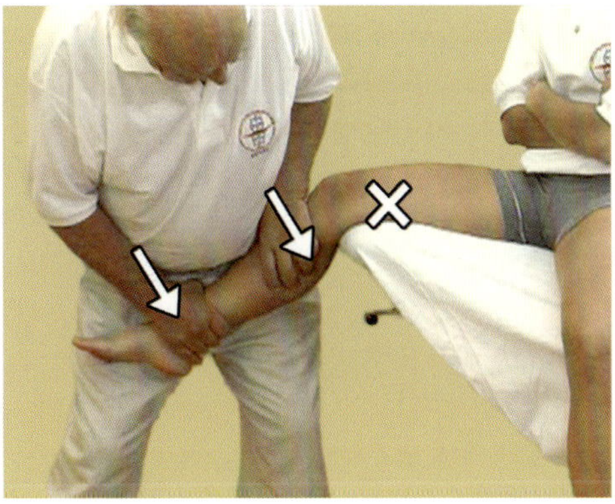

Figure 66c – mobilization in resting position, medial side

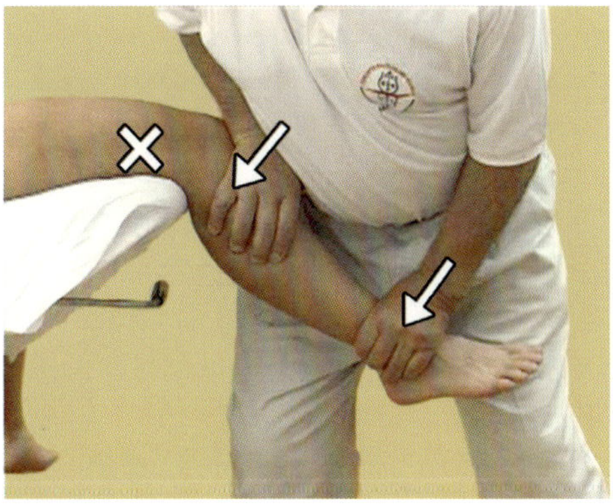

Figure 66d – mobilization in resting position, lateral side

■ Figure 66c: Mobilization in resting position, medial side

Objective

- To increase knee flexion (Concave Rule) and internal rotation range-of-motion.

Starting position

- The patient sits or lies with the lower leg over the edge of the treatment surface.
- Position the knee in its resting position.

Hand placement and fixation

- **Fixation:** The patient's thigh is fixated against the treatment surface.
- **Therapist's moving hands:** Hold the lower leg from the anterior-medial side with both hands; grip your right hand above the ankle and your left hand below the knee.

Procedure

- Apply a Grade III posterior glide movement to the medial tibia by leaning through your arms and bending your knees.

■ Figure 66d: Mobilization in resting position, lateral side

- Hold the lower leg from the anterior-lateral side.
- Apply a Grade III posterior glide movement to increase knee flexion (Concave Rule) and external rotation range-of-motion.

Note

- Knee mobilization is easier and more effective when treatment is directed specifically to the medial or lateral side.

Knee posterior glide

for restricted flexion (supine)

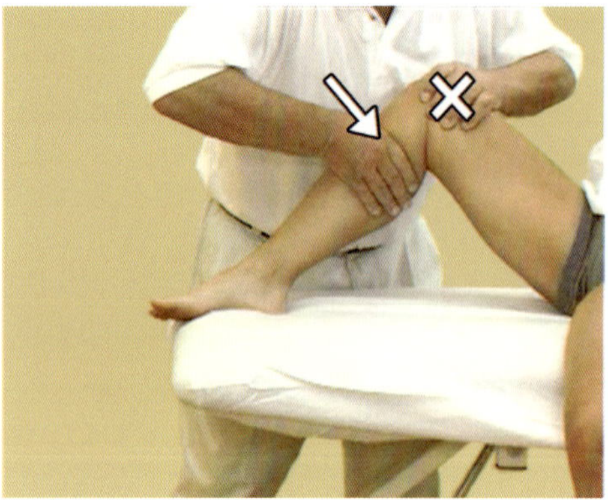

Figure 66e – mobilization in flexion, medial side

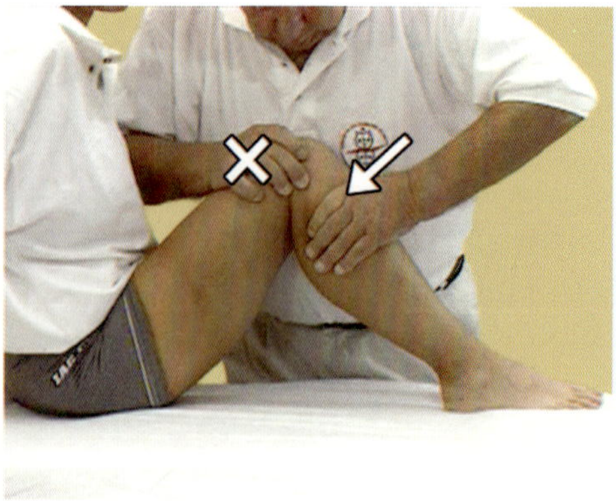

Figure 66f – mobilization in flexion, lateral side

■ Figure 66e: Flexion progression, medial side

Objective

- To increase knee flexion (Concave Rule) and internal rotation range-of-motion.

Starting position

- The patient is supine.
- Position the knee near its end range-of-motion into flexion-internal rotation.

Hand placement and fixation

- **Therapist's stable hand (left):** Hold the patient's thigh above the knee and fixate it against your body.
- **Therapist's moving hand (right):** Grip the lower leg below the knee from the anterior-medial side.

Procedure

- Apply a Grade III posterior glide movement to the medial tibia.

Note

- Knee mobilization is easier and more effective when treatment is directed specifically to the medial or lateral side.

■ Figure 66f: Flexion progression, lateral side

- Position the knee near its end range-of-motion into flexion-external rotation.
- Hold the lower leg from the anterior-lateral side.
- Apply a Grade III posterior glide movement to the tibia.
- To increase knee flexion (Concave Rule) and external rotation range-of-motion.

Knee posterior glide

for restricted flexion (prone)

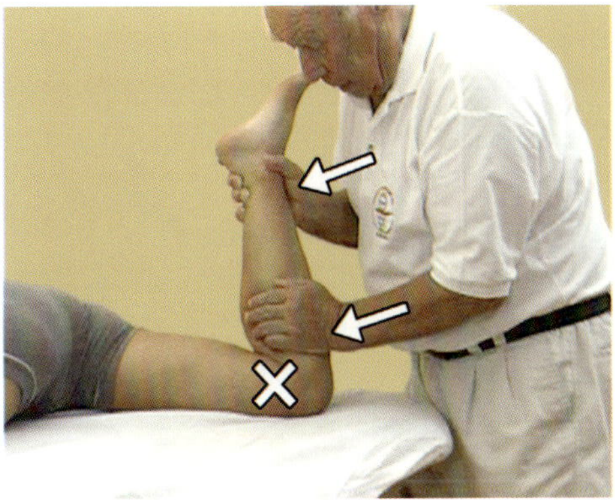

Figure 67a – mobilization in flexion, medial side

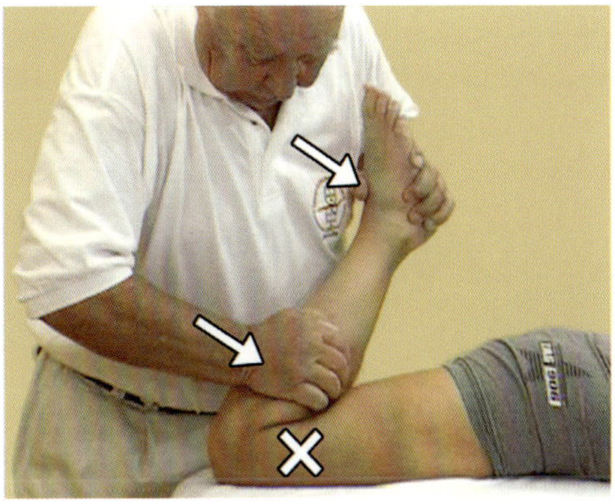

Figure 67b – mobilization in flexion, lateral side

■ Figure 67a: Flexion progression, medial side (alternate technique)

Objective

- To increase knee flexion (Concave Rule) and internal rotation range-of-motion.

Starting position

- The patient lies prone with the knee near the edge of the treatment table.
- Position the knee near its end range-of-motion into flexion-internal rotation

Hand placement and fixation

- **Fixation:** The patient's thigh is fixated against the treatment surface.
- **Therapist's moving hands:** Hold the lower leg from the anterior side with both hands; your right hand grips above the ankle and your left hand below the knee with your hypothenar eminence on the medial tibia; brace your left arm against your body.

Procedure

- Apply a Grade III posterior glide movement to the medial tibia by leaning through your left forearm; move both your hands and body together as one.

Note

- Knee mobilization is easier and more effective when treatment is directed specifically to the medial or lateral side.

■ Figure 67b: Mobilization in flexion, lateral side (alternate technique)

- Position the knee near its end range-of-motion into flexion-external rotation.
- Apply a Grade III posterior glide movement to the tibia.
- To increase knee flexion (Concave Rule) and external rotation range-of-motion.

Knee

Knee anterior glide
for restricted extension

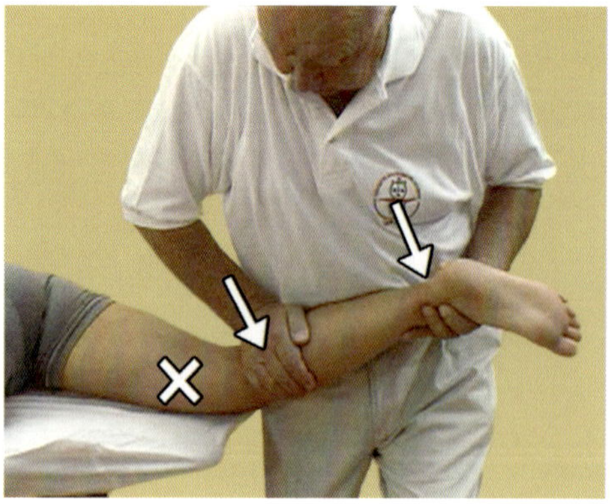

Figure 68a – Mobilization in resting position, medial side

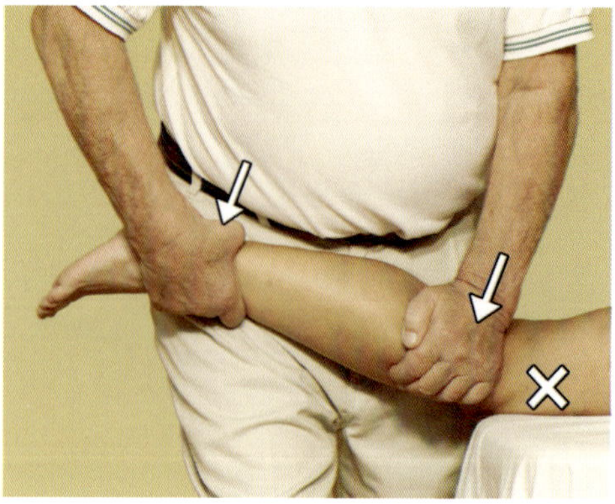

Figure 68b – mobilization in resting position, lateral side

■ Figure 68a: Mobilization in resting position, medial side

Objective

- To evaluate the quantity and quality of anterior glide joint play of the proximal medial tibia.

Starting position

- The patient lies prone with the knee near the edge of the treatment table.
- Position the knee in its resting position.

Hand placement and fixation

- **Fixation:** The patient's thigh is fixated against the treatment surface.
- **Therapist's moving hands:** Hold the patient's lower leg against your body with both hands; grip from the medial side with your left hand proximal to the ankle and your right hand distal to the knee; place your right hypothenar eminence on the tibia.

Procedure

- Apply a Grade III anterior glide movement to the proximal medial tibia by leaning through your right forearm and bending your knees; move both your hands and body together as one.

Note

- Knee mobilization is easier and more effective when treatment is directed specifically to the medial or lateral side.

■ Figure 68b: Mobilization in resting position, lateral side

- Grip from the lateral side with your right hand proximal to the ankle and your left hand distal to the knee; place your left hypothenar eminence on the lateral tibia.
- Apply a Grade III anterior glide movement to the proximal lateral tibia to increase knee extension (Concave Rule) and internal rotation range-of-motion by increasing lateral tibial anterior glide.

Knee lateral glide
for restricted flexion and extension

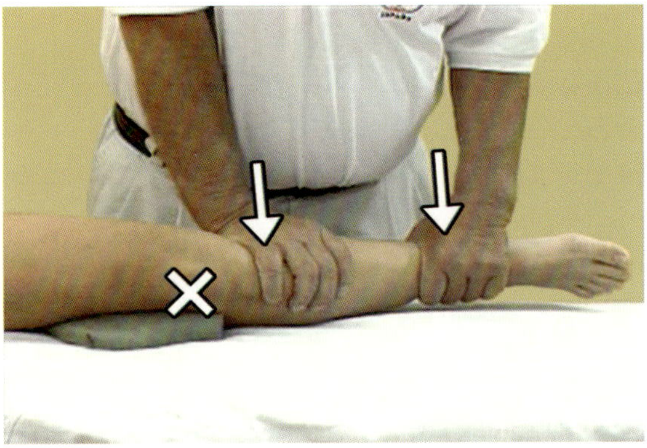

Figure 69 – test and mobilization in resting position

■ Figure 69: Test and mobilization in resting position

Objective

- To evaluate the quantity and quality of lateral glide joint play in the knee, including end-feel.
- To increase knee flexion, extension and rotation range-of-motion.

Starting position

- The patient is side-lying with the lateral side of the leg on the treatment surface.
- Position the knee in its resting position.

Hand placement and fixation

- **Fixation:** The patient's distal thigh is fixated by the treatment surface; to enhance the fixation, place a sandbag or wedge just proximal to the joint space.
- **Therapist's moving hands:** Hold the patient's lower leg from the medial side with both hands; with your left hand, grip proximal to the ankle; with your right hand, grip distal to the knee with your hypothenar eminence on the medial tibia just distal to the joint space.

Procedure

- Apply a Grade II or III lateral glide movement by leaning your body through your extended arms; move both hands and your body together as one.

■ Flexion and extension progression (not shown)

- Position the knee near its end range-of-motion into flexion (for restricted flexion) or extension (for restricted extension).
- Apply a Grade II or III lateral glide movement to the medial proximal tibia.

Knee medial glide

for restricted flexion and extension

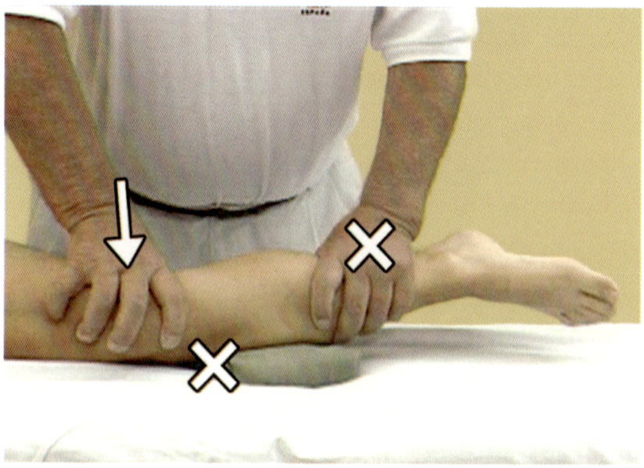

Figure 70 – test and mobilization in resting position

■ Figure 70: Test and mobilization in resting position

Objective

- To evaluate the quantity and quality of medial glide joint play in the tibia, including end-feel.
- To increase knee flexion and extension range-of-motion.

Starting position

- The patient is side-lying with the lateral side of the leg on the treatment surface.
- Position the knee in its resting position.

Hand placement and fixation

- **Fixation and therapist's stable hand (left):** Place a sandbag or wedge just distal to the knee; grip proximal to the patient's ankle and fixate it against the treatment surface.
- **Therapist's moving hand (right):** Grip around the medial side of the patient's thigh just proximal to the knee.

Procedure

- Apply a relative medial glide movement to the tibia by performing a Grade II or III lateral glide movement to the femur; lean your body through your extended right arm to produce the movement.

■ Flexion and extension progression (not shown)

- Position the knee near its end range-of-motion into flexion (for restricted flexion) or extension (for restricted extension).
- Apply a relative medial glide movement to the tibia by applying a Grade III lateral glide movement to the femur.

Patella distal glide

for restricted flexion

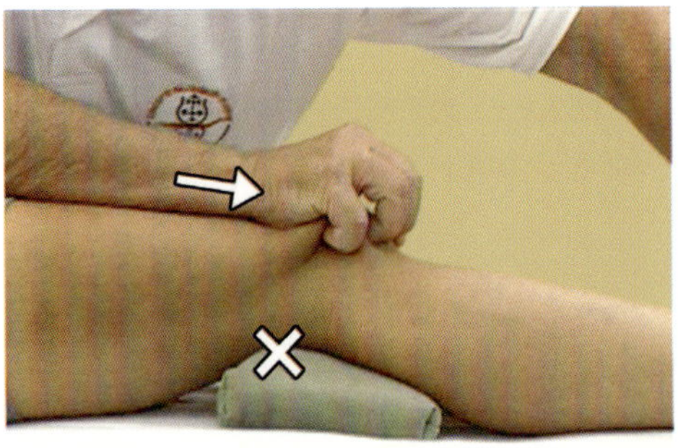

Figure 71a – test and mobilization in resting position

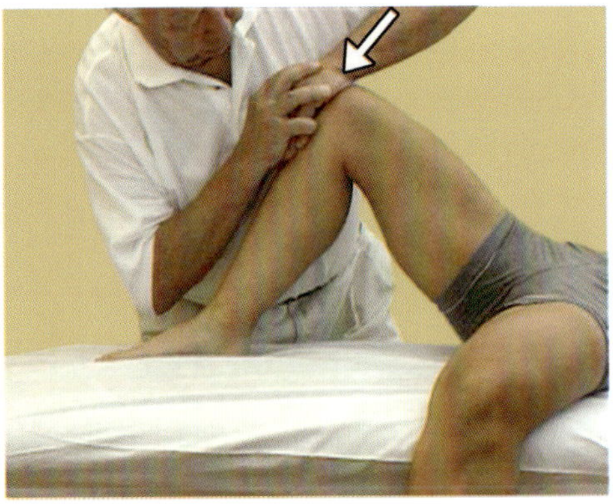

Figure 71b – mobilization in flexion

■ Figure 71a: Test and mobilization in resting position

Objective

- To evaluate the quantity and quality of patella distal glide joint play.
- To increase knee flexion range-of-motion by increasing patellar distal glide.

Starting position

- The patient lies supine.
- Use a sandbag to position the knee in its momentary resting position; adjust the size of the sandbag to control the amount of knee flexion.

Hand placement and fixation

- **Fixation:** The knee is fixated by the sandbag.
- **Therapist's moving hand:** Grip with the heel of your right hand over the proximal edge of the patella and your fingers around the distal aspect of the patella; rest your right forearm along the patient's thigh; you may place your left hand over your right hand to enhance your grip.

Procedure

- Apply a Grade II or III distal glide movement to the patella; keep your forearm parallel to the thigh to avoid dorsally-directed compression forces to the patella. Use your grip on the patella to simultaneously apply a Grade I traction to avoid pain during the gliding movement.
- Apply a Grade III traction movement to the patella using the fingers of both hands to grip firmly around the patella (not shown).
- When restricted distal glide of the patella restricts knee flexion, it is important to increase patellar mobility before using knee joint mobilization techniques.

■ Figure 71b: Flexion progression

- Position the joint close to its end range-of-motion in flexion. Apply a Grade III distal glide movement to the patella.

Knee

Patella medial and lateral glide
for hypomobility

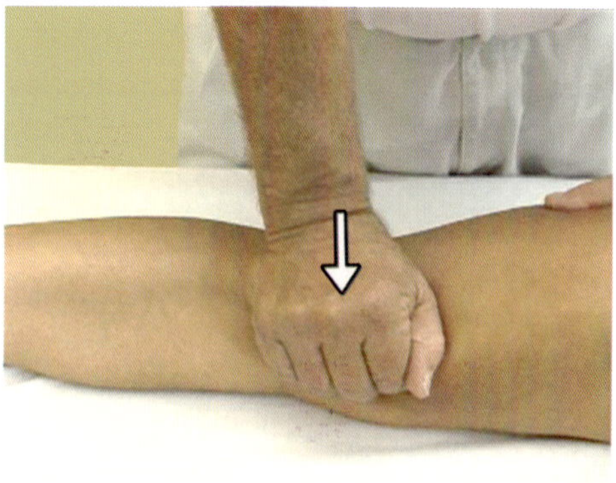

Figure 71c – mobilization in resting position medial glide

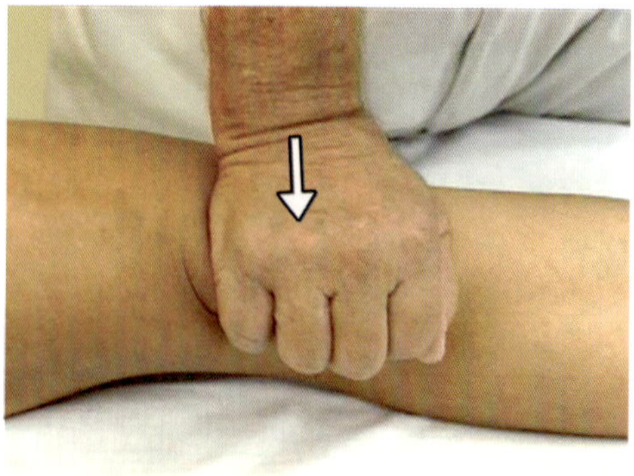

Figure 71d – mobilization in resting position lateral glide

■ Figure 71c: Mobilization in resting position, medial glide

Objective

- To increase knee movement by increasing medial glide of the patella.

Starting position

- The patient lies supine. The leg is rotated medially.
- Position the knee in its resting position. If necessary, use a sandbag to position the knee in its momentary resting position.

Hand placement and fixation

- **Therapist's stable hand (right):** Grip around the thigh above the patella from the anterior side.
- **Therapist's moving hand (left):** Grip with the heel of your hand and fingers over the lateral and medial edges of the patella with a simultaneous Grade I traction.

Procedure

- Apply a Grade II or III medial glide movement to the patella.

■ Figure 71d: Mobilization in resting position, lateral glide

- Adapt the same technique with the patients's leg rotated laterally.
- Apply Grade II or III lateral glide movement to the patella.

CHAPTER 20

HIP

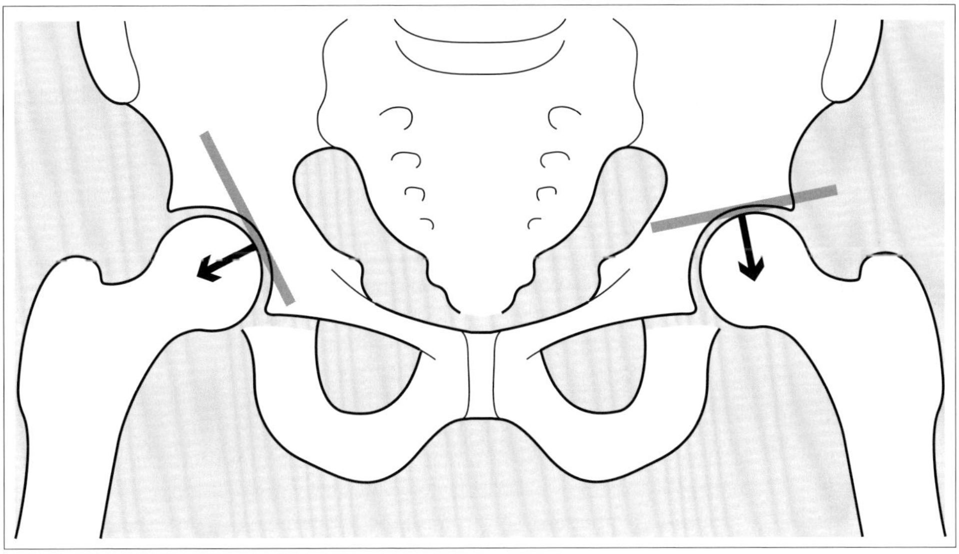

Hip

20 Hip

(art. coxae)

Functional anatomy and movement

The hip joint is an anatomically and mechanically simple, triaxial ball-and-socket joint (unmodified ovoid).

The convex articulating surface is formed by the head of the femur (*caput ossis femoris*). The head of the femur is about two-thirds of a sphere on the neck of the femur (*collum ossis femoris*), which is itself approximately five centimeters long. The neck of the femur forms an angle of approximately 126° with the longitudinal axis of the femoral shaft (angle of declination) and an angle of approximately 12° with the frontal plane (angle of femoral torsion). The head of the femur faces the acetabulum in a medial, cranial, and slightly ventral direction.

The ilium contains the acetabulum (a lunate-shaped, concave articular surface) and the non-articular floor of the cavity, the acetabular fossa. The acetabular labrum is continuous with the acetabular rim; the transverse acetabular ligament running across the acetabular notch completes the circle. This ligament converts the notch into a foramen through which vessels and nerves pass in the ligament of the head of the femur.

The acetabular fossa is occupied by an articular fat pad (*pulvinar acetabuli*, or *corpus adiposum fossae acetabuli*), which can be pushed out or sucked in through the acetabular notch by variations in pressure.

Bony palpation

Ventral
- Hip joint
- Anterior superior iliac spine
- Anterior inferior iliac spine
- Iliac crest
- Symphysis pubis
- Lesser trochanter

Dorsal
- Iliac crest
- Posterior superior iliac spine
- Posterior inferior iliac spine
- Ischial tuberosity

Lateral
- Iliac crest
- Greater trochanter

Figure 20.1
Ligamentum capitis femoris

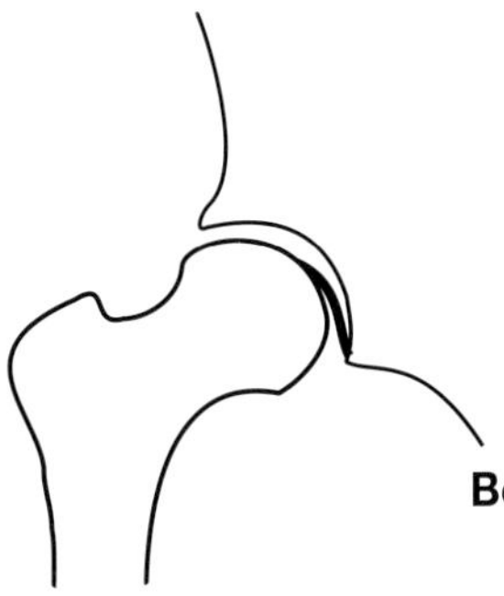

Ligaments

- Iliofemoral ligament (ventral)
- Pubofemoral ligament (caudal)
- Ischiofemoral ligament (dorsal/cranial)
- Zona orbicularis
- Ligament of the head of the femur (*lig. capitis femoris*) is not palpable. This ligament is taut when the hip is in adduction, and relaxes during hip abduction and during a hip traction mobilization.

Bone movement and axes

- Flexion - extension: around a transverse axis through the head of the femur
- Abduction - adduction: around a sagittal axis through the head of the femur
- Internal - external rotation: around a longitudinal axis through the head of the femur and the knee joint

End feel

- Firm

Joint movement (gliding)

- Convex Rule

Treatment plane

The deep, spherical concave contour of the acetabulum functionally has multiple treatment planes, depending on the position of the joint and the direction of the mobilization force.

- One treatment plane for the hip lies on the concave surface of the weight-bearing portion of the superior acetabulum; i.e., distal traction mobilization is at a right angle to this treatment plane.
- Another treatment plane lies on the concave surface of the anterior-lateral facing portion of the acetabulum; i.e., lateral traction mobilization is at a right angle to this treatment plane.

Zero position

- Thigh in the frontal plane
- The following two lines lie at right angles to each other:
  ... between the anterior superior iliac spine and patella
  ... between the two anterior superior iliac spines

Resting position

- Hip flexed approximately 30°, abducted approximately 30° and slightly laterally rotated

Close-packed position

- Maximal extension and medial rotation and abduction

Capsular pattern

- Medial rotation - extension - abduction - lateral rotation

Hip

Hip examination scheme

(Refer to Chapter 3 and 4 for more information on examination)

Tests of function

1. **Active and passive movements, including stability tests and end-feel**

Transverse axis	
Flexion	130 °
Extension from zero	15 °
Extension in abduction	40 °
Dorsal-ventral axis	
Abduction	45°
Adduction	20°
Longitudinal axis	
Lateral rotation	45°
Medial rotation	40°

2. **Translatoric joint play movements, including end-feel**

Traction - compression	(Figure 72a)
Gliding	
Lateral	(Figure 74a)

Hip

3. Resisted movements

	OTHER FUNCTIONS
Flexion	
Iliopsoas	Lateral rotation
Rectus femoris	Knee extension
Tensor fascia latae	Abduction, internal rotation; knee extension, external rotation
Extension	
Gluteus maximus	Lateral rotation
Biceps femoris	Knee flexion, external rotation
Semimembranosus	Knee flexion, medial rotation
Adductor magnus	Adduction
Abduction	
Gluteus medius, minimus	Medial rotation
Tensor fascia latae	Flexion, medial rotation; knee extension, external rotation
Adduction	
Adductor magnus	Medial rotation
Adductor longus, brevis	Flexion, lateral rotation
Pectineus	Flexion, lateral rotation
Gracilis	Flexion, medial rotation
Lateral rotation	
Iliopsoas	Flexion
Gluteus maximus, minimus	Extension
Obturators, gemelli	Extension
Quadratus femoris	Flexion, adduction
Piriformis	Extension, abduction
Medial rotation	
Gluteus minimus, medius	Abduction
Adductor magnus	Adduction
Tensor fascia latae	Flexion, abduction; knee extension, external rotation

4. Passive soft tissue movements

Physiological

Accessory

5. Additional tests

Trial treatment

Traction (Figure 72b)

Hip techniques

Figure 72a	Distal traction for pain and hypomobility
Figure 72b,c	Distal traction for hypomobility (alternate technique)
Figure 73a,b	Distal traction for restricted flexion
Figure 73c	Distal traction for restricted extension
Figure 74a	Lateral traction for pain and hypomobility
Figure 74b,c	Lateral traction for restricted flexion and extension
Figure 75a	Dorsal glide for restricted flexion
Figure 75b	Ventral glide for restricted extension

Hip distal traction
for pain and hypomobility

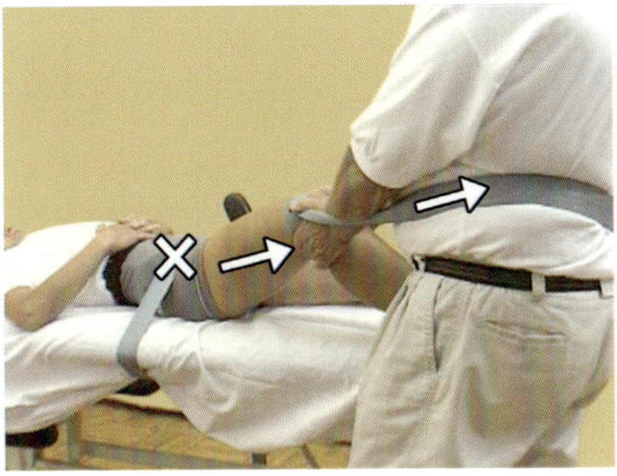

Figure 72a – test and mobilization in resting position

■ Figure 72a: test and mobilization in resting position

Objective

- To evaluate the quantity and quality of distal traction joint play in the hip, including end-feel. Distal traction movement tests the weight bearing area on the upper surface of the acetabulum.
- To decrease pain or increase range-of-motion in the hip.

Starting position

- The patient lies supine with the knee in flexion.
- Position the hip in its resting position.

Hand placement and fixation

- No fixation is needed to test movement without end-feel.
- Fixation is required to test end-feel, for treatment with traction-mobilization, and for manipulative thrust techniques. Use a pommel (pictured) or stirrup around the right ischial tuberosity to prevent caudal movement of the right innominate; use a strap around the pelvis just below the anterior superior iliac spines to prevent side-bending of the spine.
- **Therapist's moving hands:** Grip around the distal thigh with both hands; use a traction strap over your hands and around your body to reinforce your grip for longer treatments; adjust the strap so that when the strap is taut your arms are nearly straight.

Procedure

- Shift your body backward and pull through your extended arms to apply the Grade I, II, or III distal traction movement.
- Suitable for early training in manipulative thrust techniques. Shift your body weight backward to take up the slack and apply the thrust with your arms.

Hip distal traction

for hypomobility (alternate technique)

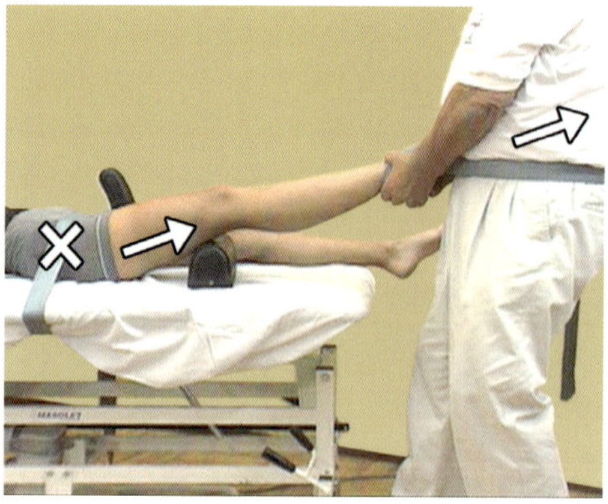

Figure 72b – mobilization in resting position

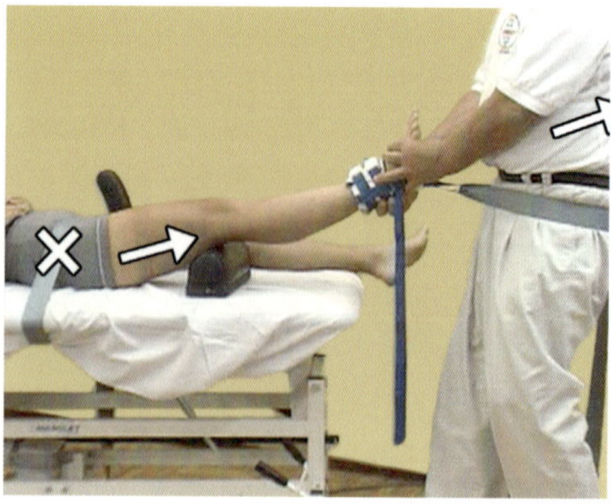

Figure 72c – mobilization in resting position

■ Figure 72b: mobilization in resting position, alternate technique

Objective

- To increase range-of-motion in the hip. Distal traction movement primarily affects the weight bearing area on the superior surface of the acetabulum.

Starting position

- The patient lies supine with the knee in full extension.
- Position the hip in its resting position.

Hand placement and fixation

- **Fixation:** Use a pommel (pictured) or stirrup around the right ischial tuberosity to prevent caudal movement of the right innominate. Use a strap around the pelvis just below the anterior superior iliac spines to prevent side-bending of the spine.
- **Therapist's moving hands:** Grip above the patient's ankle with both hands; use a traction strap over your hands and around your body to reinforce your grip for longer treatments; adjust the strap so that when the strap is taut your arms are straight.

Procedure

- Shift your body backward and pull through your extended arms to apply a Grade I, II, or III distal traction movement.
- Suitable for early training in manipulative thrust techniques. Shift your body weight backward to take up the slack and apply the thrust with your arms.

■ Figure 72c: mobilization in resting position, alternate technique

- Use a traction cuff to facilitate your grip for Grade III distal traction mobilization treatments of longer duration.
- Suitable for early training in manipulative thrust techniques. Shift your body weight backward to take up the slack and apply the thrust with your arms.

Hip distal traction
for restricted flexion

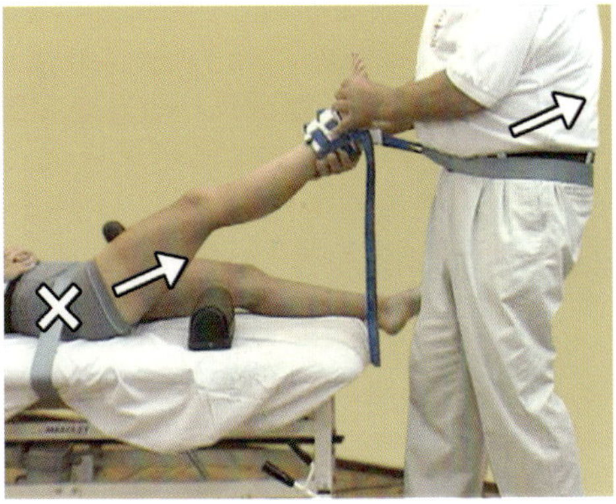

Figure 73a – mobilization in flexion

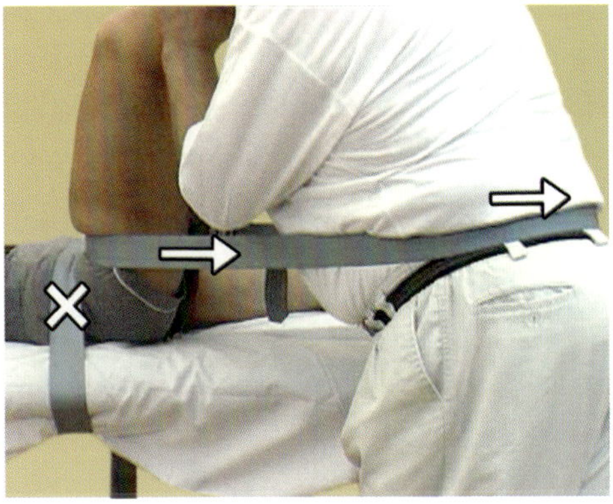

Figure 73b – mobilization in flexion

■ Figure 73a: Flexion progression

Objective

- To increase flexion range-of-motion in the hip by increasing hip distal traction joint play.

Starting position

- The patient lies supine.
- Position the hip near its end range-of-motion into flexion; adjust the height of the treatment surface to control the amount of hip flexion.

Hand placement and fixation

- **Fixation:** Use a pommel (pictured) or stirrup around the right ischial tuberosity to prevent caudal movement of the right innominate; use a strap around the pelvis just below the anterior superior iliac spines to prevent side-bending of the spine.
- **Therapist's moving hands:** Grip above the patient's ankle with both hands; use a traction strap over your hands and around your body to reinforce your grip for longer treatments; adjust the strap so that when the strap is taut your arms are straight.

Procedure

- Shift your body backward and pull through your extended arms to apply a Grade III distal traction movement; pull slowly and sustain each pull for a minute or more.

■ Figure 73b: Flexion progression for 90° or more

- Position the hip near its end range-of-motion into hip flexion; position the mobilization strap around the patient's proximal thigh and around your body; apply a Grade III distal traction movement to the femur.

Hip distal traction
for restricted extension

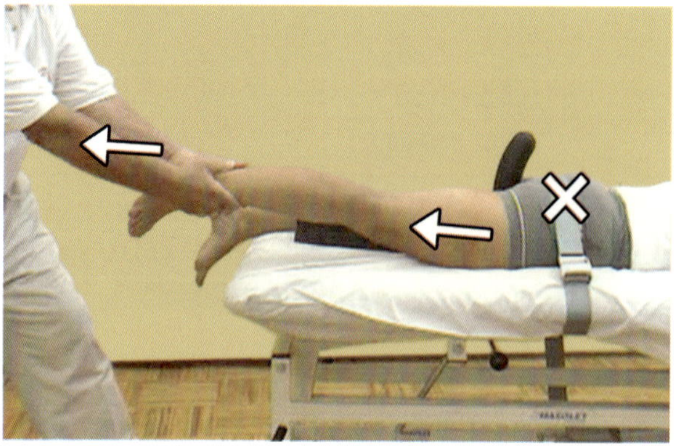

Figure 73c – mobilization in extension

■ Figure 73c: Extension progression

Objective

- To increase extension range-of-motion in the hip by increasing hip distal traction joint play.

Starting position

- The patient lies prone.
- Position the hip near its end range-of-motion into extension.

Hand placement and fixation

- **Fixation:** Use a pommel (pictured) or stirrup around the right ischial tuberosity to prevent caudal movement of the right innominate; use a strap around the buttocks to prevent side-bending of the spine.
- **Therapist's moving hands:** Grip above the patient's ankle with both hands; in the presence of knee pain in knee extension, bend the patient's knee slightly and grip above the knee.
- You may use a traction strap over your hands and around your body to reinforce your grip for longer treatments; adjust the strap so that when the strap is taut your arms are straight.

Procedure

- Shift your body backward and pull through your extended arms to apply a Grade III distal traction movement; pull slowly and sustain each pull for a minute or more.

Hip lateral traction
for pain and hypomobility

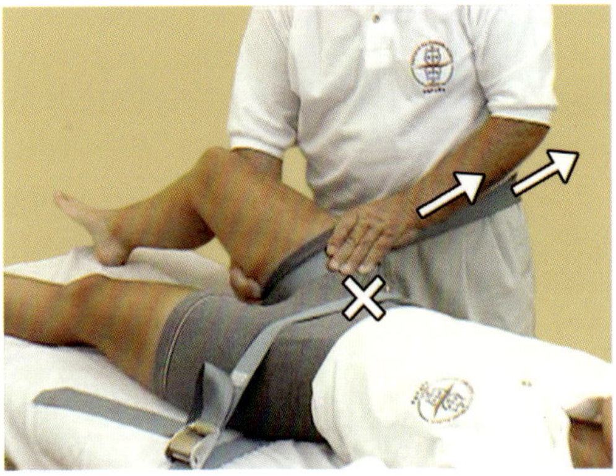

Figure 74a – test and mobilization in resting position

■ Figure 74a: Test and mobilization in resting position

Objective

- To evaluate the quantity and quality of hip lateral traction joint play.
- To decrease pain or to increase range-of-motion in the hip.

Starting position

- The patient lies supine.
- Position the hip in its resting position.

Hand placement and fixation

- **Fixation:** Use a strap around and under the patient's pelvis and attach it to the opposite side of the treatment surface. For mobilization you may reinforce the strap fixation with your left hand by pressing on the patient's lateral pelvis in a medial and slightly cranial direction.
- **Therapist's moving hands:** To facilitate mobilization, use a traction strap around the patient's proximal thigh and around your body. Support the patient's thigh with your right hand to control the hip resting position. Your left hand may be placed underneath the traction strap for better control.

Procedure

- To apply a Grade I, II, or III traction-mobilization, shift your body backward and pull through the strap in a lateral and slightly caudal direction in line with the neck of the femur. Your arms and body should move together as one. If your left hand is fixating the patient's pelvis, it should not move.
- Suitable for early training in manipulative thrust techniques. Shift your body weight backward to take up the slack and apply the thrust with your arms.

Hip lateral traction

for restricted flexion and extension

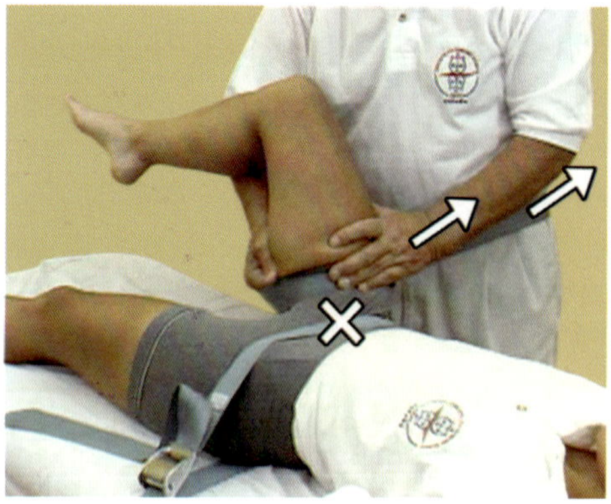

Figure 74b – mobilization in flexion

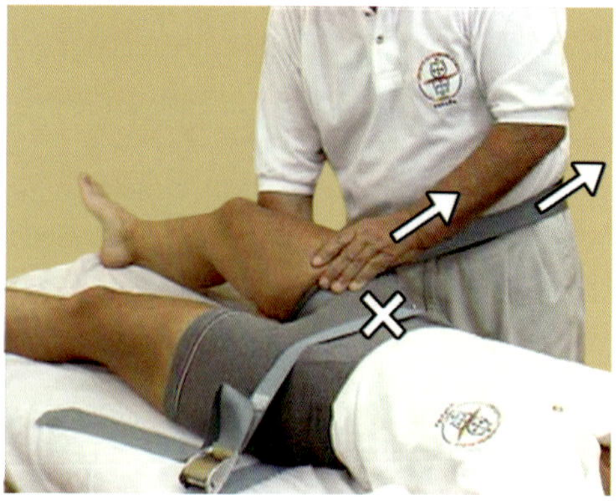

Figure 74c – mobilization in extension

■ Figure 74b: Flexion progression

Objective

- To increase hip flexion and adduction range-of-motion (Convex Rule).

Starting position

- The patient lies supine.
- Position the hip near its end range-of-motion into flexion.

Hand placement and fixation

- **Fixation:** Use a strap around and under the patient's pelvis and attach it to the opposite side of the treatment surface; you may reinforce the strap fixation with your left hand by pressing on the patient's lateral pelvis in a medial and slightly cranial direction.
- **Therapist's moving hands:** Use a traction strap around the patient's proximal thigh and around your body; with your right hand, support the patients thigh to control hip position. Your left hand may be placed underneath the traction strap for better control.

Procedure

- Shift your body backward and pull through the strap in a lateral and slightly caudal direction to apply Grade III lateral traction movement (in line with the neck of the femur); your arms and body should move together as one. (If your left hand is fixating the patient's pelvis, it should not move.)

■ Figure 74c: Extension progression

- Position the hip near its end range-of-motion in extension and adduction.
- Apply a Grade III lateral traction movement to the femur.
- Note that with greater degrees of extension restriction, the hip may still be in a position of flexion. To increase extension from the zero position, the patient lies prone.

Hip dorsal glide

for restricted flexion

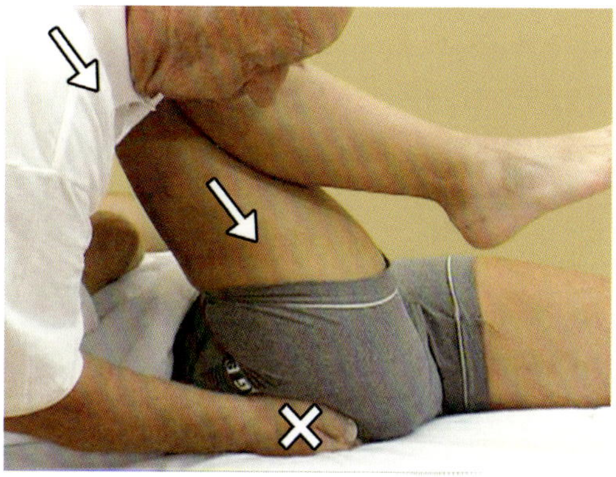

Figure 75a – mobilization in flexion

■ Figure 75a: Flexion progression

Objective

- To increase hip flexion range-of-motion (Convex Rule).

Starting position

- The patient lies supine.
- Position the hip near its end range-of-motion into flexion.

Hand placement and fixation

- **Fixation and therapist's stable hand (right):** The patient's pelvis is fixated against the treatment surface; reinforce the fixation with your right hand beneath the right side of the patient's pelvis.
- **Therapist's moving hand (left):** Hold the patient's leg against your body with your left hand; position the patient's knee against your left shoulder and chest.

Procedure

- Lean your body into the patient's knee along the line of the thigh to apply a Grade III dorsal glide movement; your left arm and body should move together as one.

Hip ventral glide
for restricted extension

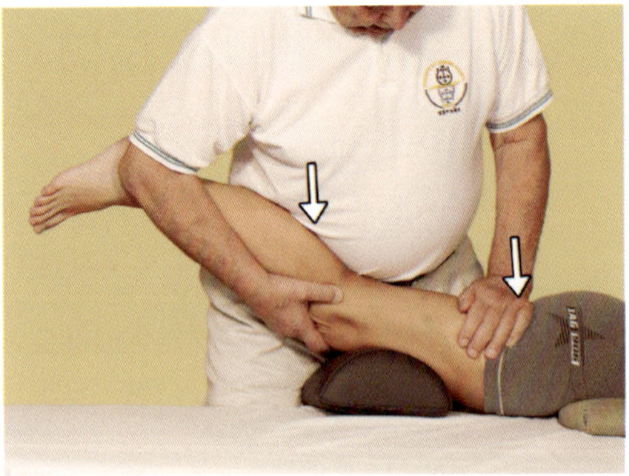

Figure 75b – mobilization in extension

■ Figure 75b: Extension progression

Objective

- To increase hip extension range-of-motion (Convex Rule).

Starting position

- The patient lies prone.
- Position the hip near its end range-of-motion into extension with a support above the knee.

Hand placement and fixation

- **Fixation:** The patient's pelvis is fixated against the treatment surface; reinforce the fixation with a sandbag or wedge under the anterior pelvis.
- **Therapist's moving hands:** With your right hand, grip the patient's lower leg and knee to control hip position; with your left hand, grip the posterior thigh just distal to the hip joint space.

Procedure

- Lean over your extended left arm to apply a Grade III ventral glide movement. Your body and both your hands should move together as one.

REFERENCE

Terminology

The lexicon of terms used in this book series evolved over many years with contributions from practitioners in many disciplines and from many countries, and may not conform to the terminology used in a particular country or clinical field.

End feel

A passive manual assessment of joint movement *quality* applied after the first stop of a passive movement. The sensation imparted to the therapist's hands at the limit of motion is described as relative degrees of resistance and elasticity.

Normal end-feel

The characteristic elastic end-feel in a normal joint. When the end-feel is released the joint rebounds back to the first stop or into the slack. Described as soft, firm or hard depending upon the anatomical characteristics of the joint and the direction of movement tested.

Pathological end-feel

When the quality and behavior of resistance after the first stop is uncharacteristic for the joint being tested.

First stop

The point in the range of joint movement where the first marked resistance begins.

Final stop

The point in the range of joint movement at the limit of palpable motion.

Glide test

A joint evaluation technique performed with a passive translatoric joint play gliding movement. Provides the most accurate information about the direction, degree and nature of a gliding restriction in a joint. Includes assessment of end-feel. Testing in all movement directions.

Grades of movement

A three-zone classification system that defines a specific range of translatoric joint play motion according to the relative looseness and resistance in the joint at various points in the range.

Grade I (loosening)

An extremely small translatoric traction force which produces no appreciable joint separation, but acts to nullify the normal compressive forces acting on the joint.

Grade II (tightening)

Translatoric movement in the range where the joint structures are on slack before the first stop. Divided into two sub-zones: 1) The slack zone (SZ) where there is little resistance to movement, and 2) The transition zone (TZ) where the tissue tightens rapidly before the first stop.

Grade III (stretching)

Translatoric movement in the range beyond the first stop, where the structure limiting joint movement are stretched.

Hypermobility

Joint movement greater than established norms. A joint can be hypermobile in one direction and hypomobile in another direction.

Hypomobility

Joint movement less than established norms. A joint can be hypomobile in one direction and hypermobile in another direction.

Joint mobilization

A general term used to describe various techniques applied to increase mobility in hypomobile joints. In this text, "joint mobilization" refers to "translatoric joint mobilization."

Joint play

Very small accessory joint movements that occur as a consequence of internal or external forces on the body. These movements are not under voluntary control.

Translatoric joint play

Linear translatoric accessory joint movements not under voluntary control. Includes traction, compression, and gliding. In this text the term "joint play" refers to "translatoric joint play."

Traction

Linear translatoric joint play movement that separates joint surfaces at a right angle to the treatment plane.

Compression

Linear translatoric joint play movement that approximates joint surfaces at a right angle to the treatment plane.

Gliding

Linear translatoric joint play movement parallel to the treatment plane. In practice, passive gliding movements are applied with a simultaneous traction component.

Joint stabilization

A general term used to describe various techniques applied to decrease mobility in hypermobile joints.

Kaltenborn convex-concave rule

A method to deduce the direction of decreased joint gliding in cases where a glide test cannot be used. Based upon the arthokinematic relationship between normal bone movement (bone rotations) and the corresponding joint movement (joint roll-gliding).

Convex rule → Opposite

In bones with a convex joint surface, restricted bone movement is associated with gliding restriction in the *opposite* direction.

Concave rule → Same

In bones with a concave joint surface, restricted bone movement is associated with gliding restriction in the *same* direction.

Kaltenborn treatment plane

An imaginary plane that passes through the joint at a right angle to a line that connects the axis of rotation in the convex joint surface to the deepest aspect of the articulating concave joint surface. For practical purposes, one can estimate the location of the treatment plane by imagining that it lies over the concave articular surface. The treatment plane remains with the concave joint partner whether the moving joint partner is concave or convex.

Manipulation, Manipulative thrust, Thrust mobilization

High velocity, low amplitude passive joint movement applied with a quick thrust of the hands, most commonly used to normalize joint movement when treating intra-articular restrictions. In this text the terms “manipulation,” “manipulative thrust” and “thrust mobilization” refer only to “traction-manipulation.”

Traction-manipulation

Translatoric high velocity, low amplitude passive thrust movement producing separation (distraction) in the joint at a right angle to the treatment plane. All points on the adjacent joint surfaces move equally apart from one another resulting in separation of the joint surfaces. There is no curvature in the movement.

Glide-manipulation

Translatoric high velocity, low amplitude passive thrust movement producing a gliding movement (translation) parallel to the treatment plane. There is no curvature in the movement. In practice, the gliding thrust movement is applied with a simultaneous traction component.

Manual mobilization, Manipulative therapy

Passive joint mobilization techniques performed with the hands, including non-thrust mobilizations and manipulative thrusts.

Non-thrust mobilization

A low velocity passive translatoric joint movement applied with the hands. Performed either within the slack (Grade I and Grade II for pain-relief or relaxation) or at the limit of motion (Grade III) for stretching.

Pain-relief mobilization (Grade I - IISZ)
Intermittent Grade I and IISZ translatoric joint movements applied in the momentary resting position to reduce symptoms such as pain or muscle spasm. Used when joint movement is restricted by joint fluids, inflammatory changes, discomfort, or muscle response rather than by shortened tissues.

Relaxation mobilization (Grade I - II)
Intermittent Grade I and II translatoric joint movements applied in the momentary resting position to decrease pain and relax muscles. Used when joint movement is limited by muscle spasm and soft tissue tone rather than by shortened tissues.

Stretch mobilization (Grade III)
A series of sustained translatoric joint stretching movements applied after the first stop to increase range-of-motion and normalize end-feel. Can be performed in the resting position and in nonresting positions for specificity.

Overpressure

A passive manual assessment of joint movement *quantity* applied at the limit of an active joint movement.

Resting position

The resting position ("least-packed position" according to MacConaill) is a joint position where articular structures are most lax and allow the greatest range of joint play.

True resting position
The resting position of a normal, healthy joint.

Momentary resting position
The resting position of a pathological joint in which it is impossible, difficult, or impractical to achieve the true resting position.

Nonresting position
Joint positions used to increase or decrease soft tissue tension in specific structures to focus an examination or facilitate treatment.

Rotation

Occurs when the path of a bone movement curves *around* an axis. The corresponding movement in the joint is called "roll-gliding". All active movements are technically rotations, however most practitioners use the term "rotation" only to refer to movements that curve around the longitudinal axis of a bone. Normal roll-gliding characteristically begins with a short curvilinear glide parallel to the joint surface followed by a rolling movement.

Translation

A straight-line (linear) bone movement *along* an axis without rotation. Translations are performed passively as traction, compression, or gliding movements in relation to the treatment plane. The corresponding movement in the joint is called "joint play."

Trial treatment

An evaluation procedure in which a treatment technique is used to confirm a diagnostic hypothesis.

■ Upper extremity joint and muscle chart

MUSCLE	NERVE	ROOT	Shoulder* 90 ABD	40 ADD	65 FLEX	35 EXT	90 INT ROT	60 EXT ROT
Pectoralis major	Pectoral (lat., med.)	C5 – T1		X	X		X	
Pectoralis minor	Pectoral (lat., med.)	C6, 7, 8						
Serratus anterior	Long thoracic	C5, 6, 7						
Trapezius	Accessory C1-C2	C2, 4						
Latissimus dorsi	Thoracodorsal	C6, 7, 8		X		X	X	
Rhomboid	Dorsal scapular	C4, 5						
Levator scapulae	Dorsal scapular	C3, 4, 5						
Deltoid	Axillary	C5, 6	X	1	X	X	1	1
Supraspinatus	Suprascapular	C4, 5, 6	X					1
Infraspinatus	Suprascapular	C5, 6						X
Teres minor	Axillary	C5, 6		1		1		X
Subscapularis	Subscapular	C5, 6, 7		1		1	X	
Teres major	Lower subscapular	C6, 7		X		X	X	
Coracobrachialis	Musculocutaneus	C5, 6, 7		1	X			
Biceps brachii	Musculocutaneus	C5, 6	1		1		1	
Brachialis	Musculocutaneus	C5, 6						
Triceps brachii	Radial	C7, 8		1		1		
Anconeus	Radial	C7, 8, T1						
Pronator teres	Median	C6, 7						
Pronator quadratus	Median	C8, T1						
Flexor carpi radialis	Median	C6, 7						
Palmaris longus	Median	C7, 8						
Flexor carpi ulnaris	Ulnar	C7, 8						
Flexor digitorum superf.	Median	C7, 8, T1						
Flexor digitorum profundus	Median, ulnar	C8, T1						
Flexor pollicis longus	Median	C8, T1						
Brachioradialis	Radial	C5, 6, 7						
Extensor carpi radialis (2)	Radial	C6, 7, 8						
Extensor digitorum	Radial	C7, 8						
Extensor digiti minimi	Radial	C7, 8						
Extensor carpi ulnaris	Radial	C7, 8						
Supinator	Radial	C5, 6						
Abductor pollicis longus	Radial	C7, 8						
Extensor pollicis (2)	Radial	C7, 8						
Extensor indicis	Radial	C7, 8						
Lumbricals (III-IV)	Ulnar	C8, T1						
Lumbricals (I-II)	Median	C8, T1						
Adductor pollicis	Ulnar	C8, T1						
Abductor pollicis brevis	Median	C8, T1						
Opponens pollicis	Median	C8, T1						
Flexor pollicis brevis, lat.	Median	C8, T1						
Flexor pollicis brevis, med.	Ulnar	C8, T1						
Interossei dorsal	Ulnar	C8, T1						
Interossei palmar	Ulnar	C8, T1						

X = prime mover or main function   1 = accessory mover or secondary function   * = with fixated scapula

Shoulder Girdle				Elbow		Forearm		Wrist				Finger				
45	7	30	20	150		80	90	80	90	30	20					
ELEV	DEPR	PRO-TR	RETR	FLEX	EXT	PRON	SUP	DORS	PALM	ULN	RAD	FLEX	EXT	ABD	ADD	OPP
		X														
	1	1														
	X	X														
X	X		X													
	X		1													
1			X													
X																
				X			X									
				X												
					X											
					X											
				1		X										
						X										
				1		1			X		X					
				1		1			X							
				1					X	X						
				1					X			X				
				1					X			X				
									X			X				
				X		1	1									
				1			1	X			X					
				1			1	X					X			
				1				1					X			
				1				X		X						
				1			X									
							1		1		1			X		
							1	1			1		X			
								1			1		X			
												X	1			
												X	1			
															X	1
														X		
															1	X
												X				1
												X			1	1
												1	1	X		
												1	1		X	

Reference

Lower extremity joint and muscle chart

MUSCLE	NERVE	ROOT	Hip					
			130	15	45	20	45	40
			FLEX	EXT	ABD	ADD	EXT ROT	INT ROT
Iliopsoas	Lumbar plexus, femoral	L1, 2, 3	X				X	
Gluteus maximus	Inferior gluteal	L5 – S2		X	1	1	X	
Gluteus medius	Superior gluteal	L5, S1	1	1	X		X	1
Gluteus minimus	Superior gluteal	L5, S1	1	1	X		1	X
Tensor fascia latae	Superior gluteal	L4, 5	1		1			1
Piriformis	Sacral plexus	S1, 2		1	1		X	
Obturator externus	Obturator	L3, 4				1	X	
Obturator internus, gemelli	Sacral plexus	L5, S1		1			X	
Quadratus femoris	Sacral plexus	L5, S1	1			1	X	
Pectineus	Obturator, femoral	L2, 3	1			X	1	
Adductor longus, brevis	Obturator	L2, 3, 4	1			X	1	
Adductor magnus	Obturator, sciatic	L2, 3, 4		1		X		X
Sartorius	Femoral	L2, 3	1		1		1	
Rectus femoris	Femoral	L2, 3, 4	X					
Vasti	Femoral	L2, 3, 4						
Gracilis	Obturator	L2, 3	1			X		1
Biceps femoris	Sciatic	L5 – S2		X		1		
Semitendinosus	Tibial	L5 – S2		1		1		
Semimembranosus	Tibial	L5 – S2		X		1		
Gastrocnemius	Tibial	S1, 2						
Popliteus	Tibial	L4 – S1						
Plantaris	Tibial	S1, 2						
Soleus	Tibial	S1, 2						
Tibialis anterior	Deep peroneal	L4, 5						
Extensor hallucis longus	Deep peroneal	L5, S1						
Extensor digitorum longus	Deep peroneal	L5, S1						
Peronei	Superficial peroneal	L5 – S2						
Flexor hallucis longus	Tibial	S2, 3						
Flexor digitorum longus	Tibial	S2, 3						
Tibialis posterior	Tibial	L4, L5						

We made some compromises to combine both joint and muscle functions in one chart. Where necessary we used the signs "X" and "1" and gave preference to joint function.

Joint Chart: Read from top to bottom. Muscles acting on the joint are listed for each anatomical movement including prime and accessory movers.

Muscle Chart: Read from left to right. Functions are listed for each muscle's main and secondary functions.

Knee				Ankle				Toe	
160	5	45	15	20	40	40	20		
FLEX	EXT	EXT ROT	INT ROT	DORS	PLANT	INV	EV	FLEX	EXT
	1	1							
1			1						
	X								
	X								
1			1						
X		X							
X			1						
X			X						
1					X	1			
1			1						
1					1	1			
					X	1			
				X					
				1		1			X
				1			1		X
					1		X		
					1	1		X	
					1	1		X	
					1	X			

X = prime mover or main function 1 = accessory mover or secondary function

Reference

Convex-concave table

The Kaltenborn Convex-Concave Rule is used to determine the direction of restricted gliding in a joint based on the anatomical shape of the joint surfaces, i.e., convex or concave. Since the therapist more commonly moves the distal joint partner when testing and mobilizing joints, we list the shape of the distal moving bone in this table.

Joint	Function	Moving bone	Shape
Fingers (PIP, DIP)	flexion/ extension	distal phalanx	concave
MCP	abduction/adduction	proximal phalanx	concave
First CM (thumb)	flexion / extension abduction adduction	metacarpal metacarpal	concave convex
Wrist	dorsal/palmar	capitate, scaphoid, lunate, triquetrum	convex
	dorsal/palmar	trapezii	concave
Radio-ulnar			
Distal	pronation/supination	radius	concave
Proximal	pronation/supination	radius	convex
Humeroradial	flexion/extension	radius	concave
Humero-ulnar	flexion/ extension	ulna	concave
Shoulder	all movements	humerus	convex
Sternoclavicular	elevation/depression protraction/retraction	clavicle clavicle	convex concave
Acromioclavicular	all movements	scapula	concave
Toes (PIP, DIP)	flexion/ extension	distal phalanx	concave
MTP	abduction/adduction	proximal phalanx	concave
Foot	all movements inversion/eversion	navicular, cuneiform cuboid	concave convex
Talocalcaneal	inversion / eversion	anterior calcaneus posterior calcaneus	concave convex
Ankle	dorsal/plantar flexion	talus	convex
Tibiofibular	all movements	fibula head	concave
Knee	all movements	tibia	concave
Hip	all movements	femur	convex
Jaw (TMJ)[1]	all movements	mandible	convex

1 The chapter on examination and treatment of the jaw appears in "Manual Mobilization of the Joints: Volume II – The Spine." Note that in earlier editions prior to 2002, the jaw chapter appeared in "Volume I – The Extremities."

Bibliography

Brodin H., J. Bang, P. Bechgaard, F. Kaltenborn, E. Schiøtz. *Manipulasjon av Ryggraden*. Oslo: Universitetsforlaget, 1966.

Cramer A. *Lehrbuch der Chiropraktik der Wirbelsäule.* Ulm-Donau: Karl F Haug Verlag, 1955.

Cyriax J. *Textbook of Orthopedic Medicine,* Vol. 1. London: Bailliere Tindall, 1982.

Drobil R. *Die aktive Bewegungstherapie*. Wien: Wilhelm Maudrich, 1945.

Evjenth O. and J. Hamberg. *Autostretching*. Alfta, Sweden: Alfta Rehab, 1989.

Evjenth O. and J. Hamberg. *Muscle Stretching in Manual Therapy*, Vols. I and II. Alfta, Sweden: Alfta Rehab, 1984.

Gray's Anatomy 35th edition, Norwich, Great Britain, 1978.

Kapandji I. *Physiology of the Joints,* Vol. III. Edinburgh: Churchill Livingstone, 1978.

Kaltenborn F. *Manual Mobilization of the Joints, Volume I: The Extremities*. Oslo: Norli, 2011.

MacConaill M.A. and Basmajian, J.F. *Muscles and Movements,* Krieger, Huntington, New York, 1977.

Mennell J. *Science and Art of Joint Manipulation,* Vol. II. London: Churchill, 1952.

Ottosson A. *Sjukgymnasten - vart tog han vägen? (The Physiotherapist - What happened to him? A study of the masculinization and de-masculinization of the physiotherapy profession 1813 - 1934.)* Historic Institution, University of Gothenborg, Sweden, 2007.

Schiøtz E. and J. Cyriax. *Manipulation Past and Present*. London: W. Heinemann Medical Books Ltd, 1975 (This book has an exhaustive bibliography).

Schiøtz E. *Manipulasionsbehandling av columna under medisinsk-historisk synsvinkel (History of manipulation)*, excerpt from *Tidsskrift for Den norske laegeforening*, 1958.

Spalteholz W., and R. Spanner. *Atlas of Human Anatomy*. Amsterdam: Scheltema & Holkema NV, 1961.

Stoddard A. *Manual of Osteopathic Technique*. London: Hutchinson, 1980.

Stoddard A. *Manual of Osteopathic Practice*. London: Hutchinson, 1983.

White A. and M. Panjabi. *Clinical Biomechanics of the Spine*. Philadelphia: Lippincott, 1978.

Notes

AFTERWORD

Manual therapy education

The ability to see and feel joint movement is important in all aspects of physical treatment and rehabilitation, whether neurological, orthopedic, sports, cardiac, or respiratory. Mastery of manual joint evaluation and treatment techniques not only insures the delivery of more effective treatment, but also trains clinicians to recognize precautions and dysfunctions requiring special handling. This book series was written expressly for this purpose. Orthopedic manual therapists should be competent in all of the basic mobilization and manipulative thrust techniques in this book series: *Manual Mobilization of the Joints - Volume I: The Extremities* and *Volume II: The Spine.*

Graduates of entry-level professional programs in orthopedic medicine and manipulative therapy should demonstrate both academic and hands-on mastery of OMT (Orthopedic Manipulative Therapy). Unfortunately in real life, entry-level programs sometimes emphasize one over the other, concentrating on academics at the expense of hands-on training or vice versa.

In clinical education today, there is a trend toward university-based curricula. The Kaltenborn-Evjenth Concept supports university-based manual therapy training in principle, as it strengthens the theoretical and basic-science foundations of future practitioners. However, it is critical for these programs to also insure that their graduates can deliver effective clinical care. Competency in OMT requires both "head and hands". It takes years of study and practice to achieve mastery in orthopedic manual therapy. Just as with mastery of a musical instrument, the theory and basic technique can be learned quickly, but it takes years of practice to play well.

A written description of a manual technique cannot adequately address the many nuances in patient handling that are critical to effective practice. For this, supervised clinical practice is essential. One of the most important factors in manual therapy training is a good teacher. An advanced clinical degree with certification in an orthopedic specialty does not guarantee skill in manual techniques.

There is no shortcut to learning manual joint treatment techniques. Only time and experience can teach this, with hands-on guidance from an experienced clinical instructor.

Our Nordic OMT training programs for physical therapists require 2000 hours of supervised clinical practice. In recent years we have been alarmed to see OMT training programs, some of them university-based, that require as little as 150 hours of supervised clinical practice. Graduates of those programs wishing to master manual techniques must continue their education in costly private post-professional courses. Short courses and textbooks alone cannot provide the supervision and time necessary to develop competence in orthopedic manual therapy.

Teaching manual mobilization techniques

Practitioners new to manual therapy are often dangerously heavy-handed. It may take much practice before a practitioner can reliably sense when they are approaching the first stop and to accurately sense the end-feel. To attempt a Grade III stretch-mobilization or manipulative thrust before mastering this skill runs the risk of injuring the patient or student practice partner with overstretching or unwanted compression forces.

We find that the practice of soft tissue treatments, especially functional massage, helps develop passive joint movement skills. After some time working with soft tissues, the student practitioner will begin to feel the presence of bones and joints beneath the soft tissues and how these structures move. Over time, the student practitioner will acquire the ability to judge how much these structures move in relation to each other and whether the quality of movement is normal. Such techniques develop handling, coordination and palpation skills that are essential prerequisites to the practice of specific joint mobilization techniques.

Student practitioners should first master joint testing techniques and Grade I and II mobilization movements before attempting Grade III stretch-mobilization techniques or manipulative thrusts. When practicing on asymptomatic subjects, we recommend student practitioners use only within-the-slack Grade II mobilization forces to avoid tissue injury and joint overstretching.

Joint movement tests and end-feel testing are excellent methods for monitoring change in a patient's physical status and for assessing a patient's response to treatment. These assessments are only as good as the therapists using them.

The skill to feel and judge specific joint movements takes time, talent, and frequent practice. Practitioners should be able to perform a manual mobilization procedure with either hand, on either side of the patient. This takes practice.

Students practitioners should demonstrate proficiency in the manual handling of normal joints before attempting manual techniques on real patients. Student practitioners should demonstrate basic proficiency in manual treatment of the extremities before progressing to manual treatment of the spine. This is especially important when learning manipulative thrust techniques.

Teaching manipulative thrust techniques

Manipulation is the most valuable technique for the treatment of intra-articular restrictions. Those who say vibrations or slow-stretch mobilizations are equally effective are mistaken, and likely do not possess sufficient manipulative skill upon which to test their assumptions on real patients.

It takes many years to develop the clinical acumen, sensitive feel and explosive speed which are the hallmark of the master manipulative-thrust practitioner. An alarming number of practitioners have the mistaken belief that manipulative skill can be acquired through reading and a few hours of instruction on a short course. This is not possible. More importantly, it is dangerous.

Students must possess the speed and coordination to apply safe and effective manipulative thrust techniques in the extremities before being taught spinal manipulation. Training in basic joint manipulation, particularly the safe traction manipulations applied in the joint resting position presented in this book series, should begin early in OMT education. However, many manipulation techniques, including most spinal manipulations, are advanced and should only be taught in long-term training programs with clinical supervision by master practitioners.

It is not unusual for practitioners skilled in joint mobilization to have difficulty with manipulative thrusts, and vice versa.

It is a paradox that the manipulative techniques that are safest for the patient and use the least force, are often the most difficult to master because they require greater palpation sensitivity, coordination and quickness. Conversely, the manipulative techniques that are easiest to learn are often the most dangerous for the patient because they incorporate longer lever arms, non-specific gross rotatory movements, and large-amplitude forces.

While gross rotatory manipulations can be effective, these techniques can also cause serious injury, including spinal paresis, cerebrovascular accidents and patient death. Gross rotatory techniques can injure both extra-articular and intra-articular structures in any part of the body and have no place in entry-level education.

In recent years we have been alarmed to see manipulation techniques presented on short weekend courses and published in texts for novice practitioners. These texts include advanced techniques that can cause harm in less-skilled hands and some techniques that are unnecessarily dangerous even in skilled hands. Advanced manipulative techniques should only be taught with hands-on training in clinical settings.

Traction thrust techniques for student practitioners

A low-force manipulation technique utilizing a quick thrust initiated from the joint's momentary resting position is safe and effective in differential diagnosis and for the trial treatment of joint conditions. An entry-level OMT skill training should include traction-thrust manipulations to insure that students have sufficient time and practice to develop the speed and quickness necessary for safe and skilled application of a manipulative thrust.

Following are the basic traction-thrust manipulations presented in this text. These techniques were carefully selected for safety in the hands of student practitioners.

Upper Extremity

Fingers	fig. 1a, 1b
Metacarpals	fig. 6a, 6b 7a, 7b
Wrist	fig. 8a, 8b
Forearm	fig. 22
Elbow	fig. 24a, 24b
Shoulder	fig. 28a, 28b
Shoulder girdle	fig. 39a, 39b, 39c

Lower Extremity

Toes	fig. 43a, 43b
Metatarsals	fig. 48 (adapt from metacarpals)
Foot	fig. 50a, 51a, 54b
Ankle	fig. 56b, 56c
Knee	fig. 64a, 64b
Hip	fig. 72a, 72b, 72c, 74a

Recommendation to abandon rotatory joint techniques

Comments by Freddy Kaltenborn in a letter to 22 IFOMT members, 2008

I have not used a rotatory technique in my practice nor taught a rotatory manipulation in over 15 years. By 1979, I no longer taught rotatory techniques for the extremity joints, and in 1991 I stopped teaching rotatory techniques in the spine. I came to these decisions based upon many years experience. It is my hope that all practitioners of manual therapy will follow my example and avoid these high-risk treatments.

I learned my first rotatory thrust techniques for the spine and extremities in 1945, while a student in Gymnastic school (physical education) in Germany. These manipulative thrusts were applied as a continuation of a restricted movement. At the time, Cyriax advocated rotatory spinal manipulation with simultaneous strong traction forces, based on the premise that this was necessary to reduce a spinal disc protrusion.

The first time I observed anterior-posterior (translatoric) joint movement and joint traction treatment, was in 1952 on a course taught by James Mennell in London. Mennell used the technique only on extremity joints. I wondered about this and began my study of joint biomechanics to gain a better understanding, especially for treatment of the spine.

As I gained experience in patient treatment, I became aware that some rotatory techniques were more painful than others and caused problems after treatment. This rarely happened with translatoric techniques, which were primarily tractions at that time. I had already begun to teach manual therapy to medical doctors and physical therapists in the Nordic countries and openly discussed my concerns about rotatory manual therapy techniques with many students and colleagues.

Olaf Evjenth, one of my students who later assisted with my teaching, joined me in my journey to develop translatoric thrust techniques, primarily tractions, that were both safe and effective.

In 1992, Gwenn Jull, as chairperson of the IFOMT Standards Committee, stated in the Educational Standards document:

"Orthopaedic manipulative therapists have developed some unique procedures, which eliminate rotatory stresses and emphasize glide and distraction movements. Rotation and extension are recognised as being movements which can provide a hazard especially when applied to the cranio-vertebral region."

It is my hope that all OMT practitioners, and especially member organizations of IFOMT, will recognize and respect the patient safety principles addressed in this document.

Evidence-based treatment and research

In an ideal world treatment decisions would be based on the evidence revealed by clinical trials. However, many variables affect accurate determinations of cause and effect in arthro-neuro-muscular disorders. The validity of clinical trials in the manual therapies is confounded by many factors.

» Valid measurement tools for manual interventions have not yet been developed.

» There are few inter- and intra-rater reliability studies for manual techniques.

» All too often a manual therapy novice performs the manual techniques in a research study rather than a master practitioner. This will impact research results. Both research and clinical practice require a concentrated focus of learning and years of practice to gain any amount of mastery.

» There are difficulties in the development of accurate and meaningful functional diagnoses and assessment measures to monitor changes in patient response and upon which to interpret findings.

» Research results are unreliable when studies do not differentiate various techniques. Not all manual mobilization and manipulation techniques are the same. Research reports should provide a detailed description of the techniques used, including:

- The precise position of the patient and the targeted joint. For example, research results using mobilization and manipulation techniques initiated from outside the resting position may not be applicable to Nordic OMT methods.
- The speed and amplitude of the movement. For example, the term "manipulation" has been used by various authors to describe any type of treatment performed with the hands, from slow stretch mobilizations to manipulative thrusts. In the Nordic System, the term "manipulation" is reserved for small amplitude high velocity thrust techniques.
- Whether the movement includes a traction component. Both Nordic System non-thrust mobilizations and manipulative thrusts include a traction component. Techniques used by others often do not.
- Whether the movement is translatoric or rotational
- The precise direction of force

Research should explore important and relevant questions, including the cellular and soft tissue effects of manipulative therapy.

We encourage experienced manual therapists to collaborate with clinical researchers to make meaningful contributions to the body of knowledge of manipulative therapy.

History of the OMT Nordic System

Early Roots

Joint traction and manual manipulation have been used for musculoskeletal treatment since early times. Woodcuts, stone reliefs, and statues illustrate traction treatments in use over 5000 years ago.

Hippocrates, the famous Greek physician and forefather of ancient medicine, utilized traction extensively. In the year 1500, manuscripts were discovered in Greece on the island of Crete, attributed to Niketas (circa 900 AD) with references to Appolonius (circa 50 AD) that refer to Hippocrates. The manuscripts included 30 drawings of various traction and manipulation techniques for the spine and extremity joints attributed to Hippocrates. Among these manuscripts are the first documented examples of manual therapy and traction for the extremity joints (see *Figure A-1* and *Figure A-2)*.

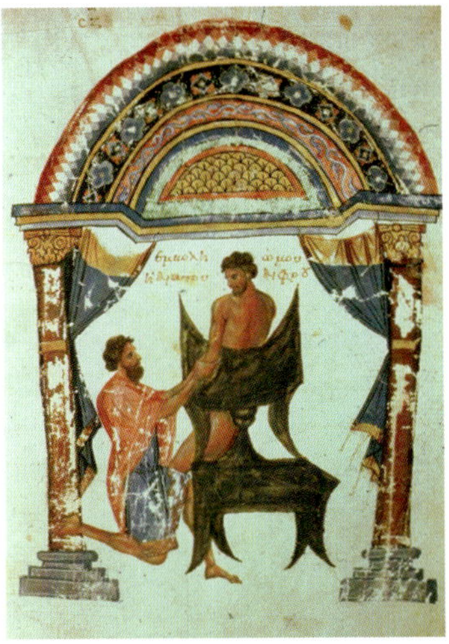

Figure A-1 [1]
Hippocrates'
elbow traction procedure

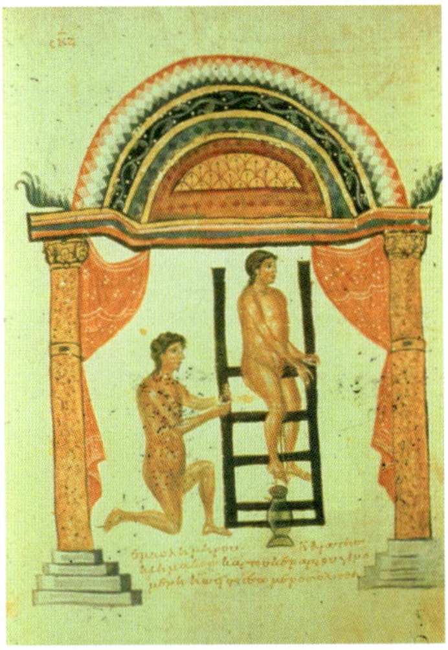

Figure A-2 [1]
Hippocrates'
hip traction procedure

During the Middle Ages (200-1500 AD), joint traction and some manual joint techniques continued to be practiced by physicians. However, many physicians abandoned treatments involving physical contact due to fear of infection following the Black Plague (1347- 1350).

1 Figure were copied with permission from Schiøtz. The original works are held as a "valuable treasure" in the library Biblioteca in Firenze, Italy, as "Codex Laurenzianus LXXXIV,7".

Dissatisfied with the musculoskeletal care provided by the medical practitioners of the time, lay people without professional training also treated joints, both with traction and manipulative thrusts. These "folk medicine" practitioners were known as "bone setters" in English-speaking countries, and as "joint setters" in Norway.

Several contemporary manipulative disciplines began in the 1800's and early 1900's, including Osteopathy, Chiropractic, Naprapathy, and Swedish Medical Directors, a branch of the Swedish Gymnastik discipline, whose practice influenced Kaltenborn's early professional training. The use of manual treatment methods by physical therapists was documented as early as 1813 in Sweden.

■ OMT Nordic System

The story of the OMT Nordic System began in the 1940's when Kaltenborn became frustrated in his attempts to treat patients with joint dysfunction. Kaltenborn's professional training, first as a physical educator and athletic trainer in 1945, and later as a physical therapist in 1949, included mobilization techniques and primitive manipulative thrusts as well as exercise. Kaltenborn recognized that these treatments had limited effect. Many of his patients reported finding greater relief from chiropractic treatment.

In Norway at that time doctors of physical medicine would only support the introduction of a new physical therapy approach if it came from within the traditional practice of medicine. Therefore, Kaltenborn turned to the work of Dr. James Mennell, a physician of physical medicine, and Dr. James Cyriax, a physician of orthopedic medicine, both at St. Thomas Hospital in London. These physicians were unusual in their commitment to bringing their experience in manual medicine to the training of physical therapists. Mennell began teaching his techniques to physical therapists as early as 1907 and wrote his first textbook for physical therapists in 1917, *Physical Treatment by Movement and Massage* (published by Churchill, London). He later published *The Science and Art of Joint Manipulation, Volume I: The Extremities* (1949) and *Volume II: The Spine* (1952). Dr. Cyriax's approach to the evaluation and treatment of soft tissue disorders, first published in 1947 in his *Textbook of Orthopaedic Medicine, Volume I: Diagnosis and Volume II: Treatment,* remains a core concept in the OMT Nordic System today.

In 1952 Kaltenborn went to London with his colleague R. Stensnes, to observe the joint mobilization techniques of Dr. Mennell and to study with Dr. Cyriax. Upon his return to Norway, Kaltenborn demonstrated his newly acquired skill at the Medical Association for

Physical Medicine, which then agreed to cosponsor the first course on the Cyriax approach taught by Kaltenborn in 1954. While there was resistance to acceptance of these techniques by the Norwegian national physical therapy professional organization, (i.e., the NFF), cosponsorship was welcomed by the local Physical Therapy Association Oslo [1], and was taught to eight physical therapists. These physical therapists had dual certification as physical educators and athletic trainers. This signalled the beginning of a significant change in the Norwegian medical establishment's view of manual therapy. Well into the 1950's, many Nordic physicians considered manual therapy outside of the practice of medicine and would not support it. Norwegian physician Eiler Schiøtz documented manual therapy's historic place in medicine in his monograph, the *History of Manipulation* (1958), which helped support the eventual inclusion of manual therapy within the scope of traditional medical practice.

In 1955, Dr. Cyriax visited Norway to oversee instruction in his approach and to examine the first physical therapists to complete those studies. Kaltenborn, together with the graduates of his courses, formed the Norwegian Medical Manipulation Group, an ongoing study group that practiced and further developed what was becoming a specialized MT approach for physicians and physical therapists.

Up to this point, the joint evaluation and treatment techniques used by Mennell, Cyriax, and the Norwegian Medical Manipulation Group were regional and nonspecific. In the mid-1950's this treatment approach changed dramatically with the contributions of Albert Cramer and Alan Stoddard, who began to incorporate specific spinal techniques from chiropractic and osteopathy into their teaching. Cramer was both medical doctor and chiropractor, while Stoddard was both medical doctor and osteopath. Cramer and Stoddard described their techniques in textbooks. These books made specific joint treatment methods accessible to physicians and physical therapists. In the late 1950's and early 1960's, Kaltenborn studied at both schools where Stoddard taught: The British School of Osteopathy and The London College of Osteopathy. Kaltenborn also studied with Cramer at the Ärzteseminar: Forschungs- und Arbeitsgemeinschaft für Chiropraktik e.V. (FAC) in Hamm, Germany. These studies led to Kaltenborn's certification as an instructor in both Osteopathy and Chiropractic.

1 At this time the Physiotherapy Association of Oslo represented practitioners in both the City of Oslo and in the County of Akershus.

Cyriax, Cramer and Stoddard worked with Kaltenborn for many years to determine which evaluation and treatment tools from orthopedic medicine, chiropractic and osteopathy should be a part of OMT for physicians and physical therapists. Cramer and Stoddard assisted Kaltenborn teaching these techniques to the Norwegian Medical Manipulation Group.

■ MT ad modum Kaltenborn

1958 - present

Kaltenborn began to develop his own theories and techniques and to incorporate these into his evolving MT system. His integrated approach became known as "Manual Therapy (MT) ad modum Kaltenborn" or "The Kaltenborn Method."[1]

Among Kaltenborn's contributions were an emphasis on translatoric (linear) joint play movements in relation to a treatment plane for evaluating and mobilizing joints, the use of grades of movement, the convex-concave rule, three-dimensional pre-positioning for joint movement, protecting adjacent nontreated joints during procedures, self-treatment, and ergonomic principles applied to protect the therapist (see *Introduction: Special features*).

During this period of time Kaltenborn's method included:

- Physical education, athletic training, physical therapy, and medical training therapy (later called MTT)
- Orthopedic Medicine (from J. H. Cyriax and J. B. Mennell)
- Chiropractic (from B. J. Palmer and A. Cramer)
- Osteopathy (from A. T. Still and A. Stoddard)
- Kaltenborn's original techniques (F. M. Kaltenborn)

Kaltenborn emphasized functional evaluation of the locomotor system and the biomechanical treatment of dysfunction. In those days patients often presented with joint stiffness due to prolonged immobilization in plaster casts for the treatment of fractures. (Modern-day treatment of these disorders incorporates joint movement to prevent post-immobilization stiffness.)

Kaltenborn's methods supplemented traditional physical medicine approaches with treatment techniques for symptom relief (especially for pain), relaxation of muscle spasm, stretching of shortened joint and muscle connective tissues.

---

1 In 1958, only Norwegian P.T.'s referred to Kaltenborn's approach as "Manual Therapy ad modum Kaltenborn." During the 1960's practitioners in other European countries adopted the term as well, as did Nordic medical doctors in 1965.

Starting in 1960, Kaltenborn presented his MT courses to physical therapists from the Nordic countries. By 1962 physicians attended as well. At this time, Dr. Schiøtz and other physicians created the Nordic Physicians Manual Medicine Association (NFMM). This association developed groups to teach Kaltenborn's MT system and appointed medical educational coordinators for the Nordic countries, including Denmark, Finland, Iceland, Norway and Sweden, for which Kaltenborn served as Nordic Educational Director for Physicians and Physical Therapists. Graduates of these training programs were known as Orthopedic Manipulative Therapists (OMT).

■ OMT Nordic System, Kaltenborn-Evjenth Concept

1968 - present

Olaf Evjenth, OMT, a skilled Norwegian clinician with a background in physical education, athletic training and physical therapy, joined Kaltenborn in 1968.

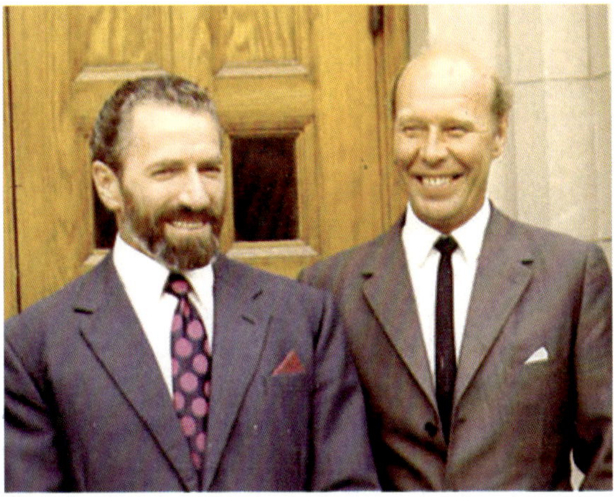

Figure A-4
Evjenth and Kaltenborn (from left) introduced their OMT concept in Canada in 1972.

Evjenth expanded Kaltenborn's approach with specialized techniques for muscle stretching and coordination training. In particular, Evjenth believed in more intensive training for patients and developed programs that, in addition to monitoring pain and range of movement, assessed performance. Evjenth also modified specific exercises for patient use at home with automobilization, autostabilization, and autostretching. Evjenth and Kaltenborn, together with members of the Norwegian Medical Manipulation Group, began to develop additional self-treatment techniques, equipment for home treatment, and ergonomic innovations including mobilization wedges, fixation belts, and grips to make treatments more effective and less physically stressful for the therapist (always a concern in the Kaltenborn-Evjenth Concept). In 1990, Evjenth introduced symptom alleviation testing as a method for localizing lesions and improved symptom provocation testing. This aided in making evaluations more specific.

Multiple treatment techniques, often performed within the same treatment session, are basic to Kaltenborn-Evjenth Concept. This approach to treatment was improved further as Evjenth and Kaltenborn began to sequence techniques for the most effective results.

Kaltenborn and Evjenth presented the "OMT Kaltenborn-Evjenth Concept" worldwide in 1973 at the first meeting of the International Seminar of Orthopaedic Medicine / Manipulative Therapy (ISOMMT). At this meeting, the ISOMMT founders administered the first international examinations in OMT.[1] At this time the concept was based upon MT ad modum Kaltenborn with contributions from Olaf Evjenth and other practitioners.

Kaltenborn's philosophy has always been to integrate useful tools from other approaches. Over the years, the OMT Nordic System benefited from the contributions of many physical therapists and physicians, both in the Nordic countries and worldwide. A few have been especially important to the Kaltenborn-Evjenth Concept:

- Herman Kabat, M.D. (USA) and physical therapists Margaret Knott (USA) and Dorothy Voss (USA) developed the proprioceptive neuromuscular facilitation (PNF) principles behind Nordic OMT active relaxation and muscle reeducation techniques
- Oddvar Holten P.T. (Norway) developed a post-professional course curriculum for medical training therapy (MTT), which had been part of MT ad modum Kaltenborn and practiced by manipulative practitioners.
- Dennis Morgan D.C., P.T., O.M.T. (USA) developed specialized exercise training programs and equipment which are now incorporated into Nordic OMT treatment programs.
- Geoffrey Maitland (Australia), a manual physical therapist with whom Kaltenborn had many stimulating discussions about their concepts and approach.

1 The founders of ISOMMT were F. Kaltenborn, O. Evjenth, J. Cyriax M.D., W. Hinsen M.D., chiropractor, and A. Stoddard M.D., osteopath.

In 1974, Maitland and Kaltenborn, together with physical therapists Stanley Paris and Gregory Grieve, founded the International Federation of Orthopaedic Manipulative Therapy (IFOMT), which later became a subgroup of the World Confederation of Physical Therapists (1978). Through IFOMT's international forums, OMT Nordic System representatives have been a major influence on physical therapy. The OMT Nordic System's continuing evolution has been aided by this opportunity for its practitioners and founders to interact with representatives of other OMT approaches worldwide.

OMT Nordic System standards formed the basis for IFOMT educational and certification standards adopted in 1975 and 1977. Many other countries in which the OMT Nordic System is taught are beginning to develop similar educational and certification standards.

To date, the OMT Nordic System is taught in the five Nordic countries, and in Australia, Austria, Belgium, Germany, Greece, Italy, Japan, Korea, Netherlands, New Zealand, Poland, Spain, Switzerland, and in North and South America.

The OMT Nordic System has expanded to encompass evaluation, treatment and research for a complete arthro-neuro-muscular approach to manual physical therapy. Education incorporates clinically supervised residencies and written and practical examinations. At the highest levels of training, practitioners are also required to conduct independent research in the field of manipulative therapy.

The best OMT practitioners do not restrict their practice to a single approach or school of thought, but rather develop expertise in many systems. Master clinicians utilize techniques derived from many sources, modifying, combining and refining their repertoire of techniques into a unique application for each individual patient. As OMT practice so evolves, the principles of treatment which encompass all schools of thought will more clearly emerge.

Perhaps the time has come for OMT practitioners to cease naming treatments according to a school of thought. The principles of treatment are far more important than the name of the practitioner who first developed the technique. It is not important that a technique, for example, was originally part of the "Kaltenborn", "Cyriax", "Maitland", or any other method. Such compartmentalization of clinical practice hinders the development and growth of the OMT profession.

❖